The Art, Science and Business of Aromatherapy

Your Guide for Personal Aromatherapy and Entrepreneurship

By Kayla Fioravanti, R.A.
Certified and Registered Aromatherapist, Cosmetic Formulator

Other Books by Kayla
How to Make Melt and Pour Soap Base from Scratch:
A Beginner's Guide to Melt and Pour Soap Base Manufacturing

Coming Soon!
DIY Kitchen Chemistry, Simple Homemade Bath & Body Projects

When I was Young I Flew the Sun as a Kite

Puffy and Blue

Selah Press

Reviews

"Kayla represents the saying, "when one door closes, God opens a window." Even though she has experienced failure, she managed to do what evades so many, and that is to get back up and start again. Kayla's knowledge of the aromatherapy world is vast, and she applies it not only in her business, but her personal life. I highly recommend this book to anyone that is interested in learning more about essential oils, from blending to incorporating them into their business safely."
Lisa M. Rodgers, Personal Care Truth

"In this book, The Art, Science and Business of Aromatherapy, Your Guide for Personal Aromatherapy and Entrepreneurship, that rightly brings aromatherapy to its next evolutionary step as a business, Kayla Fioravanti tells a story – well, two stories. One is a personal story that provides an inspirational foundation of what is possible in the business of aromatherapy. The second story provides an in-depth study necessary to develop an aromatherapy business of your own.

Kayla makes the most of her background and experience as a product formulator and manufacturer by introducing uncommon essential oil details. They include information similar to and beyond that found on an MSDS (Manufacturers Safety Data Sheet) like CAS numbers, flash point, appearance, INCI names and other aspects of ingredient classification. This vital information will help the novice, as well as seasoned aromatherapists, to become more tuned into the nuances and the vast array of detail required to become proficient at the use of essential oils. This is also valued information when purchasing your essential oils.

If you are interested in creating essential oil products for yourself or as a serious business venture, this is your learning and reference manual. What you get in The Art, Science and Business of Aromatherapy are ingredients, recipes, the facts, the myths, the cautions, the ins and outs of naturals and synthetics, brand building, marketing, sensible business practice and a vast array of aromatherapy manufacturing how-to. And if all you're interested in is keeping your kids from getting the "sickies and ickies," well, that's in here too. In her breezy, yet direct and solid style, Kayla lays down the laws of aromatherapy – and you know she means business."
Jimm Harrison, educator and founder Jimm Harrison Phytotherapy Institute and author of *Aromatherapy: Therapeutic Use of Essential Oils for Esthetics*

"After following the aromatic journey of this amazing woman for several years now in her videos, blogs, articles and more recently as a champion for protection from regulatory influences on natural product formulators and small business I am not surprised at the level of knowledge, expertise, and personal experience put into the fact packed book, The Art, Science and Business of Aromatherapy, Your Guide for Personal Aromatherapy and Entrepreneurship. Kayla Fioravanti, has put together the most useful book I have ever seen for the business of making and using aromatic products, from sourcing, formulation, crafting, soapmaking to manufacturing in general.

"Besides being a concise book on aromatherapy useful for personal or professional endeavors, the book debunks some aromatherapy myths like certain safety issues with essential oils, and pregnancy for instance. All the while this book provides details on product ingredients including essential oil characteristics not in other books such as FDA notations, FCC specifications, and physical tests such as specific gravity, refractive index, boiling point, etc. The entire variety of base materials that Kayla has used in products are detailed as well as soap making information- again material not found in other books.

Based on her experience Kayla shares Good Manufacturing Practice guidelines and formulation information with tips from experience including important information anyone making products needs to know, such as how to keep your products from being classified as a drug, and other such important information invaluable to those just going into business. Besides containing great resources such as essential oil profiles, aromatherapy schools, suppliers, crop calendar, weights and measurements, this book is packed with personality, and practical worthy tips based on Kayla's experience raising a family, and running a successful business.

This will be one new aromatherapy book you will want to add to your library. I highly recommend this book for personal and professional use and it will be required reading for my students. Thank you Kayla for making this available, job well done!"
Sylla Sheppard Hanger, Founder/Director of the Atlantic Institute of Aromatherapy, United Aromatherapy Effort, Inc. and NAHA Chair of the Safety Committee

"'Wow!' is the word that best describes how I felt while reading Kayla Fioravanti's new book: *The Art, Science and Business of Aromatherapy, Your Guide for Personal Aromatherapy and Entrepreneurship.*

I would recommend this book to anyone who already is an aromatherapist or has an aromatherapy business, and for those who want to start a new business in the wonderful field of aromatherapy. Schools that offer education in aromatherapy would also benefit by including this book on their recommended reading list.

The book was written with passion and devotion to the art of aromatherapy. I felt inspired when reading Kayla's personal story of her aromatic adventure and how it all began with the essential oil of Tea Tree. She generously shares her personal experiences and her in-depth knowledge of the oils, both of which are invaluable when it comes to having a successful aromatherapy business. Kayla's writing style is honest, understandable and refreshing.

Kayla's start-to-finish 'how-to' tips offer the reader advice and knowledge that can be used time and time again. The book includes a detailed timeline of the history of aromatics, including labeling requirements, and everything in between. A section on essential oil profiles is followed by a vast list of resources. Everything but the aromatic kitchen sink can be found in this book! And come to think of it, there even is information on what type of sink space to include in your aromatherapy business space planning too!

I think the reader will enjoy and appreciate this book as much as I did."
Kelly Holland Azzaro, RA, CCAP, CBFP, LMT, NAHA President

"A little bit business inspiration, a little bit textbook and a lot of great practical ideas on how to work with essential oils and aromatherapy for your small business are packed into this helpful, down to earth book. Kayla writes with ease and makes even the most difficult concepts easily digestible for everyone from the home crafter to the accomplished businessperson. You'll learn about how to blend essential oils, why to use certain oils, about crop growing seasons and much much more. This is a great reference book for anyone interested in essential oils."
Anne-Marie Faiola, Founder SoapQueen.com

"Through The Art, Science and Business of Aromatherapy, Your Guide for Personal Aromatherapy and Entrepreneurship, Kayla has lifted the art of aromatherapy to a new level. Not only will you find information about essential oils, but you'll also discover Kayla's warm, witty perspective. This book is comprehensive, clear and beautifully presented. I love the recipes ("Messy Cupcakes" is my favorite), and with each page I turn, my love for aromatherapy deepens and grows. This book is an indispensable addition to the library of the aromatherapist, the entrepreneur and everyone in between."
Donna Maria Coles Johnson, Founder & CEO, Indie Beauty Network

"Lucky for us, Kayla has hit another home run with her second book! Her profound gift for distilling complex scientific concepts down to their essence shines through in The Art, Science and Business of Aromatherapy. This comprehensive, insightful reference should be staple in the library of anyone interested in natural products or organic medicine and any budding entrepreneur considering a career in the personal care market. Kayla's candid recollection of her early days in business is as illuminating and inspiring a tale as any I have read. I especially appreciate the invaluable aromatherapy blending information, as well as the recipes and formulas sprinkled throughout the text. In short: this volume is a virtual goldmine brimming with wisdom from one of the brightest minds in the industry."
Lela Barker, Founder Bella Luccè and From Morocco with Love

"WOW, Kayla!!! This is truly magnificent! I really love your book, it is excellent. It is perfect for those wishing to start a business or better yet, trying to save a current one. The profiles are excellent! I also loved your explanation of the chemical constituents and basic chemistry in general. Your descriptions of scent are wonderful and I found myself craving the scents while reading them. The Biblical references are beautiful, I love them. I will want two copies, one for my desk and one at home."
Kathy Steinbock, Aromatherapist, Soapmaker

The Art, Science and Business of Aromatherapy
Your Guide for Personal Aromatherapy and Entrepreneurship

By Kayla Fioravanti, R.A.
Certified and Registered Aromatherapist, Cosmetic Formulator

Editing by Bethany Learn and Aleta Sanstrum, Ready2Publish

Cover and Text Design by Alex Badcock

Copyright © 2011 by Kayla Fioravanti

ISBN-13: 978-0615571492 (Selah Press)
ISBN-10: 0615571492

Printed in the United States of America

Published by
Selah Press

Dedication

To Dennis,

God blended some powerful synergy when He blessed me with you.

"…where you go I will go, and where you stay I will stay. Your people will be my people and your God my God. Where you die I will die, and there I will be buried. May the LORD deal with me, be it ever so severely, if even death separates you and me." Ruth 1:16-17

Acknowledgements

It took a community effort to get this book out my head, onto paper and into print. I could have never accomplished this alone. I am grateful for the team that carried me through this process.

Thank you to one of the world's leading experts in aromatherapy, Robert Tisserand for his advice and scrutiny of this book. I am honored that Sylla Sheppard-Hanger, Founder/Director of the Atlantic Institute of Aromatherapy and NAHA Chair of the Safety Committee gave so much of her time and effort to checking this book for aromatherapy accuracy. I am so appreciative to Kelly Holland Azzaro, RA, CCAP, LMBT, LMT and NAHA President for her priceless input and correction. I have the highest respect for these aromatherapists who have changed the face of the industry. I am honored to even get to play on the same ball field with the three of them.

Special thanks to my editors Bethany Learn and Aleta Sanstrum of Ready2Publish. Aleta cleaned up my grammar while Bethany took all the puzzle pieces of this book and transformed the entire flow of it. This book was a project I worked on long ago, set aside and picked back up sometime later. I am so grateful to my early editors Dana Brown and Lesley Ann Craig who helped me get started on this project in the first place. When both were otherwise committed, Bethany and Aleta effortlessly picked up the project and ran further with it than I ever imagined taking it. Thank you all!

Special thanks for the incredible insider industry information that Steven Borden, our buyer at Essential Wholesale, shared with me. I never could have even attempted this project without Ryan Mader holding down the fort in the R&D Lab. We have been especially blessed by all the employees who have crossed the door of Essential Wholesale over the years. They have supported us, taught us how to be leaders and blessed us with trust over the years. A special shout out to the Essential Wholesale leadership team of Diane Humke, Laura Badcock, Barry Weinmann, Rick Hume and Alex Badcock for consistently going above and beyond the call of duty. I am also thankful for our Essential Wholesale customers for giving us the privilege of being a part of their dreams. We never could have reached for our dreams without you.

I'd like to give a special shout-out to my Facebook "Committee" who advised me on content, the name of my book and cheered me along the way. Also to my purr-therapists Go-go and Star who sat with me through every word of this book. Thanks David Sanford of Credo Communications who removed all the barriers to publishing by sharing his insider information with me. Thanks to the creative mastermind behind the look of this book, Alex Badcock.

I am particularly grateful to my husband Dennis. He built a business around my passions and then nudged me into growth beyond my wildest dreams. I feel blessed by our three children, Keegan, Selah and Caiden, who have taught me new things about myself and life every day. My son, Keegan, was the inspiration that launched me into becoming an accidental aromatherapist. And I'm thankful that when I was six my parents bought me a chemistry set and a perfume kit, and in doing so taught me that experimenting is play. I will forever miss my mother and cherish my father.

Last, but most importantly, I am eternally grateful to my savior Jesus Christ. I am strongest when I am bowed down at the foot of the cross.

Table of Contents

About the Author

Kayla is a Certified, ARC Registered Aromatherapist and the co-Founder of Essential Wholesale and its lab division, Essential Labs. She is a wife and mother of three. She started her company along with her husband, Dennis. In 1998, Kayla started creating products in her kitchen using essential oils and a $50 investment. Over the years Dennis and Kayla turned the profit from their first batch of products into more supplies and repeated the process over and over again, remaining a debt free company.

In 2000, Dennis and Kayla started an all-natural aromatherapy based Home Party Plan. In 2002, they changed their business plan and became the distribution and manufacturing company, Essential Wholesale. This was followed by the addition of Essential Labs in 2005. The initial $50 investment from their home kitchen, combined with blood, sweat and prayers, has now become a multi-million dollar organically certified and U.S. Food and Drug Administration (FDA) compliant company.

Kayla has passionately shared her knowledge of aromatherapy, crafting, business, and formulating. She is the go-to industry specialist for formulating aromatherapy, natural, organic and pure cosmetics and personal care items. She has formulated thousands of products including: mineral make up, skin care, body care, and products for bath, spa, hair, baby, pets, aroma and much more. Through her lab division, Essential Labs, Kayla has formulated private-label personal care products for hundreds of businesses worldwide.

Kayla can be found on YouTube where she teaches a variety of do-it-yourself (DIY) recipes for the Essential Wholesale series called "Kitchen Chemistry TV." Kayla's articles can be found in dozens of publications including: Dermascope Magazine, Les Nouvelles Esthetique, Global Cosmetic Industry (GCI) Magazine, New York Metro Parent, Saponifier, National Association of Holistic Aromatherapy and Essential Wholesale's educational arm, the Essential U blog. Kayla has been featured in, and has given expert advice to hundreds of magazines including: Real Simple, Self Magazine, Prevention Magazine, Good Housekeeping, Home Business Magazine, Women Entrepreneur, Elle, Private Label Buyer, Redbook, InStyle Magazine, Woman's World and more.

Kayla wrote a chapter in the book *Millionaire Mom: The Art of Raising a Business and a Family at the Same Time* by Joyce Bone. Her quotes are featured in the 2009 and 2010 "The Woman's Advantage" calendar. Kayla has been a guest on radio programs such as Millionaire Moms Radio, The Organic View, Organic Beauty Radio, Indie Radio, KPDQ Northwest Showcase, Good Day Oregon, 104.1 The Fish, and many others.

Kayla has been an outspoken advocate for small business owners in the halls of Congress since 2007. Kayla created the Essential U blog, an educational center for aromatherapy, cosmetics, industry standards, and business ownership. She has been an expert on the website Personal Care Truth, Information Based on Scientific Facts, because of her passion to spread science-based factual information about cosmetics and the personal care industry. One of her goals is to help protect small businesses from regulatory interference which may hamper the pursuit of the American dream.

:: *Chapter 1* ::
The Accidental Aromatherapist

In the Beginning, There was Tea Tree

The story of how I got started in the aromatherapy, soap, natural cosmetics and personal care industry is very much like the story of many others who start a small business: I was fulfilling a personal need. It was the summer of 1998 when my son, Keegan, got a case of ringworm on his face that would not go away.

We tried Over-the-Counter (OTC) drugs and prescriptions to clear it up, but it kept growing. Since I was partly raised while living overseas, I had learned to go to the apothecary to find natural cures. So I headed to the tiny, local health food store where we were living in Edmond, Oklahoma as it was the closest thing I could find to an apothecary. The store clerk had nothing to do but stand in the book aisle and read books with me. Everything we read pointed to tea tree essential oil as the cure to ringworm.

At that time, our family was on a very tight student budget, so I bought the smallest bottle of tea tree essential oil and headed home to see if my eleven-dollar investment would work. Much to my surprise, within three days the ringworm was completely gone. In addition, I had expected the tea tree to cause allergic reactions because I am allergic to fragrances, but I had no problems. Because of that combination of events, I became very intrigued about this thing called aromatherapy.

Before that encounter with tea tree essential oil, I had always just assumed that aromatherapy was one of the foo-foo fluffery esoteric things out there in the market. When I thought of aromatherapy I envisioned the incense burners that make me take the long way around the hippy haven stores that line Hawthorne Avenue in Portland, Oregon.

With my new-found interest in the healing benefits of essential oils, I went to the local library and checked out every book they had on aromatherapy. After I read those, I put in a request for all of the aromatherapy books available in the state to be sent to my local library. Once I started digging into the science of essential oils, I was fully addicted to learning. It was then that I started researching and studying to become a certified aromatherapist.

At that time I was a stay at home mom, homeschooling my now-ringworm-free son, while my husband was a full-time student and working full-time! When Christmas arrived we needed to make our gifts because we couldn't afford to purchase them. So, I decided to use the tea tree from our medicine cabinet to scent the melt and pour soap we bought from the local craft store. We created an assortment of soaps with different sizes and shapes and packaged them up nicely. My husband, Dennis, has a long history of creating companies, so he decided to add re-order forms along with the gifts. In retrospect it might have been a bit tacky, but it worked!

Our friends and family loved the soap and, not only did they order more, but they referred us to their friends and family. When the orders came in we just kept making more, thinking our little hobby would be nothing more than that, but we were wrong! Bit by bit people began asking for more products and we started to expand our line at first by buying from overseas or out of Canada since no one in the U.S. made bulk natural products at the time. We started to realize that our little Oklahoma-based aromatherapy hobby was turning into a miniature micro-business.

When my mother suffered a heart attack, I felt the need to move back to the Northwest to be closer to my parents. But our hobby didn't bring in enough funds to afford us the luxury of moving. It wasn't until shortly after I totaled our car in an accident that an opportunity presented itself. When a $6,000 check came in the mail to replace our car Dennis asked if I would prefer to use it to move to Portland or to buy a new car? I jumped at the opportunity to take the money and move our family and business back to the Pacific Northwest with the car we had left.

It was a Friday, and on the following Monday Dennis was scheduled to start his training with the Police Academy – so it was now or never. So that Monday, instead of it being the first day at the Academy for Dennis, it became moving day. We loaded the back of our U-Haul with all of our earthly garage-sale possessions along with a small box filled with essential oils and soap molds. In the cab of the U-Haul we packed in one car seat with our six week-old baby Selah, one cat litter box, one beloved cat named Star, two adults and our 6 year-old son Keegan.

It was a snug fit, but we were excited. We had just enough money to get us to Portland to set up our new lives. We hitched our 12 year-old car onto the back and headed North to a land of unknowns. We had no job, no place to live, and very limited resources with only 5 days to return the truck before we got charged again…But we were full of hope, aspirations, and dreams. Anything seemed possible.

After about twenty miles, just outside Oklahoma City, the truck broke down for the first time. After a couple of hours of quick repairs, we continued our journey. Everything was going well until the next day. As we drove up a long incline in Burley, Idaho, we noticed lots of black smoke pouring of our U-Haul. This time there were no quick repairs to be made. The U-Haul guys unhooked our car, towed our U-Haul off the highway, and set us free in the Middle-of-Nowhere-Ville, Idaho. We holed up in a seedy hotel with our cat, a baby, and a 6 year-old while repairs were made, and our time and resources diminished. We were detoured, but we were not fazed – yet.

With our truck fixed three days later, the guys at U-Haul hitched our little car back onto the tow dolly and sent us on our way with promises to reimburse us for our detour sometime later. We left Burley with even more dreams. Dennis has spent the down time imagining up new divisions and exciting directions. I have to admit, our little detour sparked new ideas in Dennis' mind that—by the sheer size of those dreams—scared me.

With one day to spare before the U-Haul was due to be returned, we rolled into Portland, Oregon in need of a job and a home. We unhitched our car from the U-Haul and found that it had aspirations of its own: to roll down the hill and away from us undeterred by the constrictions of brakes. We discovered that we had literally dragged our twelve year old Toyota the five hundred and eighty six miles between Burley, Idaho and Portland, Oregon with the emergency brake engaged. The U-Haul mechanic had set it when he loaded our car back on the dolly and forgotten to release it. Still undaunted, we forked over our formally-earmarked house deposit money to have brand new brakes put on our old car. We rented a car so we could still find a place to live that day.

Traditional home rental options were out since we had no deposit funds left, no jobs, no income, no credit, and very little money. Our journey had depleted our funds for first and last month's rent, security deposit, and all the other fees those people threw at us, walking in the door. After several rejections in town, we found ourselves driving way out in to the countryside in the small town of Molalla. As we drove through a cute little neighborhood, Dennis suddenly stopped the car to talk to a man putting up a For Sale sign in the lawn.

A few minutes later, Dennis came back to the car and said, "Let's go get the truck." Despite our situation, he had convinced that man to rent us his home until it sold. He handed him a check for that month's rent and drove back to get all our worldly belongings so that we could move into our cute, new home. We were ready to unpack and settle in so we could get back to our new hobby business.

However, when we pulled the U-Haul up to the house with great anticipation, and we released the back door of the U-Haul to unpack, we found that all our life possessions and our "business in one box" was covered in thick black soot. It seemed that the black smoke that had poured out of the U-Haul truck had been going directly into the storage area of the truck. We suddenly had no clothes, bedding or furniture—nothing was spared!

A few set-backs later—and even more broke than we had planned—we got ourselves settled into the Northwest. We started homeschooling Keegan, and Dennis started school. Our Molalla home-front meant that Dennis had a 36 mile commute each way to and from school. Between his studies, though, we started building our dreams into a business.

Our kitchen became our R&D lab. I ordered more library books and, in between homeschooling and caring for our little baby, filled my mind with more information on aromatherapy and cosmetics. Business came natural to Dennis, and he began building up our mail-order aromatherapy business as we sat on the floor of our new home with our new particle-board desk furniture. We were not willing to allow the roadblocks, detours, and distractions to stop us from reaching for goals.

A few weeks later a friend noticed how enthusiastic I was about aromatherapy, so she invited me to have a product party at her house and teach what I knew about essential oils. She invited her friends over, and I taught them all about aromatherapy. Two of the women asked how they could become consultants and sell my product. I wrote down their info and promised to get back to them. I went home with $500 worth of orders and a new idea. Dennis took that idea and ran with it. He developed a multi-level business plan and manual. We signed up our first consultants that same week. As we grew our party plan, we endured yet another move to be closer to Dennis' school. Meanwhile we continued to fill the orders for our little multi-level business out of our small apartment kitchenette.

The party plan really took off, and we found ourselves supporting over fifty consultants after only a few months. As we raced around trying to fill orders we realized that we had to move the business out of our two-bedroom apartment kitchenette to a "huge" 600 square-foot building to keep up with our growing need for ingredients and supply space. We were very scared because that was a huge investment for us with absolutely no guarantee of success. I thought, "Well if we fail, at least we can move into our manufacturing space until our lease is up."

In the middle of all of this, our family expanded with the birth of our daughter Caiden, and we were determined to keep everyone with us while we grew our business. Dennis focused on growing the business while I made the products. We were completely overwhelmed as we worked night and day toward a vision that was not very clear at the time and changed often. We contacted all of the cosmetic manufacturing companies in search of someone who would private label for us or custom formulate product that met our needs. It was then that we discovered that the industry purchase minimums were either 4 drums (220 gallons) or 10,000 pieces and we couldn't afford or store either one. With new challenges facing us, Dennis and I decided to re-invent how "natural" cosmetics were being made, so I went back to the library to do more research, and the journey continued.

This was long before there were craft books on how to make bath and body products. I read all of the copyrighted recipes of the chemical companies in order to better understand the chemistry of cosmetics. Once I gathered enough knowledge to understand the concept of emulsion and preservation, I became a research and development queen. I ordered samples of ingredients, and by trial and error I created our own cosmetic formulas that were safe, stable, and made with naturally-derived ingredients.

Once we had perfected our formulas, Dennis realized that there was a giant niche in the industry that was wide open. No one was offering "natural" bulk bases to the small businesses, crafters, or hobby-level consumers. He also determined that it would be much easier to manufacture in bulk and sell to thousands of small businesses than it was to make one retail product at a time.

I was terrified. I knew Dennis would succeed and I couldn't imagine making hundreds if not thousands of gallons-worth of product. I was making all of our products in two-gallon batches! I remember clearly the sheer panic that overtook me when Dennis announced that we were going to change our business model in the midst of our original aromatherapy party plan company. I had worked so many hours writing training material, formulating products, doing parties, training consultants, making product, and doing everything else it took to build our party plan business from scratch. We were busier than you could imagine, growing substantially while working our tails off.

Dennis had this bright idea to start a new company and call it Essential Wholesale. He wanted to shut down the party plan and become a wholesale manufacturer of the cosmetic bases, using the formulas we had developed. It seemed counter intuitive to me to shut down something that, for all intents and purposes, was working. He was totally sold out on his new vision for our future, but I was scared of the change. What I didn't know—but what Dennis could see clearly—was that the party plan business was about to implode because its growth was unsustainable given our lack of capital resources.

The reality was that we were working around the clock, and nothing about our business model left an opportunity for that to ever change. Our mistake was that when a customer attended one of our parties they had the ability to order a customized aromatherapy product for their exact needs. That meant that every product had to be scented and mixed by me, because the use of the correct dose of each essential oil in a given product could only be determined by a trained aromatherapist—and I was it. We were working until two or four a.m., only to go back to our office by nine a.m. and do it all again. It was insane, but I was afraid that if we changed I would have to pay the same dues to succeed in the new company.

Dennis had the forethought to change our business model so that someday our jobs would be able to be duplicated. Our organically-grown business that had started with only fifty dollars, combined with a significant investment of time and effort, needed a makeover.

I was emotionally hanging onto all the time and energy we had invested into our party plan. Dennis was using logic and striving for a better future for us. I was frightened of the change. Dennis talked about one day making thousands of gallons of product in one batch, and I wondered how I could physically do that, given that I was killing myself to produce the few gallons we produced per week at that point.

Thankfully I let go of my worries and grasped onto the dreams of my husband. I made the leap with my eyes wide open, hands shaking, heart palpitating, and my vision firmly focused on Dennis' dream. Once I made the successful leap to his dream, it became mine. I thank God that I was able to set aside my fear of change and let go of a faulty future that would have held us back from our greatest potential.

Our original business, FCP Parties, ran from 1999 to 2001. In 2001 we began the early stages of launching Essential Wholesale, and we were exclusively supported by that division by October of 2002. And 2003 was our first year of having only Essential Wholesale sales and customers. So for four years, from 1998 through 2002, we transitioned from one idea to another, blindly weaving our way toward an idea that had yet to be discovered. Finally, in 2003 we embarked on our continuing journey with Essential Wholesale.

We created Essential Wholesale with no minimum dollar amount for bulk wholesale product and 2 gallon minimums for custom formulating. Essential Wholesale hit the ground running. We quickly outgrew our 600 square-foot facility and moved to a 2,500 square foot space. We outgrew that space within five months but still managed to operate there for one and-a-half years. We are currently housed in a 35,000 square-foot, certified organic, and FDA registered facility. However, Essential Wholesale is once more out of space and will be moving in 2012 to a 58,000 square-foot, state-of-the-art manufacturing space.

Imagine if I had allowed my fear of change to stifle the dreams that Dennis had for Essential Wholesale and, later, Essential Labs! Now, we have over 4,000 gallons worth of tanks in our tank farm, and when I walk through it and remember all the small batches that I killed myself making, I have to smile. I was afraid of the growth ahead because I envisioned myself making *every ounce of product* when in reality, business growth freed me up and I haven't made an ounce of product outside of the R&D lab for years. Thank God I got myself out of the way of our potential.

Our labs division, created in 2005, and known as Essential Labs, became the private label and contract manufacturing division that specializes in creating custom natural and organic cosmetics, mineral make-up, and personal care items to companies big and small around the world.

We are passionate about clean and natural products. We have loved being a part of people's hopes and dreams. Every day we have had the opportunity to support small start-up companies and have watched hundreds of them become big companies. We have seen thousands of people create a comfortable income that allows them to stay home with their families. Plus, when a "big" company decides to partner with us to create a new "natural" alternative line to what they have been selling, we get *really* excited!

Shouldn't our everyday lives be centered on what we are passionate about? Shouldn't we spend our time consumed with what we love, believe in, and cherish? We have loved working on Essential Wholesale because it was never work to us. Dennis enjoyed building and developing this business. I loved the researching and developing of products.

As a couple, we managed to create a business that allowed us to be creative in our own ways and to work together toward a common goal. This business gave me an outlet for my creative passions which include creating new things and writing the Essential U blog, writing articles for countless industry and consumer magazines, all while feeding the science nerd in me. It has opened the door for me to write this book and my first book, *How to Make Melt and Pour Soap Base from Scratch*.

If I look back even further, I can find the roots of Essential Wholesale and my passion for this industry in my childhood. My parents have said that they should have known what my brother and I would grow up to be, based on our interests as children. We both followed our passions. My brother Kevin loved to watch Mutual of Omaha's Wild Kingdom and Jacques-Yves Cousteau. He watched these shows with great interest and curiosity and his career led him to the top of Discovery Channel and National Geographic.

As we grew up, I sat beside him and studied the color variations of the shag carpet. I was unable to focus in on the T.V. program itself. I found myself lost in my environment and wondering how things worked. I preferred to sit in my room playing with my chemistry set or perfume set over watching a television show of any kind. I conducted all sorts of experiments and never followed the directions. I lived outside the box, always striving to see what would happen if I mixed my chemistry set ingredients with my perfume kit ingredients. I also spent hours digging through my mother's bathroom cupboards in search of things to smell, touch, and experience.

In fourth grade I fell in love with putting my words down on paper. I set my pen free to scribble every thought and every expression that bounced around in my mind. I wrote "Dear Diary" in endless journals accompanied by volumes of poetry. I wrote out my joys, tears, goodbyes, life lessons, and my love. I scribbled down notes to remind myself of how a string of words sounded as they bounced off of each other.

I remember the day poetry came alive for me, I was sitting on the bleachers in Stuttgart, Germany waiting for another softball team to finish playing so that my game could start. With pen and paper in hand I watched a spider crawl across the bleachers and right then and there wrote my first poem. On that day, words came alive on paper, and ever since then, I have dreamed of being a famous poet. I have written thousands upon thousands of poems since then. I spent years transcribing the music that I heard inside my mind into poetry. In college, when I traveled home for vacations, I carried a military duffel bag filled with all the poetry that I had written in my lifetime. Today, a young woman like me, overflowing with words, only needs to carry her laptop computer or smartphone to hold as many of her poems.

I never imagined that all those years of writing would someday become part of the modern American graffiti known as blogging. I never dreamed that I would use my love for words to scrawl out my life across the computer screens of America. I imagined my words contained within the covers of a poetry book but never as a blog, free to travel the digital world. I wonder how many from my generation and older dreamed of publishing books and how many from my children's generation will realize the freedom that the internet has given the creative mind. Significant changes in the publishing world have made it easy to place my books into online bookstores.

By the time I reached adulthood, my passions had increased to creating in the kitchen, making my own perfumes and beauty products, and writing words on paper. But there was no congruency and no plan of how to pull together a lifestyle that would allow my creativity to earn me a living. My husband, Dennis, brought the missing link to my world. His vision to build Essential Wholesale was a perfect fit to my passions.

In my thirties, I gathered up my creative skills and my science abilities along with my knowledge of how the human brain and body works, and I became an aromatherapist and cosmetic formulator. However, it took until I was forty years old for me to experience the most fulfilling years of my life. I have combined all of my passions: perfume (aromatherapy), chemistry (cosmetic formulating), color art (make-up) and poetry (newsletter, blog and books) along with my love of my family.

I am the person who will jump into a freezing river or push my body past exhaustion to reach the top of a mountain on my hands and knees just for the experience. And I am the person who will start a business on a shoestring budget. I will chase giant dreams with my husband into overwhelmingly fast-paced business growth. I am the person who will fail, experience utter defeat and then jump right back into the same raging river of business. And I'm okay with that now. I'm not bothered by the people who are standing on the banks of the river shaking their heads in disapproval. I love the rush, love the experience, and I thrive in the growing and painful experiences of it all.

That said, we must remember that behind every business success story is at least one or more business failure story. Dennis and I are no different. As a matter of fact, many investors are hesitant to invest in someone who hasn't failed yet. Our business success story has two major business failures that both preclude and are intertwined with our story.

Failure #1 - PB&J's Live

The setting was in the kitchen of PB&J's Live on a busy Friday night. It was the winter of 1996. Dennis and I were friends and business partners. Keegan, my son, was four years old and I was a single mother. Dennis was single and a budding serial entrepreneur. The stress level at our restaurant, PB&J's Live, was high. The business was surviving from week to week on the income brought in on Friday and Saturday Comedy nights. I ran the kitchen, and Dennis was in charge of everything else.

Finances were too tight to have a babysitter, so Keegan was tucked in a safe corner within my line of sight. When the orders started coming in that Friday evening, I handed Keegan a box of markers and gave him directions to stay on the milk crate. I could swear that I had also handed him paper to write on, but given what happened next, maybe I forgot? It is likely that I had it in my mind to give him paper and markers, but I had too much on my mind, and the small details must have escaped me. From Keegan's perspective, the only thing missing in the scenario was upon which to color.

Keegan was always content as long as he was near me. He was especially quiet that night and never left the milk crate. At one point, I glanced over and noticed that Keegan was writing on his hand. I thought to myself that I would go stop him once I got the orders started. I was always rushed to get dinner on every table before the comedy act started.

The hours rolled on, and with each glance at Keegan, I noticed a growing marker tattoo expanding on his body. I kept thinking there would be a break in the dinner rush, which would provide the opportunity for me to go stop his body art, but I didn't have a moment to spare as order after order after order piled in. I sent plate after plate out to the dining room. PB&J's Live was hopping, and Keegan was quiet. By the time the final dessert left the kitchen, and I had time to take a hard look at Keegan, I found him, colorful and quiet on the empty milk crate.

Keegan had taken the free opportunity to not only decorate himself from head to toe, but to do so with gusto. He had colored every inch of skin he could reach without taking off his shorts. He had been so detailed in his work that he had colored behind his ears and even inside of them. He was a walking masterpiece. I couldn't be mad because I had watched him do it and hadn't stopped him. I simply had to smile while he explained each detail of his design. It was washable ink, so "no harm, no foul" was my thought.

Sometimes we have to make a judgment call on the things that we give the power to upset us. I could have beaten myself down believing that I had neglected my son. I could have been angry at my circumstances as our business was barely surviving. I could have been mad that I worked all day at a regular job and all night at our business and still didn't have enough money to get a babysitter for my son. But in reality my son was happier with me no matter what I was doing. I had chosen to start a business when I was already financially struggling. I had made choices that resulted in all the events of the night and I chose to not regret the circumstances I found myself in.

However, our business did eventually fail by circumstances outside of our control. Packing our restaurant on Friday and Saturday nights was great for us, but it did not go over well with the other restaurant and a video store with which we shared our parking lot. Our customers took over every space and then some. Not only did we share the same parking lot with these businesses, but we also shared the same landlord. The long-term relationships that the other two businesses had with our landlord outweighed her loyalty to us, and just before Christmas her lawyers sent us a cease-and-desist order. It stated that we could no longer serve hot food, that we couldn't be open at dinner time and that we could no longer provide live entertainment.

The cease-and-desist order was a business killer for us. We had sunk every penny and more into starting up PB&J's Live and had nothing left over to fight for our business or even open our doors for another meal without our menu, dinner service and live entertainment. We had made fatal errors in our contract and our location. We simply had to close our doors, auction off our equipment and walk away with a huge business loss and debt.

Dennis and I may have failed at that business but our friendship led to marriage. We all laugh at the stories of the experiences we had at PB&J's Live now. The markers washed off of Keegan. We all remember how Keegan felt like just as much of an owner of our restaurant as we did - minus the financial stress. He loved to greet people, seat people, and sing on stage before we opened. He was sad to say goodbye to his PB&J's family, and we learned a very expensive business lesson. But in the end, Keegan grew up with Dennis and I as we built, failed, rebuilt, started over, and grew our family businesses.

Failure #2 - von Natur

When we left Essential Wholesale's 2500 square foot space to move into our current space, we still had a year left on our lease. Dennis had an idea to convert the vacant building into a store, which lead to the idea of a mini spa. Since I was in quite an ambitious phase of my life, I immediately jumped on the band wagon. Between being a wife, mother and business woman, I had felt separated from my creative side, so I saw a mini-spa as an opportunity to give my artistic side a new creative outlet.

Converting an empty warehouse into a store front and mini-spa took an enormous amount of creativity, sweat and labor. In the end, the space was amazing. A local television station even did a feature on the design of the store. The layout was exquisite. The staff was great. The products were selling like gangbusters. Yet, the store was a bottomless money pit that demanded constant time, money and energy. We expanded, redeveloped and redesigned, and around the clock we worked. The spa was eating up our time and Essential Wholesale was suffering from our divided attention.

We tried everything to stop the hemorrhaging. Finally, Dennis called a halt to it all and we shut down the von Natur store and spa. I was devastated because I had invested so much emotional energy into the creative side of the building, the products and into the lives of the people that worked for us. I had to lay everyone off, admit defeat and leave behind the piece of art I had made the building into. Mentally, the spa was eating us alive. Emotionally, I was crushed.

With the spa closed, we put all of our focus into branding a product line. We launched a new look for the product and took it to trade shows. I would describe the look as "one of those things you thought was a good idea at the time." The graphics were splashy, colorful and expensive. In reality, I think the stress we were under made us go a little extreme on our look. Buyers loved our product at trade shows, and they loved the concept of our product line, but they hated our look. Our extreme packaging was a shiny, foil disaster.

On top of that, the product line itself was in chaos. There was no relationship between our packaging and the high quality of the product inside. We had not developed clear product lines, so customers were left guessing which cleanser to use with which toner. We were mid-stream, getting notice from the press and enjoying serving thousands of loyal customers. The products themselves were amazing, but we had packaged them inappropriately. We finally decided to end the product line too. To do this, we had to let go of history and wipe the slate clean.

I could not believe we were starting over again. I dreamed up many creative ways that we could use up the packaging and not lose the money we had invested, but there was no option but to scrap what we had and to start from the beginning. We went back to square one to start fresh and new, licking our wounds and learning from our mistakes. That time around, when we revamped the products, we surrounded ourselves with experts and leaned heavily on their advice and counsel. Our employees helped us redefine the product line from the inside out. They shared our burden and made it bearable.

So why did I run a private label manufacturing company, a bulk manufacturing company and launch a retail store/mini-spa along with a product line, all while trying to be a wife and mom at the same time? Well, I suffered from the "super woman complex." I have been prone to think that I could and should do everything myself. I learned from the experience to delegate, to entrust others with my dreams, my vision and my burdens.

I thought Dennis and I could do it all. Together, we had started Essential Wholesale by ourselves while homeschooling one child, with another child in a back-pack and one in my belly. We worked around the clock for that dream because we had to. Our saving grace is that, when we failed—not once with von Natur, but twice—we were surrounded by a team of people who chose to walk beside us.

We did not open the spa with the intention of learning so many hard lessons. In failure, I was humbled. I learned to let go and embrace the experience and all that it taught me. I learned that failure in business is just that: business failure. It does not equal personal defeat.

We embraced the opportunity to reinvent ourselves, but the opportunity for reinvention only came after financial, physical and emotional breaking. I had created a "whole new me" many times in life. But this time was different. In the case of the spa, I had lost sight of the ultimate goal by only focusing on the playing field that I was on. The spa was the playing field comprised of the employees, the building, and the customers. The goal was to have a successful business. We were not even heading toward the goal, but I was so emotionally wrapped up in the playing field that I fought Dennis when it was time to let go.

I was like a drowning woman flapping frantically for something to stop me from drowning, all the while fighting against the rescue. When I surrendered to the rescue I was so relieved. The burden had been so extreme that even the heavy task of laying people off and closing our doors was a massive relief. Closing the spa was the most logical move we had ever made. Level-headed as I am, I still needed a moment to grieve the failure and the broken relationships and let go. The night before the spa closed I wept privately, but by morning I was all business.

Our lives were changed dramatically in the process of the spa and product lines' multiple false starts, wrong directions and new beginnings. Since we are a married couple in business together, we have had to walk through this process without laying blame on each other. We have had to fail together, change together, start over together and - above all - put our relationship first.

I have been blessed with a husband who has always seen a very big picture. Yes, I was terrified in the beginning of our business because his vision was so huge! I could only see the orders that were in front of me each day. He would talk about our future, and it seemed so unrealistic when it was just the two of us barely making ends meet. I had to let go of my misdirection and follow Dennis' lead toward our mutual vision. We had done that once before when we morphed Essential Wholesale out of our previous business model, and I had the faith in him to follow his lead and stand by his side as we put in the labor and hard work each day.

The spa failure was very painful, though, because it was out in the world for everyone to see. I am extremely private while in pain, but this failure, this forced reinvention, was so very public. At first, I resisted being reinvented because it meant a public admission of failure. It meant that my business which others depended upon for income was going to fold underneath them. I was humiliated by the thought of letting other people down and not meeting their expectations.

The Lessons Learned in Failure
The biggest thing I learned while going through the process of failure is to not fight against it, so my philosophy is to be open to change. Be open to opportunities that come your way. Learn as much as you can from other people's mistakes, and from reading business magazines and books whenever possible. When things aren't working, don't hold onto an idea, a business, or the certain way you did things before.

Sometimes you get side-tracked and lose your focus on the goal. Don't beat yourself up, just allow yourself to refocus and change directions. You have to take a moment to have a pity party, but then let go and get on with the business of starting over.

Equip yourself with the lessons of others, your own life lessons, and a heavy dose of reality. One of the great lessons that I learned from failure was to become vulnerable. There are times in business that you make mistakes. You can't put your failures and mistakes in a bag and carry it around with you, occasionally using them to beat yourself up. The people that I laid off embraced me and faced their new jobless challenge. Many of them are still in my life.

More than anything, don't make any excuses that stop you from changing. For instance, if you want to lose weight you might excuse yourself from your workout one day by saying, "I'm too tired to exercise." However, until you start exercising, you will remain too tired. Once you follow through on your decision to start moving, your energy will be boundless.

My decisions got me to where I am in life. I took ownership of them, and the bitterness that could have grown out of discontent died for lack of nourishment. Don't trip yourself up or hold yourself back with excuses that you invent and hold on to for comfort or for fear of change. Forgive yourself, forgive others, and forgive your circumstances, so that you can be free to move forward and enjoy your journey.

Allow yourself to blossom right where you are and stop waiting for all of your ducks to be in a row. Maybe your ducks won't come together in a straight line at first. I know mine don't. The reality is that tomorrow my ducks could be scattered everywhere, but when I move in one direction, they will follow me. They won't do so in an orderly fashion, and there will be a lot of quacking, but my metaphoric ducks will eventually fall into line behind me as I paddle toward my goals. If I hang back, they hang back; if I throw my hands up in the air and surrender, they scatter. The very best thing for you to do is to move toward your goals and allow your frenzied ducks to follow.

Of course, we all want to move forward and succeed, but what if we could go back? If I found myself back at the beginning, and if I was starting out *then* with what I know *now*, I would live my life exactly the same. However, I wouldn't beat myself up for the chaos I create around me. I wouldn't allow others' disapproval of my creative energy to bother me.

I've never done anything halfway or without passion. If I choose to do something, it is wholeheartedly while I jump in with both feet. I've been known to jump into deep waters with my eyes closed, trusting that not only will I survive, but that I will thrive in the crisis.

I tend to over-commit myself and be stretched thin. I have friends who shake their heads and say, "I don't know how you do it." Well, I don't know how I *wouldn't* do it. If my plate wasn't already full of today's challenges, I would gather up other challenges. It is just my nature.

What is balance to me, is bedlam to another. I've allowed myself to embrace my own sense of balance. At times, there are tipping points that steal my laughter, and I have to fight back to reach my personal equilibrium. As the saying goes, "If mama ain't happy, ain't nobody happy." If I stop laughing and can't find humor even in the chaos, then my life is tipped out of balance, but when I am still laughing, there is still hope in every situation.

As I balance business and family in my own unique way, some might see my life as a state of constant chaos with varying degrees of out-of-control pandemonium. But I have discovered that I blossom right there in the middle of the self-imposed chaos. I operate well inside a world that many wouldn't enjoy. I know that is the case with most entrepreneurs. Rather than reaching for a life vest when we are drowning, we grab onto more of life. When our lives overflow, we are energized and renewed by the experience.

I believe it is healthy to accept who I am and allow myself to be everything God has created me to be even if I'll never fit into a conventional mold. In fact, I've realized that I can't make my life fit into the world's mold - it doesn't fit. How liberating it was for me to understand that my dreams and aspirations don't have to fit into another person's vision of success! Accepting and loving the person that I am has freed me to experience success beyond my wildest dreams.

When I stopped fighting against myself and my situation, I was free to succeed. For example, our family's focus on business places our children right in the middle, and that is not wrong or right, just different. It is the right path for our family, even if it is different. It is okay to be different.

I have learned to love living out loud, with failure alongside success, experiencing the strain of trials, all while walking beside my husband as we shoulder the burden together of the life we have chosen. I have learned that:

- When my circumstances are not like I imagined they would be … to find peace.
- When my fairy tale image of family is different than I expected… to rejoice in the details of the unexpected.
- When I am in the midst of failure … to get up and start again.
- When life feels like it is spinning out of control … to find my equilibrium and enjoy the adrenaline rush.

I have also learned that my creativity is mobile and not tied to the location in which I create. My creativity is a gift that I can use as a Cosmetic Formulator and Aromatherapist, as an artist and a writer. I don't have to hold on to one piece, one building, or one vision. It is an ever constant source of motivation that can flow into all aspects of my life.

Business and life are both like a canvas. You can wipe it clean and start over again. If you are like me and your strokes are heavy, your canvas will show the evidence of what you have done before. Even a scarred canvas can become something new and beautiful. I am so glad that my canvas can be used and that I can speak from my experienced journey of failure and success to better guide you around the pitfalls and trapdoors in this business.

It is never too late to succeed! Although I am in my forties now, I don't believe I am done growing up. I don't believe I am done succeeding. I still might be that famous poet I've always dreamed of becoming! It is early yet, and I still have a long and adventurous journey ahead of me.

Never be afraid of dreams so big that they cast a giant shadow of fear and doubt.

:: Chapter 2 ::
The Genesis of Aromatherapy

The Plant Apothecary

The word "aromatherapy" simply means: treatment with scent. It is the use of essential oils for the treatment of mind and body. The term "essential oil" comes from the Latin word, *essentia*, which means: essence or pertaining to essence. Essential oils are volatile because they are able to" fly" or evaporate since they are a liquid that quickly becomes gaseous. "Aroma" refers to: the naturally occurring scent of the essential oils and "therapy" refers to: the physical and psychological treatment imparted from essential oils.

Essential Oils are highly concentrated, potent oils produced by plants. Plants draw their energy from light, darkness, sun, and soil. They synthesize this energy into molecules of carbohydrates, proteins and fats in their own "chemical factories." The essential oils produced in this process are extracted from the plants, trees, seeds, shrubs, flowers, fruit peels or leaves. Plants are the crude fuels that humans and animals break down to produce adenosine triphosphate, known as the energy currency of life. Essential oils are, therefore, high-grade fuel that the plants themselves create when they absorb plant foods.

That said, the term "oil," in reference to essential oils, can sometimes be misleading. Essential oils are not actually oily like vegetable oils that are expressed from nuts and seeds. Essential oils are not oily at all. In fact, most essential oils are actually very light and appear watery. Most essential oils have a low viscosity while only a small handful has a high viscosity (e.g. sandalwood). According to the International Organization for Standardization, essential oils are a "product made by distillation with either water or steam, by mechanical processing of citrus rinds, or by dry distillation of natural materials. Following the distillation, the essential oil is physically separated from the water phase."

Essential oils provide a concentrated dose of nature's vast pharmacologically active ingredients in a single drop of oil. Essential oils are the most concentrated form of any botanical. Essential oils are the purest form of the plant's living structure. It takes an estimated one pound of any given plant to create one drop of essential oil, however some essential oils require much more than a pound of product per drop. For example, it takes about 1.3 lbs. or 125 rose buds, to produce one drop of rose absolute.

One hundred-percent pure unadulterated essential oils are distinguished by extraordinarily diverse substances that only nature can produce. But even though they are natural we teach that, to be completely safe, it is recommended to never apply undiluted essential oil to your skin. Essential oils should be diluted in carrier oil, lotion, soap, bath salts or other modes of application. A little bit of essential oil goes a long way. It only takes four to five drops of essential oil per ounce of unscented product to scent at the common level of one percent.

Aromatherapy Around the World and Through the Ages

Aromatherapy has developed and expanded from one culture to the next as it has spread throughout the world. There are thousands of essential oils on the market today but only about 300 are commonly used. The reasons for the differences in approaches from country to country can be explained by exploring the history and sources of aromatherapy. When we understand how aromatherapy has crossed many continents, cultures and centuries, we can better understand its roles in present times.

Egypt: The Egyptians were the first true aromatherapists. They are believed to have been first to use the essential oils of plants which they infused into carriers. They used fragrances in all aspects of their lives. Essential oils were used in their cosmetics, in their daily baths, in massages, and to fumigate sick rooms.

Essential oils were important in Egyptian religious ceremonies as well. They burned frankincense at dawn as an offering to the sun, and myrrh at dusk as an offering to the moon. Hieroglyphics in Egyptian temples depict the blending of oils and describe oils recipes. An ancient papyrus discovered in the Temple of Edfu contained medical formulas and perfume recipes for rituals performed by the alchemist and high priests.

Essential oils were significant in the embalming process of mummies. Beautiful alabaster jars and ebony coffers, filled with oils in preparation for the arrival of their dead into the "next world," were left in the tombs. The essential oils were used in the mummification process because of their antibacterial and antiseptic properties that helped prevent decay and decomposition of the bodies.

The tombs of the Pharaohs were filled with jars of essential oils they believed rendered the skin of the deceased supple when they arrived in the next world. In 1922, when archaeologists entered the tomb of Tutankhamen (King Tut), there was still a lingering fragrance from the pots of essential oils that had been there for over 3,000 years. The quality and expense of the essential oils used in burial were symbolic of the class and wealth of the dead.

For centuries, Egypt was well-regarded as the perfume capital of the world. In 48 BC, when Julius Caesar returned to Rome with Cleopatra VII after conquering Egypt, perfume bottles were tossed to the crowds to demonstrate his total domination of Egypt.

The Bible: During the exodus from Egypt, the Israelites took with them the knowledge of the Egyptians. The ancient Hebrews valued plants for medicinal, perfume and religious purposes. The Bible makes 231 references to various plants, herbs, anointing and holy oils and perfumes in both the Old and New Testaments.

In one reference, God gives a recipe for anointing oil: "Then the Lord said to Moses, 'Take the following fine spices: 500 shekels of liquid myrrh, half as much (that is, 250 shekels) of fragrant cinnamon, 250 shekels of fragrant cane, 500 shekels of cassia - all according to the sanctuary shekel - and a hin of olive oil. Make these into sacred anointing oil, a fragrant blend, the work of a perfumer. It will be sacred anointing oil.'" Exodus 30: 22-25.

We are told that frankincense and myrrh were offered by the three wise men to the infant Jesus, which again, gives a reference point of the value of essential oils in ancient times. "And when they were come into the house, they saw the young child with Mary his mother, and fell down, and worshipped him; and when they had opened their treasures, they presented unto him gifts: gold, and frankincense, and myrrh." Matthew 2:11

The significance of frankincense and myrrh being given to Jesus Christ at his birth is that both were known as embalming materials used by the Egyptians for Kings. The gift of frankincense and myrrh at his birth meant that Jesus was born to die for this world. In fact, myrrh is mentioned in the telling of the burial of Jesus as well. "He was accompanied by Nicodemus, the man who earlier had visited Jesus at night. Nicodemus brought a mixture of myrrh and aloes, about seventy-five pounds." John 19:39. Not only was Jesus born to die, but was the awaited Messiah King of Israel. "Then Nathanael declared, "Rabbi, you are the Son of God; you are the King of Israel." John 1:49

The following scripture in the Bible again mentions essential oil and its worth at that time: "Then Mary took about a pint of pure nard, an expensive perfume; she poured it on Jesus' feet and wiped his feet with her hair. And the house was filled with the fragrance of perfume. But one of his disciples, Judas of Iscariot, objected. 'Why wasn't this perfume sold and the money given to the poor? It was worth a year's wages.'" John 12:3-5.

Nard, today known as spikenard, was holy anointing oil that was used at the time for anointing, consecration, dedication and worship. It was worth about $2,200 in today's currency, which was equivalent to a year's wages for a common laborer at the time. The significance of nard being used just six days prior to Jesus being crucified can be seen in Jesus' response to Judas, "Leave her alone," said Jesus. "Why are you bothering her? She has done a beautiful thing to me. The poor you will always have with you, and you can help them any time you want. But you will not always have me. She did what she could. She poured perfume on my body beforehand to prepare for my burial. I tell you the truth, wherever the gospel is preached throughout the world, what she has done will also be told, in memory of her." Mark 14: 6-9

In Hebrew the word nard translates to "light." "When Jesus spoke again to the people, he said, "I am the light of the world. Whoever follows me will never walk in darkness, but will have the light of life." John 8:12

Greece: The first documented history of distillation was recorded by Herodotus, known as the Father of History, when he documented the method of distillation for turpentine in 425 BC.

Between the second and third centuries, the philosopher, Theophrastus, was Aristotle's pupil and later became his successor in the Peripatetic school. His botanical works, *Historia de Plantis* and *De Causis Plantarums*, were some of the earliest of their kind. Theophrastus is known as the Father of Botany, and in his scientific treatise *On Odors*, he covered the blending of perfumes, shelf-life, substances that carry scent, the use of wine with aromatics, and the effect of odor on the mind and body. *Historia Plantarum* formed the basis for all succeeding studies of plants and classifications until the Linnaean system was established in the 1750s.

The Greek physicians, Hippocrates, Galen, and Dioscorides all used essential oils for medicinal purposes and wrote texts that remained in use throughout the Middle Ages. Hippocrates developed herbal medicine into a scientific system by basing prescriptions upon accurate observation and diagnosis of the patient. He believed in daily aromatic baths and massages for wellness.

Galen, the physician to the Gladiators, sent the soldiers out to battle with a first aid kit containing myrrh.

Dioscorides noted that drancunculus oil can keep cancer in check, is an abortifacient, cures gangrene, and is good for eyesight. He also discovered the first source of salicylic acid from the willow tree, now used in aspirin.

When Alexander the Great defeated King Darius of Persia he threw out the King's box of ointments and perfumes. However, his interest in plants and aromatics later grew as he traveled in Asia. He dispatched deputies to both

Yemen and Oman in pursuit of the source of Arabian incense. Alexander the Great is said to have been in the habit of anointing his body with oils and having incense continuously burning by his throne.

Around the third century, history reports that Maria the Jewess, also known as Maria Prophetess, made a huge impact in alchemy with the invention of the double-boiler and the first true still, known as the tribokos. Her water bath, originally known as the balenim Maria, bain-Marie or "Maria's bath," but now known as a double-boiler, is still used today in kitchens and laboratories around the world to maintain temperature or to slowly heat a substance. Her tribokos was made of copper tubing, ceramic pottery and metal. The tribokos worked when plant material and water were heated up, creating vapors in the still. These vapors would condense on the inside of the still, and then trickle down to be collected in a bottle. These techniques and tools, plus other inventions of Maria's, are still used today.

Cleopatra VII, who was the last and most famous monarch of the dynasties established in the East by Alexander the Great, was a fragrance fanatic. According to history, she was seductive and striking, but not a great beauty. She is said to have used perfumes and cosmetics to her advantage. To this day, women still use cosmetics and perfumes to their advantage. Cleopatra certainly was a trend setter.

Rome: In the first century AD, Rome was said to be using 2,800 tons of imported frankincense and 550 tons of myrrh per year. The extravagant Emperor Nero had the first air conditioning system built in order to deliver the scent of rose throughout his entire palace. In 54 AD, Nero gave the ultimate "aroma party" when he spent the equivalent of $100,000 to scent just one of his infamous extravagant events.

The Roman historian, Pliny, mentioned plant-based remedies in his book *Naturalis Historia*, Latin for Natural History. He gave 32 remedies created from rose oil, 21 from lily, 17 from violet, 25 from pennyroyal, and a spikenard ointment for coughs and laryngitis.

The Romans planted herb and rose gardens in the foreign countries they invaded and settled. Those Roman crusades helped spread the knowledge and techniques of herbalists and perfumers. The famous English Gardens are the legacy of the conquering Romans.

By 3 AD, Rome was the bathing capital of the world. There were more than a thousand fragrant baths located throughout the city. After their baths, the Romans treated themselves to luxurious and aromatic massages. The Romans used essential oils for cosmetics, hygiene and medical treatments. They used three different types of perfumes: solid unguents (salves and balms), scented oils, and perfumed powders.

Claudius Galen was a Greek physician under Roman employ who treated the wounds of the Gladiators. He used medicinal herbs, and it is said that no gladiators died of battle wounds when treated by Galen. He became the personal physician to the Roman Emperor Marcus Aurelius and he conducted extensive research in herbal medicine.

India: The historic use of aromatics in India is vast. Aromatherapy was used in every aspect of life and included baths, cosmetics, perfumes, seduction, medicinal purposes, and religious ceremonies. Ayurveda, the traditional Indian medicine, has been practiced for over 3,000 years and incorporates aromatic massage. During Indian Tantric ceremonies, participants were anointed with oils of sandalwood for the men, jasmine for the women on their hands, patchouli on the neck and cheeks, amber on the breasts, spikenard in the hair, musk on the abdomen, sandalwood on the thighs, and saffron on the feet.

Abhyanga, a fragrant massage used for seduction, is still popular today. The Abhyanga massage is not only practiced on humans but is used to encourage the mating of male and female elephants: the female elephant is given a bath and covered in fragrance as a means to excite the male bull.

India played a prominent role in the spice trade, offering seventeen different types of jasmine alone. The Muslim ruler Barbur, one of India's Mogul kings declared, "One may prefer the fragrances of India to those of the flowers of the whole world."

By the 18th century, the British took control of India. The British published *The Wealth of India*, a set of volumes on the medicinal and fragrant botanicals of India.

China: In 2800 BC, Shen Nung, legendary ruler of China and herbalist wrote, the first drug directory known as, *Pen Ts'ao Ching, Divine Husbandma's Materia Medic*). It covered 365 herbs and appears to have incorporated aromatherapy into traditional herbal practices.

Between the 7th and 17th centuries AD, the Chinese upper class lavishly used fragrances for their bodies, baths, clothing, homes, temples, paper, ink, sachets, statues, fans and cosmetics.

The Chinese Taoist believed that the extraction of a plant's fragrance liberated the plant's soul. The Chinese word "*heang*" means perfume, incense, and fragrance collectively. As there was little distinction between spices, drugs, incense and perfume, heang is classified according to the mood it induces. A heang can be tranquil, reclusive, luxurious, beautiful, refined or noble. Likewise, substances that nurtured the mind were treated the same as those used for the body. The Chinese have said, "Every perfume is a medicine."

Marco Polo journeyed to China to convince the Orient to trade directly with Genoa. Enormous quantities of spices were needed in Europe to disinfect cities against the plague and other maladies. The Muslim taxes had become an enormous liability, and Marco Polo wanted to bypass the 300 percent markup the Muslim middlemen were imposing on them.

Arabia: Mohammed is said to have loved children, women, and fragrances above all else. Rose water became popular for use in many areas of the Muslim culture, including use in foods to flavor sherbet and Turkish delight, to scent gloves, and to purify the mosques.

The Arabs played a leading role in the development of aromatic healing by creating an advanced level of chemical and pharmaceutical technology. They had established extensive trade routes, which connected India, China, the Mediterranean and Indonesia with the Arab world.

Spices and essential oils were sold and used as precious commodities. Through the trade routes, these spices and essential oils were made available to the entire civilized world. Without the Arab world, the knowledge of the Greeks and Romans may have been lost forever. Several essential oils are described in Yakub al-Kindi's *The Book of Chemistry of Perfume*.

Arabic scientists made great improvements in the technique of distillation and established a vast body of research literature regarding essential oils. They created the first solid soap, which was scented with aromatics.

Ibn-Sina, known in the West as "Avicenna," was an Arabic alchemist, astronomer, philosopher, mathematician, physician, and poet and wrote the famous *Canon of Medicine*. He used essential oils extensively in his practice and dedicated one of his 100-plus books solely to the use of medicinal plants. Ibn-Sina is credited with making significant improvements in the art of distillation of plant material by adding a water-cooled jacket around the cooling coil. This improved technique was used by the Arabs to distill ethyl alcohol from fermented sugar, creating a new solvent for the extraction of plant material.

Europe: When the Roman Empire fell in the fifth century AD, little of the knowledge of the Romans and Greeks was left in Europe. Centuries later, returning crusaders and merchants brought back the knowledge from the East. During the Middle Ages, the healing arts and sciences were left in the hands of monks cloistered away in monasteries. The Catholic Church governed European medicine in the 13th and 14th centuries. The standard of care was prayer because the church believed illness was a punishment from God.

Between the 10th and 13th centuries, the University of Salerno in Italy reached the height of its glory as a center of learning. Its School of Medicine combined Greek, Latin, Arabic and Hebrew medical practices. The University drew scholars from the East and the West. Italy became the leader of aromatics, cosmetics, and perfumes in Europe.

In the 12th century the Abbess of Bingen, known as Saint Hildegard, produced notes in a medicinal handbook about using herbs, *Liber compositae medicinae* (later known as *Causea et Curae*). She wrote about the use of lavender water, and many credit her with the launching of today's popular lavender hydrosol.

By the late Middle Ages, apothecary guilds were being established in northern Europe. Essential oils from the East were being used again to enhance the quality of life and improve the average European's chance of survival. It was the apothecaries and the perfumers, who worked daily with essential oils, that escaped the plagues and epidemics that swept through Europe.

During the 16th century, Europeans believed that bathing was unhealthy, so perfumes were used to cover the person's offending odor. The Italian influence swept through France with the help of Caterina de Medici's marriage in 1547 to France's Prince Henri II. She brought with her a personal alchemist and her perfumer, who both set up shop in Paris.

France began to predominate over Italy in the perfume world. During the reign of Henry III of France, perfume use became extravagant and even wasteful. The French used fragrances in everything from public fountains, stationery, wines, drinking water, in their homes, on their clothes, bodies, and hair. By that time many of the essential oils used today had been isolated and were commonly in use.

In 1887, Dr. Chamberland in Paris published the first modern documented research of the antiseptic properties of essential oils. His research confirmed that essential oils kill viruses, bacteria and fungus.

Unfortunately, the rise of Puritanism in the 16th and 17th centuries caused religious leaders to frown upon the use of aromatics, since pagans and witches used them in their rituals. They also believed that any display of vanity or adornment detracted from spiritual purity. As late as the 18th century, the use of perfumes and cosmetics were discouraged. In Britain, a group of lawmakers proposed a law to prohibit women from wearing scents. They believed that perfumes and cosmetics gave women an unfair advantage over men and were forms of witchcraft that allowed women to seduce men and lure them into marriage while they were not in full command of their senses.

The Rise of Synthetics

In 1868, coumarin became the first fragrance produced synthetically. It was the first of thousands of synthetic fragrances that were unsuitable for medicinal use. In 1874 the chemical structure of vanillin was determined and in 1876, synthetic vanillin production began.

Before WWII, research on essential oils drew as much scientific interest as the exploration of other drugs. Identifying the components of natural essential oils became an important field of study, which was ultimately central in the development of many chemical successes.

In 1910, Otto Wallach won the Nobel Prize in Chemistry. His work sheds light on many of the $C10H16$ group terpene structures present in essential oils by utilizing common reagents such as hydrogen chloride and hydrogen bromide. In 1909, he published the results of his extensive studies in the 600 page book, *Terpene und Campher*.

In 1939, Leopold Ruzicka won the Nobel Prize in Chemistry. He developed the synthesis of nerolidol, farnesol and jasmine. His synthesis of civetone and muscone replaced the scent obtained from the civet cats and musk deer. These endangered species had been the original source of the heavy scented musky odor considered essential by many in perfumery.

Chemists isolated the active principles within plants and manufactured them synthetically. They believed that the properties of the plants should be isolated and used separately. As the science of chemistry became more sophisticated, herbs and essential oils where replaced by synthetic drugs. Synthetic drugs could be controlled and standardized, and they came to monopolize the world of perfumery.

The Rebirth of Aromatherapy

For some time aromatherapy books had the story of aromatherapy's rebirth all wrong. It is true that Rene-Maurice Gattefosse is the father of modern aromatherapy. He began to study essential oils in 1907 with a group of scientists, and it was he who first coined the term "aromatherapy."

According to the myth, in 1928 a French chemist by the name of Rene-Maurice Gattefosse rediscovered the healing properties of essential oils. While working in his family's perfumery business, an explosion severely burned his hand. He plunged his hand into the first liquid near him. That liquid turned out to be lavender essential oil that was being used for its fragrance and for cosmetic purposes. He was amazed at how quickly his wound healed, without infection or scarring. In the myth version of this story, as a result of his burn, Gattefosse turned his scientific attention to the medicinal properties of essential oils and their benefits for skin conditions.

The story of Gattefosse's famous burn is pivotal to the history of modern aromatherapy and its rebirth. Like the story of the "fish that got away," in which the fish keeps growing with each retelling of the story, the story of Rene-Maurice Gattefosse has grown in such a way that it is told differently in nearly every aromatherapy book.

However, when I was doing some fact checking a few years ago, I discovered a reference stating that, according to Robert Tisserand, the famous telling is incorrect. I went to Tisserand.com and—lo and behold—the true story was right there on his site. In reality, his treatment of his severe burn with lavender was deliberate.

According to Martin Watt, Gattefosse used deterpenated oils which were commonly used by perfumers because they have better solubility in alcohol than whole essential oils. Deterpenated oil is an essential oil that is terpene free by means of fractional distillation at a reduced pressure.

Although all accounts of his famous burn are in 1928, it actually happened in 1910. Gattefosse's findings can be found in his 1937 book, *Aromathérapie*, along with the story of the famous burn that happened in his laboratory. It was well received by others who went on to do their own research. It was originally written in French and wasn't published in English until 1993.

Gattefosse said, "The external application of small quantities of essences rapidly stops the spread of gangrenous sores. In my personal experience, after a laboratory explosion covered me with burning substances, which I extinguished by rolling on a grassy lawn, both my hands were covered with a rapidly developing gas gangrene. Just one rinse with lavender essence stopped "the gasification of the tissue". This treatment was followed by profuse sweating, and healing began the next day (July 1910)." Rene-Maurice Gattefosse in *Aromathérapie*

Gas gangrene is a serious bacterial infection which produces gases within the tissues that are gangrene, or dead. It is a very deadly form of gangrene, and in his time, would have most likely been fatal. The bacterium that causes gas gangrene can be found in soil. I agree with Tisserand's belief that he probably came in contact with the bacterium when he extinguished burning substances "by rolling on a grassy lawn." Knowing the real story makes me even more impressed with the power of lavender. I have, on many occasions, poured lavender onto burns with amazing results. I have never witnessed the results of it on gas gangrene.

According to Gattefosse, aromatherapy was to be used to treat a symptom or a disease in the same way that conventional medicine did. He did not see a distinction between the two and believed aromatherapy to be an integral part of medicine. He was also aware of the psychological and neurological values of essential oils.

Dr. Jean Valnet, an ex-army surgeon, used essential oils during WWII to treat wounded soldiers. He discovered that they were effective in treating wounds and burns, and later he found essential oils were also useful in the treatment of psychiatric problems. Valnet's work brought credibility and authority to the practice of aromatherapy in France. He used classical methodology in his use of essential oils, and due to his diligence and devotion, many medical aromatherapists have followed in his footsteps. Valnet published *The Practice of Aromatherapy* in 1964. It was addressed to lay people as well as the medical community.

The holistic approach of aromatherapy can be attributed to the biochemist Marguerite Maury. While she was treating her patients with essential oils for cosmetic problems, she discovered that not only did their skin clear up, but they also experienced pleasant and surprising side effects. They had improved sleep, reduced symptoms of rheumatism, and increased mental awareness. Madame Maury pioneered the technique of applying essential oils with massage. In her approach she treated the body synergistically with touch and smell. This stimulated internal organs and improved the condition of the skin.

Robert Tisserand's book, *The Art of Aromatherapy*, was published in England in 1977. His book was the first non-scientific based book on aromatherapy. After 1980, aromatherapy diversified into four basic groups:

1. In England, the use of aromatherapy is from massage, an external and safety-conscious approach.
2. In France, the practice of aromatherapy comes from a medicinal, internal, and experimental approach.
3. In Germany, aromatherapy is approached from a medicinal and research-oriented point of view.
4. The United States practices aromatherapy through massage, using an external, esthetic, and eclectic approach.

Medical use of aromatherapy is completely prohibited or restricted in Western societies. The fragrance aspect of essential oils has taken the main route in the United States. In France, aromatherapy was first propagated by medical doctors, hence the integration of aromatherapy into conventional medicine. In English speaking countries the first translated book was published by a masseur in 1977, Robert Tisserand.

Thus, aromatherapy has taken a back seat as an "alternative" form of medical treatment. The reasons for the differences in approaches from country to country can be explained by exploring the history and sources of aromatherapy.

:: Chapter 3 ::
The Science of Aromatherapy

Unique Blueprints

I often hear people say that we should stop buying supplies overseas and only buy American. As patriotic as I am, that would end the supply of some of the greatest essential oils in the world. I can't imagine not being able to make blends from tea tree from Australia, jasmine from India, or cistus from Spain. Thus, where the plant is grown is critical to the overall therapeutic properties of the essential oils from the plant.

Essential oils are derived from a variety of different plant materials such as root, resin, wood, leaf, needle, citrus fruit, flower and seed from all over the world. Each essential oil has different therapeutic properties, and each has its very own unique blueprint. The combination of the plant's exclusive design and the energy of the sun, soil, air and water give each essential oil its own individual perfume and beneficial healing properties. The same species of plant can produce an essential oil with different chemical components depending on whether it was grown in dry or damp earth, at high or low altitude, or even in hot or cold climates.

Along with a unique blueprint, every essential oil has a unique name. If you are going to be in the business of aromatherapy and personal care products, it is time to get over any fear you might have of the Latin language. Latin is also the language of aromatherapy and cosmetic ingredients. Knowing the Latin name for an essential oil is actually more important that knowing the common name. Learning Latin for aromatherapy is basically learning a series of blocks that builds upon itself.

Classification of Plants

All living organisms belong to kingdoms. The kingdom of plants is Plantae, which is then broken down into divisions, which are divided into classes, which are divided into orders, which are divided into families, which are divided into genera, which is finally divided into species. Species are sometimes broken down into varieties, chemotypes, or cultivars.

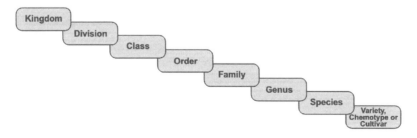

The binomial system of naming plants was developed by Dr. Carl von Linne of Sweden. The binomial system uses two identifying names including the genus and species of the plant. The proper way to write the Latin name of any essential oil is to italicize the entire name and to capitalize the first letter of the genus. The species, which is the second word, should be written in lower case. The only exception is when the species is a proper name. In some cases the variety or chemotype will follow the species by inserting the word var after the species and before the variety or chemotype, for instance, *Lavendula angustifolia var. Vera*.

Family	Common Name	Examples of Essential Oils in Family
Annonaceae	Annona Family	Cananga and Ylang Ylang
Apiaceae (Umbelliferae)	Carrot or Parsley Family	Angelica, Aniseed, Carrot, Coriander, Dill, Fennel
Apocynaceae	Dogbane Family	Frangipani absolute
Asteraceae (Compositae)	Sunflower Family	Calendula, Roman and German Chamomile, Helichrysum
Betulaceae	Birch Family	White and Yellow Birch
Burseraceae	Torchwood Family	Frankincense and Myrrh
Cannabaceae	Hemp Family	
Caryophyllaceae	Pink Family	Carnation absolute
Cistaceae	Rock Rose Family	Cistus
Cupressaceae	Cypress Family	Cypress and Juniper
Ericaceae	Health Family	Wintergreen
Fabaceae (Leguminosae)	Pea or Pulse Family	Peru Balsam
Geraniaceae	Geranium Family	Geranium and Rose Geranium
Iridaceae	Iris Family	Iris
Lamiaceae (Labiatae)	Mint Family	Sweet Basil, Catnip, Clary Sage, Hyssop, Lavender, Patchouli, Peppermint, Rosemary, Spearmint
Lauraceae	Laurel Family	Bay Laurel, Cinnamon, Litsea cubeba, Rosewood
Magnoliaceae	Magnolia Family	Champaca absolute
Malvaceae	Mallow Family	Ambrette
Myristicaceae	Nutmeg Family	Nutmeg
Myrtaceae	Myrtle Family	Bay, Clove, Tea Tree
Oleaceae	Olive Family	Jasmine absolute
Orchidaceae	Orchid Family	Vanilla absolute
Pandanaceae	Screw-Pine Family	Kewda
Pinaceae	Pine Family	Himalayan Cedarwood, Hemlock, White Fir
Piperaceae	Pepper Family	Black Pepper
Poaceae (Gramineae)	Grass Family	Citronella, Lemongrass, Palmarosa, Vetiver
Rosaceae	Rose Family	Rose absolute, Rose Otto
Rutaceae	Rue Family	Bergamot, Grapefruit, Lemon, Lime, Mandarin, Neroli, Orange, Tangerine
Santalaceae	Sandalwood Family	Sandalwood
Saxifragaceae	Saxifrage Family	Black Currant
Sytracaceae	Storax Family	Benzoin
Tiliaceae	Linden, Basswood Family	Linden absolute
Usneaceae	Usnea Family	Oakmoss
Valerianaceae	Valerian Family	Spikenard and Valerian
Verbenaceae	Vervain, Verbena Family	Lemon Verbena
Violaceae	Violet Family	Violet
Zingiberaceae	Ginger Family	Cardamom and Ginger

The essential oils of basil, cedarwood, chamomile, eucalyptus, fir, lavender, rose, rosemary, sage, thyme and ylang ylang are all prime examples of essential oils that include the chemotype. Every essential oil can have as many as one hundred components—even in the thousands, depending on the oil—and each type can have significant differences in properties and safety. That is why identifying essential oils by their proper Latin name is more important than the common name.

For example, the common name of cedarwood does not tell the whole story. There are three major essential oils that share the same common name, but yet they differ significantly. The scents of two cedars known as *Cedrus atlantica* and *Cedrus deodara* are quite different. And then there is cedar leaf, which isn't actually a cedar at all, but without the Latin name of *Thuja occidentalis*, you might miss that.

A plant in a family shares certain properties with every other plant in its family. Most families have one name, but some have two, and all have a common name as well. Latin is often the term used first in the International Nomenclature of Cosmetic Ingredients, also known as the INCI, an international designation for the declaration of the ingredients on the packaging of cosmetics. The use of INCI minimizes the language barriers that often hinder consumer understanding and international trade. The INCI names are allocated by the American Cosmetic Association, Personal Care Products Council, and they are used internationally. The adoption of INCI terminology ensures cosmetic ingredients are consistently listed using the same ingredient name from product to product.

In the United States, the Food and Drug Administration (FDA) requires that all cosmetics include a listing of ingredients using the standardized INCI name for each ingredient in descending order. INCI ingredient names on product labels allow consumers to easily compare the ingredients between multiple products, using a common language. INCI ensures transparency in cosmetic ingredient disclosure. INCI is required in America under the Food, Drug, and Cosmetic Act and the Fair Packaging and Labeling Act. In Canada, INCI is required by the Food and Drugs Act and Cosmetic Regulations. The declaration of the ingredients in accordance with the INCI system has been a legal requirement in the European Union since 1993. The declaration of ingredients in cosmetics with the INCI name is always required to be in descending order.

How Essential Oils Enter the Human Body

Essential oils can enter the human body through skin absorption and inhalation. We can understand the amazing power of aromatherapy in the human body when we start to understand the nature of the plants from which essential oils come.

We know that aromatic oils, through metabolism, are formed and stored as a by-product in the organs of a plant. Plants "smell" for two main reasons:

attraction and defense. The aromatic oils in a growing plant attract insects and animals for pollination and seed dispersal, thus aiding reproduction in a growing plant. Such plants tend to have a sweet, tempting, and attractive fragrance.

Other plants have a defense mechanism in which an unpleasant odor in the molecules of their leaves, roots or bark is unappetizing and repels predators. This security measure also protects some plants from disease by inhibiting the growth of neighboring plants, molds and fungi. Plants depend on these messages of scent to communicate through chemical signals to each other and the world around them.

The therapeutic action of essential oils is attributed to the naturally occurring chemical components within the plants. Many scientists believe that essential oils stimulate the body's own natural defense systems. Kurt Schnaubelt, Ph.D., researcher in the area of therapeutic application of essential oils, has said, "Tea tree, thyme and other oils are able to boost immunity by enhancing the body's own manufacture of gamma-globulin."

Inhalation: Psychology and Physiology

The quickest and most effective method of using essential oils for emotional issues is through inhalation. Essential oils have tiny molecules, which disperse into the air and enter through the nose. When inhaled, the scent molecules reach the olfactory epithelium, which is two groups that each has twenty-five million receptor cells at the top of the nostrils, just below and between the eyes. Odors are then converted to messages, which are relayed to the brain for processing. Inhalation provides the most direct route to the brain. Inhalation is very useful for respiratory symptoms and is as easy as sniffing drops on a tissue or cotton ball.

The average person takes about five seconds to breathe; two seconds to inhale and three to exhale. During an average year, we breathe 6,307,200 times. With every breath, we smell. The human body is capable of registering and recognizing thousands of different smells. The sense of smell is ten times more sensitive than the sense of taste. Our ability to distinguish different smells is incredibly precise, but it is almost impossible to describe a smell to someone who has never experienced it. Response to smell only takes 0.5 seconds, as compared to 0.9 seconds to react to pain.

With every breath, some scent molecules inescapably travel to the lungs. Some molecules are absorbed by the mucous lining of the respiratory pathway. Other molecules reach the alveoli and are transferred into the blood stream. Therefore, inhalation of essential oils not only affects emotions, but it also has a physical impact.

Brain activity has been observed and documented by brain scans and other imaging techniques. The lipid solubility of essential oil components applied to the skin enables the components to cross the blood-brain barrier and come in contact with the fluids surrounding the brain. Scent receptor cells transmit impulses to the olfactory area of the brain in the limbic system, which is linked to memory, emotions, hormones, sexuality and heart rate. These impulses trigger neurochemicals such as endorphins that can stimulate, sedate, relax, gratify, restore emotional equilibrium or cause euphoria, thereby bringing about a mental and physical change or response.

The limbic system of the brain plays an important role in evoking feelings and memories and assisting in stimulating learning and memory retention. It works in coordination with the pituitary gland and the hypothalamus area of the brain to regulate hormonal activities of the endocrine system. It triggers the production of hormones that govern appetite, body temperature, insulin production, and overall metabolism. This activity influences immunity, stress levels, sex drive, conscious thoughts and reactions. The limbic system includes the amygdala, which processes anger; the septum pellucidum, which processes pleasure sensations; and the hippocampus, which regulates how much attention we give our emotions and memories.

Consider the *sex drive*: One out of every four people who suffer from anosmia, which is a loss or impairment of smell, also loses their interest in sexual activity. Pheromones, which are the subtle glandular odors of each person, play a large role in sexuality. For example, women who live together have a tendency to menstruate at the same time every month. It has been seen as a natural regulation acquired when pheromones are brought in close proximity with those of other women.

Vladimir Nabokov wrote, "Nothing revives the past so completely as a smell." I know from my experience that this statement is true. My mother spent a lot of time in the hospital getting experimental radiation and chemotherapy treatments. She grew to associate the smell of the hospital with extreme pain and illness. She felt nauseous and anxious at the first whiff of a hospital.

There is a direct physical route which exists between memory and smell. Smells trigger *memory responses*, which in turn can trigger changes in body temperature, appetite, stress level and sexual arousal. Because there are no short-term memories with odors, a whiff of a familiar scent can bring back a flood of memories that are so vivid it can cause tears of joy or grief.

Smells create chemical responses to *stimuli*, hence the wave of chemical response in the stomach when confronted with a negative smell. In contrast, a yummy smell may make someone hungry because it sends a chemical response that stimulates the gastric juices.

Smells can *transport* us through time and distance: It is common for a person to walk into a room, smell the scent of their grandmother, and find themselves smiling warmly without even realizing it. Conversely, a smell can flood one with negative memories resulting in an increase in heart rate and a nauseous feeling in the pit of the stomach.

Every person has their own genetically encoded odor print that is as individual as our fingerprints. No two people smell alike, except identical twins. Mothers are able to identify their babies by scent alone. We often see animals use their sense of smell, but forget what a major role scent plays in humans as well.

Aerial Inhalation

There are so many different diffusers available on the market today. The most traditional aerial diffuser is an air diffuser or glass nebulizer diffuser. There are also true aromatherapy candles, necklace diffusers, car diffusers, reed diffusers, crystal salt diffusers, ceramic light bulb rings, tea light diffusers, room sprays, scent ball and so much more.

Citrus Reed Diffuser

1/2 cup + 2 Tablespoons Dipropylene Glycol or Jojoba Oil
1/4 cup Lime Essential Oil
1 Tablespoon Litsea Essential Oil
3 Tablespoons Orange 5 Fold Essential Oil

Directions: Pour into Square Diffuser Bottle, add reeds and use.

Well Being Reed Diffuser Recipe

1/2 cup Dipropylene Glycol or Jojoba Oil
1/4 cup + 3 Tablespoons of Essential Wholesale Well-Being Essential Oil Blend

Directions: Pour into Round Diffuser Bottle, add reeds and use.

Himalayan Salt Potpourri Recipe

Scent Portion
1 ounce Dipropylene Glycol
1 ounce Peppermint 3rd Essential Oil
Potpourri Portion
Himalayan Pink Salt (Coarse)
Dried Herbs of choice (optional)

Directions: Mix dipropylene glycol with peppermint 3rd essential oils into a spray bottle and shake. This spritz should then be spritzed onto your potpourri portion and mixed. Keep the spray bottle handy to refresh your potpourri as needed. This same recipe can be used with solar salts or coarse Dead Sea salts and any herbs of your choice.

Ingredient Information: Dipropylene glycol is a solvent used with essential oils. I have added dipropylene glycol to the glossary for further information on it.

Room Mist Recipe
½ gallon Essential Wholesale Body Linen Spray Base
1 tbsp. Polysorbate 20
1 tbsp. Essential Oil of your choice

Directions: Mix polysorbate 20 and essential oil of your choice together separately. Once they are thoroughly mixed add to Essential Wholesale Body Linen Spray base or other stably preserved base and stir.

Bed Bug Spray Recipe
1/2 gallon Essential Wholesale Body Linen Spray
1 Tbsp. Neem Tincture
1 Tbsp. Lavender Essential Oil
1 Tbsp. Lavender Distillate
1 Tbsp. Polysorbate 20

Directions: Mix polysorbate 20 and lavender essential oil together separately. Once they are thoroughly mixed add to Essential Wholesale Body Linen Spray base or other stably preserved base, add neem extract and lavender distillate and mix thoroughly.

Ingredient Information: Polysorbate 20 is a non-ionic surfactant that is used to disperse and emulsify oils into water. I have added polysorbate 20 to the glossary for further information on it.

Topical Application and Absorption
Essential oils can be added to your skin care for beautification, therapy and to scent your skincare facial and body products. Although our skin is mostly waterproof, it is still permeable to water, lipids, water soluble solutions, and other substances which have small molecular structures and low molecular weight. Substances with a molecular weight over 500 are not likely to penetrate the skin. Essential oils have a molecular weight of 225 or less (Price). In aromatherapy, molecules of essential oils applied to the skin pass through the skin's epidermis and are carried away by the capillary blood circulating in the dermis. The molecules of essential oils are then taken into the lymphatic and extracellular fluids. From there, the therapeutic components of the essential oils are broken down and used by various parts of the body.

The human body takes the most vital properties of appropriately applied essential oils, and it uses those properties to bring itself into balance and into a healthier state without side effects. After the essential oils perform their healing functions they are metabolized and eliminated with the body's other waste.

With skin being our largest elimination organ, most essential oils that are absorbed by the skin can be detected in exhaled air within 20 to 60 minutes (Katz 1947). Elimination of essential oils through saliva, urine, feces or sweat in a healthy adult body can take anywhere from 20 minutes to 26 hours. In an unhealthy adult, it can take up to 14 hours for the essential oils to pass through the body's systems.

A simple self-test can verify the claim by aromatherapists that essential oils are absorbed by the body. Lavender essential oil applied to the cheek can be tasted. Garlic essential oil can be smeared onto your ankle and will quickly be tasted. At Essential Wholesale we have tested the theory to see if inhalation would cause the same effect with garlic essential oil. We found that even a very short exposure to an open container of garlic essential oil results in a bad case of garlic breath. Blood samples taken after an essential oil is applied to the skin have proven that components of essential oils can be found in the blood stream shortly after application. (Jäger, 1992.)

Systems of the Body

- **Circulatory System:** includes the heart, blood, vessels (veins, arteries and capillaries). Essential oils that improve the circulatory system come from woods and citrus fruits.
- **Respiratory System:** includes the nose, trachea, lungs and rib muscles. Essential oils that improve the respiratory system come from leaves, needles and resins.
- **Skeletal System:** includes bones and joints. Essential oils that improve the skeletal system come from leaves and roots.
- **Urinary System:** includes the bladder, kidneys, ureters and the urethra. Essential oils that improve the urinary system come from citrus fruits and woods.
- **Muscular System:** includes the muscles and tendons. Essential oils that improve the muscular system come from leaves and roots.
- **Endocrine System:** includes glands and hormones. Essential oils that improve the endocrine system vary greatly.
- **Digestive System:** includes the mouth, esophagus, stomach, intestines, throat, liver, gall bladder, pancreas, rectum and anus. Essential oils that improve the digestive system come from roots, seeds, citrus fruits and some flowers.
- **Nervous System:** includes the brain, spinal cord and nerves. Essential oils that improve the nervous system come from flowers.

- **Lymphatic System:** includes the lymph, lymph nodes, lymphatic vessels, lymphatic capillaries and the spleen. Essential oils that improve the lymphatic system come from citrus fruits, twigs and woods.
- **Integumentary System:** includes the epidermis, dermis, hydro-dermis, hair follicles, sweat pores, sweat glands, oil glands and sensory receptors. Essential oils that improve the integumentary system come from resins and flowers.

The Top Ten Chemistry Basics for Aromatherapy

1. An atom is defined as the smallest particle of an element which can exist. Atoms consist of three types of sub-atomic particles; protons with a positive charge, neutrons with no charge and electrons with a negative charge. The number of protons determines the atomic number, which identifies a particular atom. The sum of all the protons and neutrons of an atom is called the mass number.
2. An element may be defined as a substance consisting of chemically identical atoms. There are 107 known elements, such as hydrogen, carbon, oxygen and nitrogen.
3. Molecules are composed of two or more atoms, which are the smallest · particle of any particular element that can exist alone. The chemical properties of an atom are determined by the number and arrangement of its electrons.
4. A compound is a substance consisting of elements combined together in fixed and definite proportions by weight.
5. According to The International Union of Pure and Applied Chemistry, "An atomic weight (relative atomic mass) of an element from a specified source is the ratio of the average mass per atom of the element to 1/12 of the mass of an atom of 12C."
6. The molecular weight of an atom is the sum of the individual atomic weights of the atoms that make up a molecule. Molecular weight plays a large role in essential oil blending for perfuming.
7. The chemistry of matter is divided into the sub-categories of organic chemistry and inorganic chemistry. Organic chemistry is the chemistry of carbon-containing compounds, and inorganic chemistry is the chemistry of mostly non-carbon-containing compounds. Essential oils are organic compounds.
8. An ion is an electrically charged atom, or group of atoms.
9. Chemical bonds consist of covalent bonds and ionic "bonds." A covalent bond is a true bond. It is created when two atoms share electrons and occupy the same internuclear space. Ionic 'bonds' are not true bonds, but instead an association between two oppositely charged particles. In an ionic 'bond' one atom or group of atoms gives up one or more electrons to another atom or group of atoms.

10. The property of a given molecule depends on the nature, number, position, and arrangement of atoms of the elements that it contains. The Law of Constant Composition is that all pure samples of the same compound, however prepared, consist of the same elements combined together in the same proportions by weight. This allows for analysis of essential oils to determine purity.

Elements of Aromatherapy

There are three elements in organic chemistry that are critical to your aromatherapy training: carbon, oxygen and hydrogen.

- Carbon has the atomic symbol of C, and its atomic weight is 12. Carbon always participates in a total of four bonds to other atoms in neutral organic , and it can be involved in single, double or triple bonds to another atom.
- Oxygen has the atomic symbol of O, and its atomic weight is 16. Oxygen always participates in a total of 2 bonds to other atoms in neutral organic molecules, and it can be involved in single or double to another atom.
- Hydrogen has the atomic symbol of H, and its atomic weight is 1. Hydrogen always participates in a total of 1 bond to other atoms in neutral organic molecules, and it can be involved in a single bond to another atom.

Understanding and memorizing the meaning of prefixes used in naming molecules will simplify your life. Prefixes tell you the number of carbon atoms that make up the molecule or the substituent (an atom or group of atoms substituted in place of a hydrogen atom on the parent chain of a hydrocarbon) on the molecule.

- Meth- means one carbon atom
- Eth- means two carbon atoms
- Prop- means three carbon atoms
- But- means four carbon atoms
- Pent- means five carbon atoms
- Hex- means six carbon atoms
- Hept- means seven carbon atoms
- Oct- means eight carbon atoms
- Non- means nine carbon atoms
- Dec- means ten carbon atoms

There can also be prefixes that are used tell you that multiple numbers are grouped together on the same substituent on one molecule.

- Di – means two substituents of the same type are present on the same molecule.
- Tri - means three substituents of the same type are present on the same molecule.
- Tetra – means four substituents of the same type are present on the same molecule.

Functional Groups

Essential oils can be divided into functional groups, which may be defined as a specific group of atoms in a molecule that is the part of the molecule that will most likely undergo a chemical reaction. The functional group tends to determine the chemical behavior of a molecule, but not necessarily all of the properties of the essential oils.

Alcohols and phenols are defined by the functional group OH. Alcohols can always be spotted because they end in "ol," for instance, ethanol, citronellol, geraniol, linalool and menthol. Alcohols are polar and somewhat water soluble. Alcohols have the most beneficial properties of anti-infectious, bactericidal, antiviral and are gentle to the skin.

The most common alcohols include citronellol (i.e. rose, lemon, geranium, eucalyptus,) geraniol (i.e. geranium, palmarosa) and linalool (i.e. lavender.) Essential oils containing citronellol and geraniol trigger the labeling requirements for allergens in the European Union.

Phenols are defined by an alcohol function attached directly to a phenyl ring or benzene ring. Phenols are less polar than normal alcohols and are prone to oxidation. Phenols can be identified by the endings "ol" or "phenol" for example, carvacrol, thymol and eugenol. Phenols have antiseptic, bactericidal, stimulating and anti-infectious properties. Essential oils that contain high levels of phenols should be used in low concentrations and for short periods of time. Phenols are also classified as skin and mucus membrane irritants. Despite their great antiseptic qualities, essential oils with high phenol such as cinnamon and clove oil can cause severe skin reactions.

Phenols and acids react directly with alkali to produce odorless salts. Clove oil for example, contains a large proportion of eugenol (a phenol). Phenols are actually weak acids. Other fragrant acids typically smell sour, for example acetic acid found in vinegar. The most phenols include eugenol (i.e. clove, ylang ylang), thymol (i.e. thyme,) carvacrol (oregano,) anethole (i.e. fennel,) and estragole (tarragon.) Eugenol triggers the labeling requirements for allergens in the European Union.

Aldehydes are defined by the carbon atom joined to the oxygen atom by a double bond and to the hydrogen atom by a single bond. They can be spotted by the ending "al," for instance: citral and citronellal. Aldehydes are relatively polar. Aldehydes have the properties of being anti-fungal, antiviral, anti-inflammatory, calming, tonic and anti-infectious. They also tend to irritate and sensitize the skin. Aldehydes are unstable and will easily oxidize in the presence of oxygen and even low heat.

When your nose picks up the tell-tale lemon-like aroma in an essential oil you can safely guess that it contains aldehydes, such as lemon, lemongrass and citronella. Examples of aldehydes include: aldehyde C8 (i.e. sweet orange, lemon, mandarin, grapefruit, rose, lavender) aldehyde C10 (i.e. sweet orange, mandarin, grapefruit, rose, lemongrass, lavender) cinnaminic aldehyde (i.e. cinnamon bark), citronellal (i.e. citronella,) geranial (i.e. lemongrass, litsea, lemon, lime,) neral (i.e. lemongrass, litsea, lemon, lime) and vanillin (i.e. peru balsam.)

Ketones are defined by a carbonyl group bonded to two other carbon radicals. Ketones are similar to aldehydes, but have a more pungent odor. They can be spotted by the ending "one," for instance: menthone, propanone and carvone. Ketones have the properties of promoting scar healing, helping to loosen mucus and sedating. Relatively few ketones occur as important or high constituents of essential oils.

Ketones have a bad reputation, and rightfully so when they are in high concentrations in an essential oil. But don't throw the baby out with the bathwater when it comes to ketones. The ketones that you should avoid include pulegone (found in buchu and pennyroyal) and thujone (found in mugwort, sage, tansy, thuja and wormwood.) The friendly ketones are acetophenone (i.e. cistus,) jasmone (i.e. jasmine,) fenchone (i.e. fennel,) verbenone (i.e. rosemary) and menthone (i.e. peppermint.) Ketones are known for their ability to ease congestion and loosen up mucus.

Another beneficial ketone is italidone and it can be found in helichrysum essential oil. It has amazing skin regeneration and wound healing properties. I have seen amazing results when helichrysum is blended with blue chamomile and lavender for healing wounds and even reducing old scar tissue and stretch marks. Essential oils high in ketones should be used with care in pregnancy.

Esters are formed when organic acids react with alcohols in a reaction known as esterification. They are named after both their original molecules with the alcohols dropping the "ol" and gaining an "yl" ending and the acids dropping the "ic" and gaining an "ate" ending. Esters are polar and more volatile than the corresponding acids and alcohol they come from because they lack hydrogen-bonding capacity. The properties of esters include anti-inflammatory, calming and balancing. They are also gentle to the skin.

The esters found in essential oils are normally very fragrant. They tend to be fruity and have a sedative and anti-spasmodic effect. Some esters also have anti-fungal and antimicrobial properties, such as geranium oil. Esters are gentle in their actions and can be used with great ease. An example of a well-known ester is linalyl acetate, which can be found in lavender, clary sage (*Salvia sclarea*) and petitgrain. The most common esters found in essential oils are geranyl acetate (i.e. rosemary, geranium) and linalyl acetate (i.e. *Salvia sclarea*, bergamot, lavender).

According to Kevin Dunn, when making cold processed soap esters are decomposed by the lye into an acid salt and an alcohol. The ester is often rendered odorless and the fragrant alcohol that is produced in the process was often present as one of the components of the original essential oil. Therefore, the scent of an ester containing essential oil changes in the soapmaking process in proportion to the components change, but it remains fragrant.

Lactone is an ester in which the ester functional group is part of a ring system. The other atoms of the ring are carbon atoms. They are known as cyclic esters. Lactones can be identified by the ending "one." Take umbelliferone (i.e. helichrysum) for an example. Lactones are not very significant in essential oils, but they are important to the fragrance industry as a whole. Lactones have the property of being an expectorant. They are photo and skin sensitizing. Nepetalactone is an example of a lactone. It makes up a high percentage of catnip. That's what makes it such an effective mosquito repellant. It sends off a pheromone that signals mosquitoes to go away.

Coumarins are a type of lactone. There are similarities between the actions of lactones, coumarins and ketones, including a shared neuro-toxic effect, as well as causing skin sensitization and irritation. But not all sesquiterpene lactones set off alarm bells. For instance, helenalin in arnica oil has an anti-inflammatory action.

Despite their scary introduction, the level of lactones and coumarins normally found in essential oils is very low, and so they do not cause many issues. Some coumarins, like furocoumarin-bergaptene, which is found in bergamot oil, are severely skin UV sensitive and should be used with great care in sunlight or you should chose FCF (furano-coumarin free) bergamot.

Ether is a molecule with two hydrocarbon radicals that are bonded to an oxygen atom. Ethers are the least polar of the oxygen containing functional groups. They are stable and relatively unreactive compounds. An ether molecule can be identified by the ending "ol" or "ole," for instance: anethole, thymol and eugenol. Ethers are balancing, anti-depressant and anti-spasmodic. Phenolic ethers are the most widely found of the ethers in essential oils. In aniseed there is anethol, and methyl chavicol is found in basil and tarragon.

Alkane is a saturated hydrocarbon molecule that contains carbon-to-carbon single bonds. They are generally very unreactive and non-polar. They can be recognized by the ending "ane," such as methane and hexane.

Alkene is an unsaturated hydrocarbon molecule that contains at least one carbon-carbon double bond. They are very similar to alkanes, but more reactive due to the double bonds. They can be identified by the ending "ene," for instance: ethene, 1-octene and santene.

Terpenes are alkenes that are built from two or more isoprene units. No one property can fit terpenes alone, because within terpenes there is a voluminous group of chemicals with diverse properties.

Monoterpene compounds are found in nearly all essential oils and have a structure of 10 carbon atoms and at least one double bond. The 10 carbon atoms are derived from two isoprene units. Monoterpenes readily react to air and heat sources. Citrus oils do not last well, because they are high in monoterpene hydrocarbons and quickly react to air, and readily oxidize. Some of the most commonly found monoterpenes include limonene and pinene. Limonene (i.e. most citrus) has antiviral properties and pinene (i.e. pine, frankincense, rosemary) has antiseptic properties.

Monoterpenes are very insoluble in water because it is so much lighter than water. For this reason, even with a good emulsifier such as polysorbate 20, 60 or 80, you will often have separation in a cosmetic water-based product (i.e. toner, body spray) formulated with essential oils with monoterpenes.

Sesquiterpenes consist of 15 carbon atoms and have complex pharmacological actions. They consist of three isoprene units. An excellent example is chamazulene, which is found in blue chamomile and it has anti-inflammatory and anti-allergy properties. Farnesene is a sesquiterpene also found in chamomile and rose, as well as other floral essential oils.

Alkynes contain at least one carbon-carbon triple bond. They have very similar properties to alkanes and alkenes, but are even more reactive due to the triple bonds. They can be identified by the ending "yne," for instance: 4-decyne and ethyne.

Oxides are easy spot because of the camphoraceous aroma common to them. The most common oxide in essential oils is 1,8 cineole. Common essential oils containing oxides include rosemary, eucalyptus and tea tree. Most oxides have an expectorant effect and aids in thinning mucus.

Essential Oil Types and Methods of Extraction

Distilled Essential Oil - Steam distillation is the most common method of essential oil production today. It involves the flow of steam into a chamber that is full of the raw plant material. The essential oil evaporates with the water. This evaporated oil is then carried by the steam out of the chamber and into a chilled condenser, where the steam once again becomes water. The oil and water are then separated. The oil is collected and sold as essential oil and the water, which is called a hydrosol or distillate, is often sold separately. The best essential oils are obtained by low pressure, low heat distillation.

Expressed Essential Oil - Cold pressing or expression from the peels of most citrus fruits creates expressed essential oils. Examples of this method include citrus oils from the peels of fruit; lemon, bergamot and sweet orange. This method involves the simple pressing of the rind at about 120 degrees Fahrenheit to extract the oil in the peel of the citrus fruit. This method of extraction creates essential oils that have little to no alteration from the oil's original state in the plant.

Absolute - Some plants, and particularly delicate flowers, cannot survive steam distilling. Either the plant is too delicate, or water alone cannot fully release their fragrance. Instead these plants are solvent extracted in a two-step process that creates absolutes. They are not technically considered essential oils, but they can still have great therapeutic and aromatic value. Jasmine and rose are examples of absolutes.

The processing of an absolute first involves the hydrocarbon solvent extraction of a 'concrete' from the plant material, which is a semi-solid mixture of approximately 50% wax and 50% volatile oil. The concrete is then again processed using ethyl alcohol, in which the wax is only slightly soluble. The volatile plant oil then separates into the alcohol and this mixture is removed. Next the alcohol is evaporated, which leaves you with an incredibly aromatic absolute.

CO_2 Extraction - Carbon Dioxide and Supercritical Carbon Dioxide extraction both involve the use of carbon dioxide as a solvent, which carries the essential oil away from the raw plant material. CO_2 extraction involves chilling carbon dioxide to between 35 and 55 degrees F, and then pumping the carbon dioxide through the plant material at about 1000 pounds per square inch (psi). These conditions condense the carbon dioxide into a liquid. Supercritical CO_2 extraction (SCO_2) involves carbon dioxide that is heated to 87 degrees Fahrenheit and pumped through the plant material at around 8,000 psi. These conditions make the carbon dioxide like a dense fog or vapor. When the pressure is released in both the CO_2 and SCO_2 extractions, the carbon dioxide escapes in its gaseous form, which leaves the essential oil behind.

Folded Essential Oils - Many citrus essential oils, including orange, lemon, grapefruit, lime, tangerine, mandarin and bergamot are available in as 5 fold and 10 fold forms. A folded essential oil is one that has been further distilled and is made more concentrated. Folded essential oils tend to last longer because the terpenes, which are prone to oxidation, are removed. Another benefit is that the essential oils are no longer phototoxic due to the removal of the terpenes. Folded citrus oils are the perfect choice for making cold processed soap.

Essential Oil Storage

In order to preserve the shelf life of your essential oils it is important to store them properly. You will see reference to the shelf life of each of the essential oils in the profiles section of this book with the caveat, "if stored properly." The definition of a properly stored essential oil is one that is protected from air, heat, light and moisture. It is also important to keep your essential oils out of the reach of children and pets.

- **Keep it Cool** - Most essential oils should be stored at about 65-70 °F. I say "most" because some essential oils are solid when cold including anise and rose. Citrus essential oils should be stored at the even cooler temperature of 35-40 °F. It is important to ensure that the temperature that you store your essential oils at does not fluctuate drastically.
- **Keep it Dry** - Essential oils should be kept in a dry storage area.
- **Keep it Airtight with Low Head space** - You should always keep a tightly sealed lid on your essential oils to protect them from moisture, air and to stop them from evaporating. Essential oils can even be damaged when they have a tight lid if they have a lot of headspace between the partially-used essential oil and the lid. It is good to pour your essential oils into a smaller bottle if you won't be using them up any time soon. Pay special attention to the headspace with citrus essential oils and anything with a high terpene content.
- **Keep out the Light** - Essential oils should be stored in amber, green or blue glass bottles to protect them from being exposed to light. If you buy your essential oils in large quantities, you may see them come in lined steel cans or industrial aluminum bottles which are also proper packaging materials.

:: *Chapter 4* ::
The Art of Blending Essential Oils

1:1:1 = Art : Science : Experience
Blending of essential oils is one part art, one part science, and one part experience. One key thing to keep in mind when blending for fragrance is the molecular weight of the essential oil. Essential oils that are less viscous have lighter and smaller molecules and therefore are more volatile and aromatic. These lighter and smaller molecules absorb in the body and disperse into the air fast, which means that they remain on the body for a shorter time period. Essential oils that are more viscous have heavier and larger molecules and therefore are less volatile. These heavier and larger molecules absorb more slowly into the body, which means that their aroma will stick around longer. What is exciting about molecular weight is that there is a great synergy in blending essential oils that allows the heavier molecules to hang onto the lighter molecules, thus allowing the combined aroma to last long. The term "fixative" comes from this essential oil "buddy system."

The terms "top," "middle," and "base notes" come from the molecular weight of an essential oil. The molecular weight of the essential oil determines the volatility and viscosity of the oil, which determines the classification of note. Many essential oils are classified in more than one note category. In reality, all essential oils have their own top, middle and base note to them.

Top notes evaporate quickly. They are the first note that hits your nose in a blend. Middle notes give your blend body and evaporate at a medium rate. Base notes evaporate very slowly and are fixatives to a blend.

One of the keys to making great aromatherapy blends is to determine if you are blending for scent, therapeutic properties, or both. If you are blending for therapy, start out with the essential oils that have the therapeutic properties that you want for your blend and then blend, using the essential oils that support those properties, to create an appealing aroma. The key is to embrace the subtlety of single aromas in the finished product.

Beware of Hijacking Scents
Citronella, clary sage (*Salvia sclarea*), lemongrass, petitgrain, spearmint, carrot seed, palmarosa, rosemary, thyme, and vetiver can all overpower a blend. Always start out by adding these essential oils in a low age so that they don't hijack the aroma and take over your blend.

Blending Methods

Blending by **Essential Oil Type** uses the categories of relaxing, stimulating, balancing, or euphoric types. Generally this means that you combine relaxing with balancing types, or stimulating with euphoric types, or relaxing with euphoric types.

Relaxing Essential Oils: benzoin absolute, cedarwood (*Cedrus deodora*), chamomile, cypress, frankincense, lavender, mandarin, neroli, sweet orange, sandalwood, vetiver, and ylang ylang.

Stimulating Essential Oils: basil, black pepper, cardamom, cinnamon, citronella, clove, eucalyptus, fennel, ginger, grapefruit, juniper, lemon, lemongrass, nutmeg, peppermint, rosemary, spearmint, spruce, and tea tree.

Balancing Essential Oils: bergamot, frankincense, geranium, lavender, palmarosa, rose, and rosewood.

Euphoric Essential Oils: clary sage (*Salvia sclarea*), grapefruit, jasmine absolute, myrrh, patchouli, rose, and ylang ylang.

Top, Middle, Base Note Method is when you choose at least one top, one middle, and one base note. I have found that the perfect blends using this method use have a blend of base notes that make up 45 to 55%, middle notes that make up 30 to 40% and top notes that make up 15 top 25% of the blend.

Top Notes		Middle Notes		Base Notes	
Allspice	Lavender	Allspice	Jasmine Absolute	Benzoin Resin	Litsea
Anise	Lemon	Black Pepper	Juniper Berry	Calendula	Myrrh
Basil	Lemongrass	Calendula	Lavender	Cedarwood	Oakmoss Absolute
Bergamot	Lime	Cardamon	Litsea	Cinnamon Leaf	Patchouli
Blood Orange	Mandarin	Carrot Seed	Neroli	Cistus	Peru Balsam
Cinnamon Leaf	Orange	Chamomile, German	Nutmeg	Clove	Rose Absolute
Citronella	Peppermint	Chamomile, Roman	Palmarosa	Frankincense	Vetiver
Clary Sage	Petitgrain	Cinnamon Leaf	Rose	Ginger	Ylang Ylang
Eucalyptus	Ravensara	Clary Sage	Rosemary	Helichrysum	
Fennel	Spearmint	Clove Bud	Rosewood		
Grapefruit	Tangerine	Cypress	Spruce		
Laurel Leaf		Fennel	Tea Tree		
		Geranium	Thyme		
		Ginger	Ylang Ylang		
		Hyssop			

Plant Part Blending is when you chose essential oils from one plant part, such as flowers, roots, or woods with complimentary plant parts. For instance, citrus fruits are complimentary to almost all other plant parts; woods blend great with spices; resins blend well with woods.

Synergy Blending is how you would create an essential oil with a therapeutic action. First blend for therapeutic value and then use complimentary aromas to create a pleasant aroma. This is how I blend essential oils.

Family Blending is when you chose essential oils from the same botanical family.

Family	Common Essential Oils in Family
Citrus	bergamot, grapefruit, lemon, lime, litsea, mandarin, orange, tangerine
Floral	geranium, Roman chamomile, rose, lavender, ylang ylang, neroli, jasmine
Herbaceous	basil, Roman chamomile, lavender, peppermint, rosemary, clary sage (*Salvia sclarea*)
Camphoraceous	eucalyptus, rosemary, peppermint, tea tree
Spicy	black pepper, ginger, cardamom, cinnamon
Resinous	frankincense, myrrh
Woody	cedarwood, sandalwood, pine, cypress
Earthy	patchouli, vetiver

Whichever method you chose, there are a few tricks of the trade that can help you along.

1. Blend by the drop so you can work your way out of any stinky aroma blend.
2. Don't give up on a blend too soon. You might be on the verge of an amazing breakthrough.
3. Use middle notes to bridge top and base notes together.
4. Add base notes as a fixative for your blend, even if none of the base notes are your favorite aromas. I promise you, they all blend well.
5. If your blend gets too heavy, lighten it up with top notes.
6. When you use absolutes and extremely fragrant essential oils, add only one drop. It will help with the overall cost of your finished blend. Add a special touch and keep you from drowning out the other players in your blend. If you determine that you need to add more, don't rush – add just one more drop and check your aroma.
7. Clear your palate with a whiff of strong coffee beans. When your nose becomes overwhelmed, you can make mistakes in blending.
8. Don't be afraid to walk away from a blend that is giving you problems and come back to it with a fresh nose.
9. Let your blend sit for a few hours, or even overnight, because blends change over time. What smells good today, might not smell good tomorrow.

Common sense and blending knowledge are both helpful, but ultimately it all comes down to the delicate aromas that can be picked up by the nose. Before I start blending anything, I take a moment to sniff all ingredients. Not only does that offer a last-minute quality control check of the distillates, but it awakens my senses to add the creative touch that simple book knowledge cannot lend to the artistic process of aromatic blending.

Scent Descriptions

Allspice: Warm clove-like sweet spicy fragrance.

Anise: The smell of licorice. Warm and sweet.

Basil: Sweet, spicy, warm and fiery. Somewhat licorice-like.

Benzoin Resin: Sweet, light vanilla-like aroma, used as a fixative of scent.

Bergamot: Fresh, sweet and refreshing, but with slightly spicy floral undertones.

Black Pepper: Pungent, spicy, warm, herbaceous, peppery aroma.

Blood Orange: Citrus with a green note.

Calendula: Herbaceous, pungent, and strong.

Cardamom: Fresh, sweet, green, spicy, balsamic.

Carrot Seed: Earthly, pungent aroma.

Cedarwood (*Cedrus deodora*): Soft, sweet, warm, woody, and fruity with honey overtones.

Chamomile, Roman: Sweet, herbaceous, fresh, and fruity.

Chamomile, blue: Herbaceous, sweet, heavy.

Cinnamon Leaf: A sweet, spicy hot fragrance. The aroma is smoky and warm.

Cistus: Rich, sweet and dry.

Citronella: Grassy, fruity, and slightly herbaceous with a citrus undertone.

Clary sage (*Salvia sclarea*): Nutty, heady, herbaceous, warm, and mildly intoxicating.

Clove: Warm, spicy, and slightly fruity.

Cypress: Fresh, woody, clear, light, slightly spicy with a clean scent.

Eucalyptus: Pungent, sharp, strong, and camphor-like with woody sub notes.

Fennel: Herbaceous, sweet honey, very licorice-like, and warm.

Frankincense: Soft, balsamic, heady fragrance, warm, sweet, and incense-like.

Geranium: Flowery Rose, sweet, dry citrus undertone.

Ginger: Peppery, sharp, fresh, pungent, earthy, aromatic, and warm.

Grapefruit: Warm, sweet and fresh citrus with a slight floral undertone.

Helichrysum: Green, earthy, sweet aroma.

Hyssop: Woody, earthy, sweet, and warm.

Jasmine Absolute: Rich, warm, floral, and sweetly exotic with floral honey-like aroma.

Juniper: Fresh, fruity, woody, spicy, and herbaceous.

Lavender: Fresh, floral, light, powdery, and sweet.

Lemon: The most well-known citrus scent, clean, sweet, sugary, and light.

Lemongrass: Citrus, herbaceous, and smoky. Kind of like a hay field type aroma.

Lime: Fresh, citrus scent, sweet, and candy-like.

Litsea: Strong, sweet, citrus aroma.

Mandarin: Warm, citrus, and fruity with floral overtones.

Myrrh: Warm, smoky, slightly musty, and earthy.

Neroli: Floral, powdery, spicy, and sweet with highly radiant fragrance.

Oakmoss: Dry earthy aroma used as a fixative.

Orange, Sweet: Fresh, fruity, tangy, and sweet. A perky and lively scent.

Palmarosa: Sweet, rosy, floral, herbaceous, and lemony.

Patchouli: Earthy, heavy, musty musk, penetrating, herbaceous, and smoky.

Peppermint: Minty fresh, slightly camphor-like, and candy-like.

Peru Balsam: Sweet vanilla-like aroma.

Petitgrain: Floral, fresh, and revitalizing with a hint of orange.

Ravensara: Spicy, herbaceous, clear, sweet, and licorice-like.

Rose Absolute: Intense, sweet, and floral. The queen of flowers.

Rosemary: Woody, fresh, herbaceous, powerful, and sharp.

Rosewood: Sweet, woody, and powdery soft with an underlying rose scent.

Sandalwood: Warm, rich, sweet, woody, and soft.

Spearmint: Minty, cool, candy-like, and fresh.

Spruce: Sweet, fruity, woody aroma.

Tangerine: Sweet, sparkling fresh citrus.

Tea Tree: Sharp, spicy, warm with medicinal tones.

Thyme: Powerful, warm herbaceous aroma.

Vanilla Absolute: Sweet, honey-like, distinctive. Scent said to be most like mother's milk.

Vetiver: Earthy, musty with softness and full body aroma, and sweet woody aroma.

Ylang Ylang: Sweet, intense, floral, tropical, and heady with an overtone of banana.

Candle Aromatherapy

The key to choosing essential oils for candles is matching the flash point of the essential oil to the melt point of the wax that you are using. See your supplier for wax melt points. If the flash point of your essential oil is significantly lower than the melt point of your wax base then your essential oil aroma will burn off. This will leave your candle with little to no aroma no matter how much you put in.

Wax	Melt Point	Percentage Scenting
Soy	125.8°F	6 - 8%
Paraffin	140 - 190°F	1 - 3%
Beeswax	150°F	1 - 3%
Palm	139°F	5 - 6%
Gel	180 - 220°F	3 - 5%

Essential Oil	Flash Point °F	Essential Oil	Flash Point °F
Anise	194	Lavender 40/42	160
Basil	176	Lemon	115
Bay	140	Lemongrass	169
Bergamot	136	Lime	122
Carrot Seed	138	Mandarin	129
Cedarwood	>212	Myrrh	>212
Chamomile, Roman	135	Neroli	126
Chamomile, German	140	Orange, Sweet	115
Cinnamon Leaf	194	Palmarosa	199
Cistus	>212	Patchouli	>212
Citronella	135	Pepper, Black	129
Clary Sage	174	Peppermint	151
Clove	>212	Petitgrain	151
Cypress	102	Ravensara	117
Eucalyptus	117	Rose Otto	140
Fennel	158	Rosemary	104-109
Frankencense	109	Rosewood	167
Geranium	176	Sandalwood	>212
Ginger	135	Spearmint	151
Grapefruit	109	Spruce	122
Helichrysum	118	Tangerine	124
Hyssop	138	Tea Tree	135-142
Jasmine Absolute	142	Vetiver	>212
Juniper Berry	106	Ylang Ylang	192

Carrier Oils, Butters and Bases

If you are wondering how much essential oil to add to a product, this chart will help you decide.

Essential Oil Scenting Guide	
Up to 40%	
Reed Diffusers	40%
Perfume	20%-40%
Up to 30%	
Eau de parfum	10-30%
Up to 20%	
Eau de toilette	5-20%
Up to 5%	
Eau de cologne	2-5%
Massage & Body Oil	0.5%-5%
Balm/Ointment/Salve	0.5%-5%
Shower Fizz Tabs	3%-5%
Room Sprays	1%-5%
Up to 3%	
CP Soap	3%
Oil/Butter Body Scrubs	1% - 3%
Body Butters	0.5% - 3%
Lip Balm	0.5% - 3%
Lotion & Creme	0.25% - 3%
Body Mist	1% - 3%
Up to 2%	
Hair Conditioner	0.5% - 2%
Organically Preserved Bases	1% - 2%
Up to 1.5%	
HP Soap 1% - 1.5%	1% - 1.5%

Up to 1%	
Bath Bombs 1%	1%
M&P Soap 0.5% - 1%	0.5% - 1%
Jelly 0.25% - 1%	0.25% - 1%
Masques 0.25% - 1%	0.25% - 1%
Shower Gel & Shampoo	0.25% - 1%
Astringent, Toner	0.25% - 1%
Bath Salt, Soak & Powder	0.25% - 1%
Household & Laundry	0.25% - 1%
Up to 0.5%	
Baby Products 0.25% - 0.5%	0.25% - 0.5%
Pet Products 0.25% - 0.5%	0.25% - 0.5%
Up to 0.1%	
Mineral Makeup (not eyes)	0.1%

It is vital to be familiar with carrier oils and butters so that you can choose the right carrier oil to dilute your essential oils.

Almond Butter
INCI: *Prunus amygdalus dulcis (and) Hydrogenated Vegetable Oil*
Almond butter is derived from sweet almonds specifically from the Mediterranean area, and it is obtained by cold pressing selected fruits followed by a full refining process. The natural oil contains essential fatty acids, but also contains unsaponifiables as natural waxes or paraffin, which are collected during the refining and deodorization process. In cosmetic preparations, the feel and behavior of almond butter is somewhat similar to that of shea butter (*Butyrospermum parkii*). Almond butter exhibits excellent spread-ability on the skin, making it ideal as a massage butter or carrier for treatment products. It adds moisturizing attributes to creams, lotions and bar soaps.

Almond Oil, Sweet
INCI: *Prunus amygdalus dulcis*
Sweet Almond Oil is pressed from almond kernels. The almond tree is cultivated in Southern Europe, the Mediterranean countries and California. It consists mainly of oleic acid (69%), essential unsaturated fatty acids (25%), sterolins (0.5 to 1%) and vitamin E (about 10 IU per ounce.) It is a light, nearly odorless oil. Sweet almond oil is said to have great nutritional value for all skin types. It has a similar make up to baby sebum, the oil naturally produced by the skin to protect a newborn's skin, and it is easily absorbed. It contains glucosides, minerals, and vitamins and is rich in protein. Sweet almond oil has very little natural smell and can be used as a perfume base. It was highly valued by the Egyptians for cosmetic purposes.

Avocado Butter
INCI: *Persea gratissima (and) Hydrogenated Vegetable Oil*
Avocado butter has been found to significantly increase the water-soluble collagen content in the dermis skin layer. This rich and nourishing butter deeply penetrates into deep skin tissue. It is rich in vitamins A, B1, B2, and D, lecithin, and potassium as well as Vitamin E. This is one of the natural butters

that is most easily absorbed by the skin and transported deep into the tissue. It's wonderful emollient properties make it ideal for dry, dehydrated, or mature skins. Furthermore, it also helps to relieve the dryness and itching of psoriasis and eczema. It is also high in sterolins, which help to reduce age spots and help heal sun damage and scars.

Avocado butter is obtained from the fruit of the avocado tree which grows in sub-tropical regions of the world. The butter is created from the avocado fruit oil through a unique hydrogenation process, which yields a soft, greenish butter. It has a mild odor and excellent melting properties which make it suitable for skin care.

Avocado Oil
INCI: *Persea americana*
Avocado oil is excellent for dry and wrinkled skin as it moisturizes, nourishes, and softens. It has been found to significantly increase the water-soluble collagen content in the dermis skin layer. Avocado oil contains protein, vitamins A, D, and E, and some amino acids.

Avocado oil is made from the pulp of the avocado fruit. It is rich, heavy but penetrating oil that is full of nutritive and therapeutic components. Avocado oil contains more than 20% essential unsaturated fatty acids. It contains vitamins A, C, D, and E, proteins, beta-carotene, lecithin, fatty acids, and the "youth mineral" potassium. Avocado oil is high in unsaponifiables (sterolins) which are reputed to be beneficial in reducing age spots, healing scars and moisturizing the upper layers of the skin. Unsaponifiables are a large group of compounds called plant steroids or sterolins. They soften the skin, have superior moisturizing effects on the upper layer of the skin, and reduce scars. The sterolins in avocado oil have been found to diminish age spots. Oils with the highest unsaponifiables are shea butter, avocado oil, sesame oil, soybean oil, and olive oil.

A 1991 study at the Department of Food Engineering and Biotechnology, Technion-Israel Institute of Technology found that treatment with avocado oil significantly increases the water-soluble collagen content in the dermis, which effects the age of the skin. Avocado is used in many folk medicines as an aphrodisiac. Avocado oil is an emollient and very stable. According to the American Medical Association (AMA) Committee on Coetaneous Health it does help make the skin feel softer and smoother, while reducing roughness, cracking, and irritation. Avocado oil may retard the fine wrinkles of aging and is said to help protect the skin from ultraviolet rays.

Borage Oil

INCI: *Borago officinalis*

Borage oil is produced from a wildflower commonly known as the starflower. The plant is large with blue star-shaped flowers. It grows wild all over the world, but mostly throughout Europe and North Africa. Borage has been naturalized to North America as well. It is grown and harvested for herbal use, but mostly for the oil found in the seeds.

Borage oil is a rich source of the essential fatty acid gamma linolenic acid (GLA). The GLA of borage oil is 24% which makes it the richest known source in the world. Borage oil contains polyunsaturated essential fatty acids which aid in the flexibility of the cell membranes and helps normalize trans-epidermal water loss.

In skin care, borage oil is useful because it has a cooling, calming, and diuretic effect on the skin. It soothes damaged, irritated and inflamed skin which makes it a prime candidate for blemished, mature, sun-damaged and troubled skin. Borage oil is emollient and promotes healthy skin. It contains tannins which gives borage oil a minor tightening effect on the skin while restoring moisture without leaving an oily barrier on the skin.

Borage oil capsules is highly recommended for consumption due to the fact that consuming linoleic acid (LA) gives the body the starting material to produce on its own gamma linolenic acid (GLA). Biochemically LA is converted into GLA by the enzyme Delta-6-Desaturase and further transformed into prostaglandin 1 which is beneficial to maintaining healthy skin and suppresses inflammation of the skin. Inflammation of the skin equals diseased skin and only healthy skin can look radiant.

Broccoli Oil

INCI: *Brassica oleracea italica*

Broccoli seed oil is a perfect ingredient in formulas in which you need exceptional lubricity with a non-greasy feel. The oil is a good emollient in cosmetic products including lip balms, skin creams, and hair care products. Broccoli seed oil can effectively be used as an all-natural alternative to silicone in shampoos and conditioners. It has a unique feel as well as a penetrating ability to impart a natural, healthy shine to skin and hair. The fatty acid composition of Broccoli seed oil by weight is: palmitic 3.25%, oleic acid 13.5%, linoleic acid 11.4%, linolenic acid (alpha) 9%, eicosenoic 6% and erucic acid 49%.

Carrot Oil

INCI: *Daucus carota*

Carrot oil has regenerating and toning effects, which is excellent for mature and congested skin, psoriasis, eczema, and for sensitive, couperose skin. It contains vitamins B, C, D, and E, minerals, beta carotene and essential fatty acids which is a rich source of vitamin A. It is excellent for sensitive skin. It is reported to tone skin, stimulating elasticity, and reduce scarring. Carrot oil helps to balance the moisture in our skin and conditions hair.

Castor Oil, USP

INCI: *Ricinus communis*

Castor oil, USP is a vegetable oil extracted from the seed of the castor plant. It is used commercially in 50% of lipsticks in the United States. Castor oil creates a protective barrier on the skin and is soothing. It is a triglyceride that is mainly composed of ricinoleic acid (87%), a fatty acid with an unusual molecular structure. Ricinoleic acid is a monounsaturated, 18-carbon fatty acid that has an unusual hydroxyl functional group on the twelfth carbon. It is this functional group makes castor oil unusually polar. Castor oil is a colorless to very pale yellow liquid with mild or no odor nor taste.

Castor Oil, Sulfated

INCI: *Ricinus communis*

Castor oil, Sulfated is commonly known as "Turkey Red." It is a sulfated castor oil which is created by adding sulfuric acid to castor oil. The resulting oil is water-soluble. Sulfated castor oil is the only oil that completely disperses in water which makes it an ideal carrier for essential oils in bath oil.

Cocoa Butter

INCI: *Theobroma cacao*

Cocoa Butter is a very rich butter, with excellent emollient properties and is used with great effect on very dry, dehydrated, and flaky skin. It easily absorbs into the skin and imparts sheen. Cocoa butter is the solid fat expressed from the roasted seed of the cocoa seed (beans). The cocoa tree is cultivated in most tropical countries and is native to South America. It is highly protective and acts as water repellant. Cocoa butter contains about 5 IU of vitamin E per ounce. Cocoa Butter softens and lubricates the skin. It has the aroma of chocolate. Some people find the scent overwhelming in recipes and prefer to use deodorized cocoa butter.

Coconut Oil

INCI: *Cocos nucifera*

Pure coconut oil has a small molecular structure which allows it to be easily absorbed by the skin. It leaves the skin feeling soft and smooth but not oily. Coconut oil is great for the skin because of its antioxidant properties, which gives it a long shelf life. The antioxidants in coconut oil stop the chain reaction of free-radicals creating more free-radicals. Because of the antioxidants, coconut oil not only softens your skin but protects it from further damage, while promoting healthy skin. Coconut oil is also the richest source of good, medium-chain fatty acids, which our sebum also produces as a protective layer on the skin to kill harmful germs.

Coconut oil is vegetable-sourced oil that is naturally free of the need for pesticides and other chemicals to grow and harvest. Some of the myths about coconut oil come from the belief in post-World War II times that coconut contained high levels of cholesterol, which internally or topically would result in acne. Current research on the chemical composition of coconut oil has proven that it does not contain cholesterol at all. Coconut oil contains lauric acid, which actually supports the antibacterial activity of the skin's cells.

Coconut oil is the number-one oil used to make surfactants and castile soap because it produces a nice lather. Coconut in its pure form—when it has not gone through a chemical synthesis with another ingredient—does not dry the skin. Some surfactant-based cleansers that are formulated to strip the skin do leave it feeling dry, and that is wrongly blamed on the coconut. Cleansers that are formulated for oily skin are typically designed to strip away the oily layer on the skin. Many consumers feel that their skin is truly clean in this state. However, the skin produces more oil when it is dry and a vicious cycle of oily, dry, oily, and dry is created. Soaps and cleansers can wash away the protective layer of oil and acid on our skin, leaving it feeling tight and dry. Using a coconut-based moisturizer helps make the skin feel better and helps reestablish the protective layer of oil.

Coconut oil contains the fatty acids caprylic acid, capric acid, and lauric acid. Many of the coconut-derived ingredients can be identified easily by these fatty acids. Coconut oil consists of 90% saturated fat. It is made up mostly of medium-chain triglycerides which are 92% saturated fatty acids (44.6% lauric acid, 16.8% myristic acid, 8.2% palmictic acid, 8% caprylic acid), 6% monounsaturated fatty acids (oleic acid) and 2% polyunsaturated fatty acids (linoleic acid). Coconut melts at 76 degrees Fahrenheit, but if it is stored at a cooler temperature it is solid. Coconut oil resists rancidity because it is slow to oxidize.

Coconut Oil, Fractionated
INCI: *Cocos nucifera also-known-as Caprylic/Capric Triglyceride*
Many people are familiar with whole coconut oil which is a solid a room temperature but do not have experience with fractionated coconut oil. But if you haven't tried it you are missing out on a truly great carrier (fixed) oil product.

All carrier oils consist of a class of molecules called fatty acid triglycerides which means they contain three, long-chain fatty ester groups. Most all plant-derived carrier oils consist entirely of what are called "unsaturated" fatty acid triglycerides which means they have one or more carbon-carbon double bonds in their long, fatty, ester side-chains which are typically 16 to 20-plus carbon units long. The double bonds in these side chains are susceptible to oxidation over time, and their reactions with oxygen are what produce the rancid odor that you may have noticed in your carrier oils when they get old.

Whole coconut oil also has some quite long unsaturated fatty acid triglycerides (which is why it is a solid at room temperature). But fractionated coconut oil is special in that it has a relatively high percentage of shorter length (C8, C10), completely saturated (no double bonds) triglycerides. These smaller fatty acid triglycerides are separated from the whole coconut oil to give us what is known as "fractionated coconut oil."

The separation process is non-chemical and involves a simple physical separation process, so there are no chemical residues to worry about. Fractionated coconut oil has an indefinite shelf life and is light, non-greasy, non-staining, liquid oil. It is great for use in massage, toiletries, aromatherapy and soap. Fractionated coconut oil is a very good choice for use with essential oils, as it helps carry therapeutic oils under the skin. Fractionated coconut oil can be used in creams, lotions, bath oils, bath salts and soap. Fractionated coconut oil is especially useful in face creams where light oil is desired. It is a good substitute for sweet almond oil if you are concerned about rancidity or a short shelf life. My favorite use for fractionated coconut oil is as a base for massage oil because it does not leave the sheets smelling rancid.

Cranberry Seed Oil
INCI: *Vaccinium macrocarpon*
Cranberry seed oil is essential fatty acid oil recently introduced into the supplement industry. It is the only available oil with a one-to-one ratio of omega-6 (linoleic) to omega-3 (alpha-linolenic) fatty acids. Cranberry seed oil has oxidative stability and contains 70% essential fatty acids making it a superb emollient, lubricant and conditioner for the skin. It is excellent for use in skin, hair, lip, and baby care. Cranberry seed oil contributes to the lipid barrier protection of the skin and assists in moisture retention. The oil also contains high concentrations of tocopherols, tocotrienols, phytosterols, phospholipids, and vitamin A, redefining performance and stability standards for highly polyunsatruated oils.

Evening Primrose
INCI: *Oenothers bennis*
Evening primrose oil is extracted from the seeds of a plant native to North America. However, it grows in Europe and parts of the Southern Hemisphere as well. The evening primrose plant has yellow flowers that bloom only in the evening, hence the name. Each blossom lasts only one day, blooming as the sun sets and withering after the sunrise. It can grow to be up to eight feet tall. Interestingly enough, evening primrose is considered a "weed" in most gardens. However, the oil that it produces is highly valuable both topically and orally.

Evening primrose oil is rich in the essential fatty acids linoleic acid (74%), gamma linoleic acid (9-10%) (GLA) and contains polysaturated omega-6 fatty acids. Evening primrose capsules are commonly taken orally for eczema, breast pain, lowering cholesterol, menopausal symptoms, PMS, osteoporosis and decreasing the risk of heart attack. Evening primrose oil is used topically for acne, eczema and psoriasis; it is the perfect addition to a formula designed to moisturize and soothe damaged skin.

Grapeseed Oil
INCI: *Vitis vinifera*
Grapeseed oil is pressed from the seeds of *Vitis vinifera* grapes, which are typically wine grapes. Since grape seeds are not used in the wine making process, the extraction of the seeds into oil has become profitable byproduct of the wine industry. Grapeseed oil is perfect for formulations that require a light, thin oil that is slightly astringent. It leaves a glossy but not oily film on the skin. Grapeseed oil contains an average of 11% saturated fat, 15% oleic acid, 69% linoleic acid, and less than 1% alpha linolenic acid. It is the lightest of oils, and it is virtually odorless. It is widely used in hypoallergenic natural products because it does not often cause allergic reactions in the highly allergic.

Hazelnut Oil
INCI: *Corylus avellana*
Hazelnut oil is extracted from hazelnuts. It penetrates the skin easily. It has some vitamin E content. Cold pressed hazelnut oil is a wonderful, light, penetrating oil that is slightly astringent making it good oil for acne prone skin. It is high in the essential fatty acids and is soothing and healing to dry irritated skin. Studies have shown that it can filter sunrays and is therefore commonly used in sun care products. A good oil for massage, hair care and cream/lotion formulas.

Hemp Seed Oil

INCI: *Cannabis sativa*

Hemp seed oil is extracted from the seeds of the *Cannabis sativa* plant. To most people *Cannabis sativa* is synonymous with marijuana; the Latin name translates to "useful hemp." Because of this we are often asked if our hemp oil is legal. The oil itself is perfectly legal. There is no tetrahydrocannabinol in the final product of hemp oil.

Hemp contains proteins and high quality fat, and it has a remarkable fatty acid profile. It is high in omega-3 and a 1.7% gamma-linolenic acid. It is 57% linoleic and 19% linoleic acids. This oil has the lowest amount of saturated fatty acids and the highest amount of the polyunsaturated essential fatty acids (linoleic and linolenic acids). Hemp is wonderful oil for dry or mature skin since it is said to help stimulate cell growth.

Hemp seed oil is an emollient. According to the AMA's Committee on Coetaneous Health, emollients help make the skin feel softer and smoother, reduce roughness, cracking and irritation and may possibly retard the fine wrinkles of aging. Hemp seed has a lot of minerals and is good for the skin and hair. Use this in your soaps, lotions and lip balms. It also makes a great lotion bar with almond oil and cocoa butter.

Hemp Seed Butter

INCI: *Cannabis Sativa Seed Oil and Hydrogenated Vegetable Oil*

Hemp seed butter is produced using the fatty fractions and unsaponifiables (natural waxes/paraffin's) which are collected during the refining processes which are blended with hydrogenated vegetable oil to produce a butter-like material suitable for use in cosmetics and toiletries. Hemp seed butter is made from expeller-pressed non-sterilized and non-fumigated seeds of the hemp plant.

Hemp seed oil has a high content of essential fatty acids, which help the action of hydro lipid coat, thereby reducing trans-epidermal water loss. Hemp seed oil possesses one of the highest PUFA contents of all the natural oils. It provides the four essential fatty acids beneficial to the skin: LA, GLA, LNA, and SDA— one of the highest EFA contents.

Hemp seed butter is often used in body care, soaps, facial creams, lotions, and sunscreens to impart moisture, particularly for dry, damaged skin. Hemp seed oil is one of the "driest" natural oils which are absorbed quickly into the skin, and hence the butter produced from it also exhibits a relatively dry feel. It provides excellent lubrication without being greasy.

Illipe Butter
INCI: *Shorea stenoptera*
Illipe butter is a harder butter with a higher melting point than most other exotic butters, yet it still melts on contact with the skin. The first inhabitants of Borneo (the Dayaks) have been making "butter" from illipe nuts for many centuries for therapeutic and cosmetic purposes. Illipe butter has long-lasting moisturizing attributes. It is most renowned for its skin-softening quality.

The illipe tree grows in the forests of Borneo. The tree grows from 5 to 15 meters in height, with 5 centimeter seeds. The seeds are enclosed in a thin shell with wing-like attachments that enable the seed to fall away from the mother tree. The seeds are collected from the ground and dried in the sun until the shells are sufficiently brittle to be separated from the seeds by pounding in rice mortars.

Illipe's chemical composition closely resembles that of cocoa butter, yet with a slightly higher melting point, making it ideal for use in bar soaps, lip balms, lip sticks, and other stick-type applications where a higher melting point is desired.

Jojoba Oil
INCI: *Simmondsia chinensis*
Jojoba oil is cold pressed from the nuts of the jojoba tree. The jojoba tree is cultivated in California, Arizona, Mexico, and Israel. Jojoba is pronounced *Ho Ho Ba*. Native Americans have been using jojoba for centuries. The first record of jojoba is from 1701. Father Junipero Serrra found that Native Americans were using Jojoba to treat sores, cuts and burns, and as a conditioner and for all over skin and hair treatments.

Jojoba is technically not oil, but a liquid wax ester with a long unsaturated carbon chain. Chemically it resembles sperm whale oil or spermaceti oil. It was a popular ingredient in creams. The United States banned all sperm whale products in the 1970s because they were contributing to the extinction of sperm whales. In 1977 domestic commercial jojoba oil cultivation began because it is the natural substitute for spermaceti which, in other cases, has been replaced by synthetic products.

Jojoba esters are composed of straight chain alcohols. The acid and the alcohol portions have 20 or 22 carbon atoms and one unsaturated bond. It resembles human sebum, the natural coating our body produces to protect the skin and keeps it supple. Our skin loses sebum with age, sun, wind, cold, and the environment. It contains protein, minerals and a waxy substance that mimics collagen.

Jojoba is perfect skin therapy for any skin type. It has a large molecular structure. Jojoba can help dry or oily skin. If your skin has an over-production of sebum, jojoba oil will dissolve clogged pores and restore the skin to its natural pH balance. The reason jojoba oil works so well that it actually penetrates the skin is because it is accepted as sebum.

Although jojoba oil is very expensive, it does have a long shelf life; it will never break down or go rancid. Jojoba is expensive because it takes 1,200 whole jojoba nuts to add up to a pound which has a 50% yield of oil. Because jojoba has very little scent it works as a wonderful natural perfume base. Jojoba is not greasy and absorbs right into the skin. JMC Technologies has conducted scientific research proving that jojoba can increase skin softness by up to 37%, it reduces superficial lines and wrinkles up to 25% upon application and up to 11% after 8 hours. Jojoba oil is considered to be hypoallergenic oil.

Meadowfoam Seed Oil
INCI: *Limnanthes alba*
One of my favorite oils is meadowfoam seed oil because it is probably the single, most unique oil available on the market today. Meadowfoam seed oil comes from a low-growing herbaceous winter annual that gets its name from the fact that fields of meadowfoam in full bloom appear to look like a meadow of foam. It is native to the Pacific Northwest. Meadowfoam has a good, stable shelf life because it contains over 98% long chain fatty acids. Its unique chemical properties make it one of the most stable of all of the carrier oils.

Refined meadowfoam is virtually odorless which makes it a prime candidate for use in aromatherapy products. It is rich in antioxidants and penetrates the skin easily. The stability of meadowfoam seed oil actually works to extend the shelf life of less stable ingredients in a formula. Meadowfoam is such unique and valuable oil that it is currently being studied by scientists at Oregon State University and the US Department of Agriculture.

When added to cosmetics and creams, meadowfoam re-moisturizes the skin like no other oil. In shampoos and soaps it helps add shine and moisture to the hair and scalp that are otherwise made dry and brittle by the harsh process of daily washing. In lipsticks and balms, it helps revitalize dry, cracked lips, and it helps retain moisture all day long. In many natural formulations, meadowfoam seed oil is often used in place of jojoba oil or sperm whale oil. Its texture, stability and ability to adhere to the skin makes meadowfoam a good candidate to replace castor oil lip formulations.

Meadowfoam oil, when applied to the skin, forms a moisture barrier which prevents moisture loss from the skin. Meadowfoam oil has a non-greasy feeling and soaks immediately into the skin. An added bonus to meadowfoam is that the quality that makes it adhere to the skin also acts as a binder to retain scent longer for aromatherapy-based products. Meadowfoam oil adds a good slip and lubricant value to massage products and will not turn treatment sheets rancid. Meadowfoam has a high molecular weight, but it does not winterize in cold temperatures like jojoba or avocado oils.

The research and development of meadowfoam began in the late 1950s when the United States Department of Agriculture (USDA) was in search for plants that had potential as a renewable source of raw materials for industry. Commercial development began in 1980 on an experimental 35-acre farm-scale operation in Oregon. Meadowfoam has never reached its full potential for use in industry due to the lack of consistent funding which slowed the development of the potential aspects of this unique renewable oil resource. However, the cosmetic industry has fully embraced this fabulous oil due to its unique texture, slip, moisture retention, and shelf life.

Along with the breakthrough of meadowfoam oil came the discovery of three unknown long chain fatty acids. Meadowfoam oil contains over 98% fatty acids with over 20 carbon atoms. The majority of the fatty acid composition of meadowfoam oil comes from C20 (63%), C21 (1 to 16%) and C22 (2 to 17%) fatty acids. Meadowfoam oil is found in the seeds of the plant which contain 20 to 30% oil. The high euric acid content of meadowfoam is most similar to that of rapeseed oil, however rapeseed is slightly more saturated than meadowfoam oil. Much like rapeseed oil, the by-product of meadowfoam oil produces a meal that can be used as a feed source for livestock.

All around, meadowfoam is the definition of a green product. It was developed to replace sperm whale oil in order to protect the species. It is renewable, sustainable, serves multiple industries, and the fields of meadowfoam flowers provide habitat for birds, insects and other creatures that thrive in the fields. It is grown as a rotation crop for grass seed farming which eliminates the need to burn fields in between grass seed planting and gives the farmer an off-season income. Meadowfoam also has less need for fertilizer and pesticides.

Meadowfoam oil is available cold pressed and refined. The refined version is expeller expressed, and it is virtually odorless. It has a pale yellow color. Cold pressed meadowfoam oil has a distinct herbaceous grassy odor and has a dark orange color that comes from the powerful antioxidant known as 3-MBTU, which holds a US Patent. The cold pressed is a virgin triglyceride oil that is clarified using only filtration. It is rich in the delicate active materials such as tocopherols, carotenoids and phystosterol. Use of the cold pressed oil can be problematic due to the strong natural aroma, but with proper formulating it can be used successfully.

Rosehip Seed Oil

INCI: *Rosa mosqueta*

Rosehip seed oil is extracted by cold pressing the seeds of the bright red bud (hip) of a wild rose bush native to Chile. The rosehip seed pod is what is left after the rose petals fall off of a rose. I find that, in nature, nothing is wasted; the power packed oil that comes from rosehips is a great testament to that fact.

Rosehip seed oil has a high content of unsaturated essential fatty acids (80%). It is made up of monounsaturated omega-9 fatty acid oleic acid (15-20%), unsaturated omega-6 fatty acid linoleic acid (44-50%) and linolenic (30-35%). Rosehip seed oil contains bio-available trans-retinoic acid which is highly compatible and easily absorbed into the skin. It also has high vitamin C content.

Rosehip seed oil is highly regarded for the properties it brings to the skin care industry. It is known as a very reparative oil that revitalizes dry, rough, damaged, scarred and dull skin. It is used in the treatment of wrinkles, sun damage, dry skin, scars, and it is restorative for all skin issues. It is quite absorbent and almost instantly hydrates tissue and brings moisture balance to winter skin in arid climates. It is well-known for its use in treatment after radiation. It is also known to accelerate the healing of burns and all known effects of aging including brown spots, wrinkles, and deep lines in the skin. At least one or more of your serious anti-aging and face-oriented products should have this key oil.

Safflower Oil

INCI: *Carthamus tinctorius*

Safflower oil comes from the seeds of an herbaceous thistle-like annual flower. Safflower oil is polyunsaturated oil that is similar to sunflower oil in nutritional value and shelf life. Safflower and sunflower are relatively unstable when exposed to high heat, light or oxygen. Both safflower and sunflower are good to use in low-heat or no-heat formulas. Safflower oil contains the monounsaturated omega-9 fatty acid oleic acid (78.9%), unsaturated omega-6 fatty acid linoleic (11%), palmitic acid (6.2%), and linolenic (.02%).

Sunflower Oil

INCI: *Helianthus annuus*

Sunflower oil is extracted from the seeds of the sunflower. It is made up of predominately linoleic acid (48-74%), monounsaturated omega-9 fatty acid oleic acid (14-40%), palmitic acid (4-9%) and stearic acid (1-7%). There are several versions of sunflower produced, ranging from high linoleic, high oleic and mid oleic. The variations in the unsaturated fatty acid profile are factors of both the growing climate and genetics of the plant. All sunflower oil has high vitamin E content.

Sunflower oil is used primarily in the food industry but has applications in the cosmetic industry as well. It helps form a seal that retains moisture yet allows the skin to breathe. An interesting study found that sunflower oil used as a treatment for low birth weight pre-term infants lowered the rate of infections by 41 percent. The theory is that pre-mature babies have underdeveloped skin which leaves them more susceptible to infections and that sunflower oil created the much needed barrier on the skin.

Opinion of Mineral Oil and Petroleum
Mineral oil and petroleum are the by-products of the distillation of petroleum in the manufacturing of gasoline. Both are very commonly found in your cosmetics. Take a moment and check the ingredient deck of what you have around the house.

Petroleum jelly interrupts your own skin's ability to moisturize itself. Petroleum jelly is often used to correct dry skin, but in fact it creates more problems by interfering in the natural cycle of the skin which leads to excessive dryness and chapping. It creates a vicious cycle of dryness. Breaking the cycle will create only a few days of dry skin until your skin can rebound.

My opinion is that soda pop is to water what petroleum is to plant butters. Soda pop is full of empty calories and often, caffeine, and this creates a long-term dependence on the drink. Water hydrates and restores the body. Petroleum offers nothing of value to the skin and comes up empty every time in addition to creating a long term addiction. Plant butters are rich, soothing, and feed the skin, allowing it to restore itself. Petroleum used for dry skin creates more dry skin which creates a vicious cycle. Plant butters nourish dry skin and work synergistically with the natural process of the skin.

While many soda pops often include naturally sourced ingredients, petroleum is a byproduct of drilling for petroleum, which is then further refined. Just like many soda pops the natural origins of petroleum are lost in its ill effects on the body. The refining process of petroleum also makes it unappealing to vegans due to the fact that is processed and filtered through bone-char.

:: Chapter 5 ::
Practical Aromatherapy

Create Your Story

As you build your aromatherapy business, you will encounter many skeptics and critics who do not understand the value of this ancient form of natural healing. If you are passionate about your products, then you understand that part of your role as an aromatherapist will be to educate your clients. You are reading this book because you want to soak up as much information as possible so that you're prepared to answer any question with authority.

In the first chapter, I shared my personal story. You learned how using essential oils became a way of life for me many years ago when my son developed ringworm. I invested in a bottle of tea tree oil that wiped out the parasite in three days, and that one incident led to our family starting an aromatherapy-based business, and to me becoming a Certified and Registered Aromatherapist.

What is your aromatherapy story? Are your own personal care products and medicine cabinet full of essential oils? In this book, you will learn a great deal of history and chemistry about the use of essential oils, as well as safety, regulatory and political fundamentals. Your clients, however, will not always be interested in all those cold, hard facts. They will want to know how your products work for you and other people. Sharing your personal experiences along with providing good, solid information will help you stand out among your peers and connect with your customers.

You also need to be ready to hear your customers' stories. Being a successful product provider involves listening to the needs of potential buyers. Once you understand what they are looking for, what they need help with, and what conditions they are struggling with, then you can show them how essential oils can benefit them, their clients, their friends, and their families.

Essential Sk-information

In aromatherapy, molecules of essential oils applied to the skin pass through the skin's epidermis and are carried away by the capillary blood circulating in the dermis. With good care, the skin renews itself every 28 days. Mistreated skin can take up to three to four months to rejuvenate through aromatherapy. Essential oils applied to the skin can stimulate circulation of the surface skin cells and encourage cell regeneration and the formation of new skin cells.

Factors that affect the rate of absorption of essential oils:

1. *The area size of skin matters.* Even if a set amount of essential oil is applied to the skin via carrier oil, less is absorbed if it is only applied to small patches of skin. The beauty of skin is that we have a lot of it, which allows for application over a generous portion of the body.
2. *Different areas of the skin* are more permeable than others. The palms of the hand, soles of the feet, forehead, scalp, behind the ears, inside the wrists and armpits are more permeable than the legs, buttocks, trunk and abdomen for the water soluble components of the essential oil.
3. *Subcutaneous fat has a poor blood supply* which means essential oils applied to these areas may take longer to be absorbed.
4. *Type of skin makes a difference.* Mature or dehydrated skin slows the absorption of essential oils.

Using Essential Aromatherapy in Skin Care

The largest organ in our body is our skin, weighing in at about nine pounds. It is the packaging that holds us together, keeps us warm, and acts as our first defensive warning system by constantly alerting the brain to varying conditions in our surroundings. As our environment changes, and as we change, so does our skin; it requires different care at various times in our lives.

When we are born our skin is perfect, yet day by day we begin to age. It isn't until puberty that we can clearly see those changes because they are so slight in our early years, and youthful skin is forgiving.

Overnight a child seems to transform into being a teenager. It is important to understand the changes that a teenager's skin is going through, however teens are not the only ones with skin problems and trouble areas. Babies get rashes, and the elderly get wrinkles, but aromatherapy can help with everything in between.

In our teen years, hormones change the way we need to care for our skin. At this point, raging hormones and over-production of oils can cause acne to become an issue. However, in their twenties, many are still plagued with the same skin-care issues they faced in puberty. This is an important time to talk to people about taking care of their skin. Many struggle with proper skin care in their teens and then pay the price for that poor skin care in later years.

Aromatherapy and Acne

The most common skincare mistake is using products that dry out the skin in response to oily skin. However, drying the skin up in response to it being oily simply influences it to respond to this unhealthy state by producing more even oil. Talk to your customers about drinking plenty of water and eating whole foods. The best way to healthy skin is by being healthy from the inside out. Proper skin care on the outside includes using organic and natural products that feed the skin and allow it to breathe. Talk about using gentle products, protecting the skin from the sun, and cleansing, toning and moisturizing every day and night. Tell clients to always use upward gentle strokes in all steps of their skin care regimen.

In our early thirties, hormones begin to balance out. However, many people will suffer from adult acne when their hormones begin to change in their thirties, even if they did not have adolescent acne. Stress and hormones are the key factors to adult acne. To address the blemishes and eruptions that your clients are dealing with, you must first break down the myths:

Myth #1: Acne is caused by poor hygiene. In reality, washing the skin hard and frequently can actually make acne worse. Acne is not caused by dirt or surface skin oils. Vigorous washing will actually irritate the skin and make acne worse. The best approach to hygiene and acne is to gently wash your face twice a day with a mild cleanser, pat it dry and follow up with a light moisturizer.

Myth #2: Acne is caused by diet. Extensive scientific studies have not found a connection between diet and acne. In other words, food does not cause acne, but eating a balanced diet always makes sense. Vitamin deficiency (which you can get from the lack of a balanced diet) can definitely contribute to acne problems.

Myth #3: Acne is caused by stress. The ordinary stress of day-to-day living doesn't cause acne; it just amplifies what's already there. Stress generally will elevate our hormone levels, and hormones have a direct connection to acne. Severe stress that needs medical attention is sometimes treated with drugs that can cause acne as a side effect. If you think you may have acne related to a drug prescribed for stress or depression, you should consult your physician.

Myth #4: Acne is just a cosmetic disease. Yes, acne does affect the way people look and is normally not otherwise a serious threat to a person's physical health. However, acne can result in permanent physical scars. Plus, acne itself, as well as its scars, can affect the way people feel about themselves to the point of affecting their lives.

Myth #5: You just have to let acne run its course. The truth is that acne can be cleared up. If the acne products you have tried haven't given you the results you desire, keep trying. Remember to relax with life's stresses and eat a balanced diet, while drinking plenty of water for hydration. This will all help to maintain a corrected pH balance and hormone levels.

Myth #6: Popping and squeezing acne makes it clear up faster. In fact every time you pop or squeeze a pimple, zit, whitehead, blackhead, or cyst, you cause matters to worsen. Envision squeezing a balloon in between your hands right in the middle. Now some of the air will cause pressure and expansion on the top of the balloon but notice that some of the air moves to the back of the balloon. The same is true when you pop a zit: some of the pus and bacteria releases from the top and some bacteria are forced deeper into the skin.

Myth #7: Pimples and acne are the same thing. They are related, in that pimples can occur during acne, but acne itself can be a very painful disorder of the skin caused by inflammation of the skin glands and hair follicles. Pimples, however, are generally found on the face and are a small, solid, usually conical elevation of the skin.

Myth #8: Drying out the skin will make it less oily, therefore helping with acne. In fact, products that dry the skin cause the skin to produce more sebum in order to address the overly dry condition of the skin. Your skin sends a message to your brain to inform it of the dry conditions it is encountering, and then your brain sends a message back to produce more oil.

Myth #9: Using scrubs will reduce the appearance of acne. Your skin actually becomes irritated from most scrubs, which causes inflammation of the skin and leaves the skin open to infection or disease.

Myth #10: You will outgrow acne. In fact 25% of all adult men and 50% of adult women suffer from adult acne at some time in their adult life.

Products developed for teen skin should focus more on the therapeutic value than on the overall aroma. A product that works will be used and reused more regularly than a product that smells good but is ineffective. Teens want their skin to look good above all else. Many issues of teen skin can be addressed with aromatherapy. The single most useful essential oil for teens is tea tree. It has a powerful, natural topical antimicrobial quality that not only kills germs on the surface of the skin but also penetrates the skin, making it more effective than a surface cleaner. According to Jeanne Rose, tea tree, "has the property to penetrate pus and by mixing with it, the pus liquefies which causes it to slough off, leaving a healthy surface." That's right: Tea tree essential oil has the unique property of being able to liquefy pus.

Grapefruit essential oil is another useful essential oil that works as a natural astringency. Lavender essential oil is the most commonly used essential oil in aromatherapy. Despite the floral aroma, it has useful applications in both men's and teen products. It can be used in combination with other essential oils to change the aroma. Lavender essential oil is useful to reduce inflammation, take the red out of inflamed skin, and to soothe the skin. Blue chamomile essential oil is very useful to quickly heal the skin as well. Essential oils that decongest pores are good for both men and teen products including Himalayan cedarwood, lemon, and rosemary.

Aromatherapy and Aging

Whatever the age of your clients, each one needs to be informed that if he or she hasn't been taking care of his or her skin, the time to start is now. Many people in their twenties take their skin for granted because they are not suffering the signs of aging yet. It is in our thirties that we begin to show signs of aging. Many will start to develop fine lines around their eyes. The severity of the lines can be influenced by the previous years of their lives. Smoking, drinking alcohol, consuming caffeine, and sunning during the younger years suddenly leave their mark on once youthful skin.

Other factors like using harsh abrasives to exfoliate and rough treatment of the skin (pulling and tugging while applying makeup) begin to make their mark on skin in the thirties. Many begin to see what a lifetime of good or poor exercise, diet, and sunscreen application does to the skin. In our forties, our skin starts to dry out. Most people will find that their acne is gone, the oily T-zone vanishes, and more fine lines are joined by some deeper lines.

In our fifties another hormone shift changes a woman's skin again. When menopause hits, many women experience dry skin from head to toe. The skin begins to thin out much more noticeably than in the decades before. Those who drank plenty of water, ate healthy, and consumed alcohol and caffeine in moderation will find their skin looking years younger than their counterparts.

It's the truth: Diet and hygiene are the only facets of skin care that we can use to control these changes. Tell people to feed their skin from the inside and the outside. Healthy, youthful skin radiates from a healthy body which can be gained by consuming organic foods, drinking plenty of water, taking whole food supplements, and avoiding things that destroy the immune system like caffeine, processed sugar, excessive alcohol consumption, fast food, and cigarette smoke.

Three Basic Skin Care Steps:

- *Step One: Cleanse your face and neck every morning and night with a good facial cleanser.* Always use circular, upward motions with a gentle touch on your face. Don't help gravity by tugging down on your skin and remember that the skin on your face, especially around the eyes, is very delicate. You do not need heavy pressure to cleanse, and you don't need to use anything but your hands. Washcloths are optional.

- *Step Two: Tone your skin every time you wash your face and neck with a good toner or natural astringent.* It is one of the most forgotten yet important steps in your skin care regimen. When you tone, you are adjusting the pH of your skin back to normal which is critical to keep your face balanced and healthy. Toning will also remove any stubborn dirt left on your face and prepare your skin for moisturizing. For best results, gently use a cotton ball in upward motions.

- *Step Three: Using a natural crème, serum, or lotion, moisturize your face and neck every morning and night after you cleanse and tone.* Always moisturize your face and neck in upward motions. Step three is important for all skin types. Take note that this is the step that feeds your face.

Three Extra Pampering Steps:
- *Extra Step One: Exfoliate your skin no more than every three to five days.* Exfoliate your face and neck in circular upward gentle motions with very gentle products. Remember that you are simply exfoliating off dead skin which takes very little pressure, so abrasive loofahs or shell powder-based exfoliants are just not necessary. You would never take a scouring pad to your fine china so please don't do it to your far more precious face. I recommend only using natural exfoliants that use jojoba beads and avoiding other harsh products on your facial skin.

- *Extra Step Two: When you apply eye crèmes, always use your ring finger or pinky to apply products around the delicate area of your eyes.* Your pinky and ring finger are weak by nature and force you to apply gentle pressure. Eye crèmes are designed to super moisturize the finest skin on your face.

- *Extra Step Three: Mask on a weekly or bi-weekly basis to detoxify, renew, and tighten your pores.* Before you mask, it is important to cleanse and tone. Be sure to leave the mask on your face and neck for five to twenty minutes depending on the mask type. Gently and thoroughly remove the mask with warm water. And after you mask always tone and moisturize your face and neck.

Aromatherapy Tip: The best "food" to feed your skin from the outside contains essential oils, antioxidants, and natural ingredients. Products containing oils like carrot, jojoba, avocado and rosehip contain naturally occurring nutritious food for your skin. Avoid applying chemicals to your skin that will inhibit your skin's natural functions and impede your immune system. Aging is a natural process, but a healthy body and immune system will allow you and your clients to age gracefully.

Tell your clients: Every day our skin is attacked by the sun, smoke, pollution, toxic air, and the march of time. Proper care and feeding of your skin will give your appearance a fighting chance. The skin care products that you use should be designed to feed your skin vitamins, minerals and nutrients. If you can't decide between a natural or chemical filled product, then imagine the difference between eating fresh fruit and eating a Twinkie. Your skin hungers for the fresh fruit options in skin care; life will always be full of Twinkies.

Note: You will find this book sprinkled with recipes, however you may notice that there are no recipes provided that contain high water activity such as lotions, crèmes, serums and so forth. Let me explain: You see, it has everything to do with preservation of products for the prevention of bacteria. Bacteria are a fact of life for cosmetics, foods, and pretty much any organism that contains even a trace amount of water.

David Steinberg has trademarked the perfect saying when it comes to bacteria, "Remember, Preservatives are Safer than Bacteria™" Believe it or not, every cosmetic that doesn't use a broad spectrum preservative and contains water has a three-day shelf life, even if it is a refrigerated and/or contains essential oils. I know this because I have run extensive tests on products on the market with those claims and tested every form of "natural preservation" out there. If a cosmetic has even a trace amount of water it must be preserved by some method. There is no such thing as a SAFE preservative-free cosmetic.

Cosmetic products containing water must be preserved for two main reasons: insurance companies would never cover unpreserved products and the FDA requires that products are not "injurious to user under conditions of customary use because it contains, or its container is composed of, a potentially harmful substance" and they may not "contain filth." Products are not required to be sterile but they may not be contaminated with a pathogen. All other counts must remain low and remain that way under foreseeable consumer use. The products must be tested for adequacy of preservation during the development of the product and each batch tested before released for sale. While you might have a testing facility in your business, the majority of my readers will not.

Bacteria are very dangerous things; it's illegal in your products, and it's a business killer if it crops up in your cosmetics. Unpreserved or improperly preserved cosmetics are a breeding ground for fungi, yeast, and molds because they prefer acid conditions (pH 5.5-6) at room temperature to multiply.

Determining the water activity of your product is the shortcut to deciding if you need a preservative or not. If you product is bone dry with no water then it does not need a preservative. Bacteria require water to grow and the majority of cosmetics contain high enough water levels to easily grow bacteria. Simply put, bacteria require water to support life, and if you have enough water it will thrive. That is why you will find that recipes I share with you do not contain water or do not require preservation.

Skin Therapy Never Involves Skin Abuse

I am an over-protective mother and that trait sometimes comes out even when I am dealing with full-grown adults. When it comes to other people's skin, I am like a mother bear protecting her young. I can't help it. "Skin Abuse" is a hot topic for me. I simply cannot sit by quietly and allow continued mistreatment of the skin.

As a Cosmetic Formulator I have been asked on many occasions to formulate alpha hydroxy acids peels that use high concentrations of glycolic acid. Over and over again I have turned down that kind of business. For many years I have had the firm belief that chemical peels and many spa facial peels are sometimes too harsh. My stance has always been that consistent and gentle use of alpha hydroxy acids and manual exfoliation from jojoba beads during regular facials at home is just as effective and far less painful.

A seven-week study by the University of Pennsylvania has proved my point. The study found that an at-home facial peel containing glycolic acid at 10% was as effective as the professional peels with 20-35% glycolic acid and was less irritating. Glycolic peels with higher concentrations leave the face red, raw and exposed. The responsible spa facial, in my opinion, does not send the client home in pain.

Why peel? Alpha hydroxy acids (AHA) use glycolic, malic, citric, lactic, and/or tartaric acids to improve the texture of the skin by removing the damaged outer layers. AHA treatments are used by people that want to improve the appearance of their skin, including acne, wrinkles and uneven skin pigmentation. Medical cosmetic treatments and spa treatments vary in strength and ingredients; AHAs are commonly used but at much higher concentrations than in consumer products. AHA peels at high concentrations cause stinging, redness, irritation and crusting.

Another form of peel uses trichloroacetic acid (TCA) at varying concentrations, but is commonly used for medium-depth peeling. TCA peels are used to smooth out fine surface wrinkles, remove superficial blemishes and correct pigment problems. TCA peels require several months for your new layers of skin to heal and cause sun sensitivity for months.

Phenol peels are the strongest chemical solution used for deep peels. Phenol treatments are used to correct blotches and smooth out coarse wrinkles. A phenol peel is extremely strong and will cause you to have to protect your skin from the sun forever. It forever changes the pigment of your skin and you will not be able to tan or correct any resulting uneven pigment. Phenol peels take several months to heal from.

TCA and phenol peels may cause tingling or throbbing for several days. A crust or scab will form and significant swelling may occur. But why go through all of this pain? Using effective, but gentle treatments in the facial room will keep your clients coming back for more, rather than running home to hide their red and raw face. Also, creating AHA treatment products that your clients can use in the comfort of their own home spa is a safe and effective way to help your client resurface their skin. The end result is a healthy glow and fresh skin.

Aromatherapy Tip: If your client comes to you with a red, raw and hurting face from a chemical peel' there are essential oils that can help soothe their skin. Simply add Roman and blue chamomile, lavender, and just a touch of helichrysum to a heavy moisturizer or ointment for application one to two times per day. I've included a do-it-yourself soothing toner that would be perfect for someone needing extra care after a chemical burn, sunburn, or irritated skin.

Soothing Toner Recipe
Blend Separately
0.4 ounces Lavender Essential Oil
0.05 ounces Chamomile, Roman Essential Oil
0.05 ounces Chamomile, blue Essential Oil
0.05 ounces Helichrysum Essential Oil
0.5 ounces Polysorbate 20
Add to
6.4 ounces Hyaluronic Acid
64 ounces Aloe Vera Juice

Directions: Blend the essential oils and polysorbate 20 together separately. The polysorbate will emulsify the essential oils into the water portion of this recipe, which will protect the skin from accidental neat (directly on the skin) application of free-floating essential oils. Then add the essential oil mixture to the hyaluronic acid and aloe vera juice.

Aromatherapy for Women
The menstrual cycle of a woman is comparable to a giant roller coaster. It brings us up and down, upside down and around again. Our hormones send us on a variety of loops that are sometimes scary and other times exciting and creative.

The female human body is so amazing that it even will tell you what it needs at any given time in your cycle by being unusually attracted to certain scents and unexplainably repulsed by others. For instance, I have never met a pregnant woman who did not find ylang ylang essential oil offensive during her early pregnancy. The hormone properties of ylang ylang are too powerful for early pregnancy and your body automatically protects itself. Most women have a heightened sense of smell during their entire pregnancy which automatically protects the growing child inside.

Aromatherapy can deeply affect a variety of imbalances and hormonal swings in the female body via the aroma of the essential oil. This is because a woman's body is naturally in tune with the properties of essential oils which are the living essence of a plant. Plants that release a scent for the purpose of attraction have an almost feminine nature. Essential oils that influence the female reproductive system contain chemical compounds, known as plant hormones, which resemble estrogen. Plant hormones help balance the female body by creating physical changes that create stability in our menstrual cycles, act as aphrodisiacs, increase breast milk flow, and even strengthen contractions during labor.

For more than 13 years now, I have worked with a blend of essential oils I call the Women's Balance essential oil blend - using clary sage (*Salvia sclarea*), jasmine, rose, ylang ylang, neroli, geranium and lavender. I have witnessed amazing transformations in women's lives with this blend. Women of all ages have found balance in the same blend of essential oils because their body uses what properties it needs and discards the rest. I have spoken with women who have struggled with fertility because of irregular cycles and, after using this blend, they have become regulated and even become pregnant. Due to this blend, women suffering from severe mood swings have balanced, and menopausal women have found great relief from their symptoms.

I am not a medical doctor, but I have studied essential oils extensively through many experts, through their writings, research, and one-on-one. My experiences working with oils show a correlation between particular ailments and the essential oils that help improve them. Based on my experiences, here's a list of some major issues and the essential oils that address them:

- **Aphrodisiacs:** anise, cedarwood (*Cedrus deodora*), cinnamon, jasmine, lemon, neroli, patchouli, rose, rosewood, sandalwood, ylang ylang

- **PMS:** bergamot, chamomile, cedarwood (*Cedrus deodora*), citronella, cypress, geranium, clary sage (*Salvia sclarea*), fennel, grapefruit, lavender, lemon, jasmine, juniper, neroli, orange, pine, ravensara, rose, sandalwood.

- **Hormone Havoc:** bergamot, chamomile, clary sage (*Salvia sclarea*), fennel, geranium, lavender, ravensara, sandalwood, spearmint, ylang ylang

- **Endometriosis:** clary sage (*Salvia sclarea*), cypress, eucalyptus, geranium, ravensara

- **Menopause:** basil, bergamot, cypress, chamomile, clary sage (Salvia sclarea), fennel, geranium, jasmine, lavender, orange, sandalwood, ravensara, rose

- **Hot Flashes:** clary sage (*Salvia sclarea*), chamomile, fennel, geranium, lavender, peppermint

- **Labor and Delivery:** clary sage (*Salvia sclarea*), geranium, lavender, jasmine, neroli, rose, ylang ylang

- **Postpartum:** bergamot, clary sage (*Salvia sclarea*), fennel, geranium, grapefruit, lavender, patchouli, ravensara, rose

Speaking of women's issues, did you know that eating chocolate is believed to be an unconscious attempt to keep hormone levels more steady? During PMS, most women crave chocolate. The long-standing debate is whether the cravings answer the body's physical or psychological call for chocolate. Some believe that is all in our minds and we are feeding a guilty pleasure at our weakest moment. Others believe that our bodies crave some of the more than 400 chemicals found in chocolate, many of which affect mood.

The chemicals in dark chocolate affect the body's mood-affecting chemical levels, including serotonin, endorphins, theobromine, and phenylethylamine. Serotonin is a chemical messenger in the brain that affects emotions, behavior, and thought. Endorphins are chemicals in the brain that are responsible for positive moods. Theobromine is a stimulant found in cocoa which gives chocolate its mood-elevating effects. Phenylethylamine is a naturally occurring neuroamine which has been shown to relieve depression, increase attention, and promote energy. Your body releases phenylethylamine in response to romance.

So next time you feel the urge to eat some dark chocolate while soaking your worries away in an aroma-therapeutic bath, you can know that you are only listening to your body, and blame me for the advice. Pair this soak recipe with a very fine dark chocolate and let the balancing begin.

Luxurious Goat Milk Bath Soak Recipe
Dry Ingredients
0.5 lbs. Sodium Bicarbonate
0.4 lbs. Sea Salt
0.1 lbs. Goat Milk
1 Tbsp. MSM
Wet Ingredient
¼ tsp. Women's Balance Essential Oil Blend or your own blend

Directions: Add all dry ingredients to a food processor first, then add your essential oils. Turn on your food processor for under one minute to thoroughly blend the essential oils into your soak.

Aromatherapy for Men

When formulating products for men, there are completely different aromas to consider than what you would choose for other product lines. Aromatherapy for men should be based around aromas that both appeal to them and satisfy the therapeutic needs of their skin care.

In general, men's products should not only use different scents, but they should also be scented half as much as typical products. More than anything else, men tend to dislike a product based on scent. Men tend to not be attracted to floral aromas for their own use, but the therapeutic value of many floral essential oils can be captured by blending them with spice or woody essential oils, so that the aromas of the floral oils are covered up by the spicy and woody essential oils.

In my many informal studies, which I carried out as a cosmetic formulator to develop products for men, I found that when given a variety of aromas to choose from, men tended to pick peppermint essential oil above all other single notes and essential oil blends. Peppermint essential oil has a universally popular aroma. Peppermint oil is good for circulation, stimulation of the heart rate and brain waves, and it can be used as an analgesic, decongestant, aphrodisiac, and a coolant.

Aromatherapy Tip: Peppermint combined with tea tree essential oil has an appealing aroma, and the synergy between the two oils make a perfect blend for men's care products. Other popular aromas chosen by men include citrus, woody and spice essential oils.

No Bump, No Razor Burn Shaving Soap Crème Recipe
2 tsp. of Tartaric Acid
3 tsp. of Malic Acid
3 tsp. of Glycolic Acid

¼ of a cup of Kosher Vegetable Glycerin
1/3 cup of Certified Organic Multiple Fruit Blend Tincture (Essential Wholesale)
2 cups Castile Soap
½ of a gallon Essential Wholesale Basic Concentrate Crème
15 drops Tea Tree Essential Oil
30 drops Lavender Essential Oil
3 Tablespoons Peppermint 3rd Distilled

Directions: Add tartaric, malic, glycolic acids, kosher vegetable glycerin, multifruit tincture and liquid castile soap together and stir to dissolve. Next, add Essential Wholesale Basic Concentrate Crème, tea tree, lavender and peppermint essential oil. Now you are ready to mix with an immersion blender.

Ingredient Information: Tartaric, malic and glycolic acids are alpha hydroxy acids which are used to create a "no bump" product. I have added each of these ingredients to the glossary for further information on them.

Aromatherapy for Infants and Children
When creating aromatherapy products for infants and children it is best to determine the age of your market in order to choose the safest essential oils and the correct percentage in your product. This simple chart gives a good rule of thumb to guide you.

Age	%	Safe Essential Oils
Newborn	up to 0.2%	Chamomile Roman, Chamomile German, Lavender, Mandarin, Dill
2-6 Months	up to 0.2%	Same as above, Neroli, Tea Tree, Laurel Leaf, Geranium, Rose Otto
7 Months – 1 Year	up to 0.4%	Same as above, Palmarosa, Petitgrain, Tangerine, Cardamom
2- 5 Years	up to 1%	Same as above, Ginger, Lemon, Grapefruit, Ravensara, Helichrysum
6-8 Years	up to 1.25%	Same as above, Bergamot, Eucalyptus, Myrrh, Orange
9-11 Years	up to 2%	Same as above, Frankincense, Cypress, Ylang Ylang

Nurseries, daycares, and schools are a breeding ground for a whole assortment of "sickies and ickies." We instruct them to wash their hands with soap and water every chance they get at school. In addition, we advise them to use the paper towel they used to dry their hands to grip the handle of the door as they exit the bathroom. After all, freshly cleaned hands can quickly become covered in new germs on the way out of the bathroom. Door handles and other commonly touched areas are covered in germs.

Every school year I add another essential oil to my arsenal of therapies for dealing with the "sickies and ickies" that kids pick up at school. My kids are totally healthy all summer long, but once they hit the classroom it seems the germs accumulate overnight. With aromatherapy, we encounter less and less sick days as the years go on. There are several lines of defense a mother can take, but it takes a combination of being proactive and reactive to successfully get through a school year.

Avoiding illness is critical for my children because they suffer from asthma. Any respiratory ailment sends their asthma into overdrive. Treating the air in our car and home for their asthma relief has become commonplace in our household. I developed an essential oil blend called Breathe Green for Essential Wholesale, using sweet basil, rosemary, laurel leaf, peppermint, ginger, eucalyptus, ravensara, and lemon to respond to their immune and respiratory needs.

A few days after I first blended Breathe Green, I successfully averted an emergency room trip. I was in my car and dispersed Breathe Green by pouring some on a tissue that I wedged into the air conditioning vent of my car. That was my first indicator that I was onto something with the Breathe Green blend. Last school year we used it in combination with asthma medications to successfully avoid respiratory infections, urgent care and emergency trips which had been the norm in the past.

What about another common school "icky" that every parent dreads? Back to school haircuts are the first indicator that it's time to add tea tree essential oil to the kids' shampoo for lice prevention. My family has witnessed a lot of head lice outbreaks, but we have avoided being directly affected by adding just 2-5 drops of tea tree essential oil per ounce of shampoo and conditioner. Prevention is the best medicine for lice. In addition, whenever there is an outbreak at school I always make sure to apply tea tree through their hair. I simply put a few drops of tea tree essential oil onto my finger tips and run my hands through their hair from root to tip.

I have talked many mothers through a safe and effective lice treatment when their children have been infected with head lice, and you can, too. A quick and simple solution is to mix one cup of mayonnaise with one teaspoon of tea tree essential oil. Apply the mayonnaise to the hair from the roots to the tips and cover with a plastic cap or plastic wrap. Leave it on for 20 to 60 minutes and rinse. One section at a time, carefully and thoroughly comb through the hair while it is wet. Wipe off any lice or nits as they are found. Be systematic and pay special attention to the scalp, behind the ears, and the nape of the neck.

Don't forget to treat bedding, clothing, and any other areas where lice may be hiding with tea tree essential oil as well. Simply add two to five drops of tea tree essential oil for every one ounce of laundry soap and make a tea tree linen spray to address any areas that can't be thrown in the laundry. If you don't like the scent of tea tree, try adding some lavender to it as well.

Aromatherapy Tip: Not only can essential oils prevent and treat the classroom disruption caused by lice, aromatherapy can calm a disruptive child. I have been known to bring a bottle of lotion to my child's classroom with our "taming the wild child blend" which contains Roman and blue chamomile, lavender, tangerine, and mandarin. The lotion becomes a big treat for the kids and an even bigger relief to the teacher. There are many simple aromatherapy solutions you can share with your child's classroom in order to improve the quality of learning for the entire class. I have varied my class lotion or room spray from year to year, depending on the unique needs that every classroom has and it has made all the difference.

A simple method of helping moms and kids struggling with separation anxiety is to hand them a tissue with subtle scents of lavender transferred from your fingers. On the first day of school I have been known carry a bottle of lavender with me. Everyone knows me as the aromatherapy lady, so no one questions my lavender scented hand coming to touch the head of their teary, anxiety-ridden child. It works every time. Not only does the lavender calm the child, but the interruption of the crisis helps to dissipate anxiety. Lavender is completely safe to use in children's products, no matter what you have read on the internet. Robert Tisserand thoroughly debunked the myth in his article Tea Tree and Lavender Not Linked To Gynecomastia.

This massage oil and the massage technique below saved me a lot of headache and stress. Whenever I had a cranky baby I mixed up a little mommy and me time in a bottle.

Baby Massage Oil Recipe
1 ounce Jojoba or Meadowfoam Oil
1 drop Lavender Essential Oil
1 drop Roman Chamomile Essential Oil
1 drop Blue Chamomile Essential Oil

Massage Oil Directions: Add all ingredients into a glass or PET bottle and shake.

Baby Massage Instructions

- *Pick the right time*: About 30 minutes after eating when possible.
- *Warm up the room*: No one can be relaxed while cold -- especially your baby.
- *Make baby comfy*: Put your baby across your lap or on a soft surface.
- *Massage*: Use a soft, gentle touch from head to toes - work from the head, to the face, shoulders, arms, chest, stomach, and to the legs and feet. Your touch should be as gentle as you would use to rub your own eyelids without discomfort.
- *Eye Contact*: Communicate to your baby through your loving gaze directly into their eyes.

Aromatherapy Emergency Kit

No home is complete without at least two essential oils in your medicine cabinet. Lavender and tea tree essential oils are the most popular and most common essential oils on the market. These two essential oils will be the antidote for most everything you will need. They are also the only two essential oils that can be used occasionally neat (straight on the skin) in most cases. All other essential oils must be diluted into carrier oil, lotion or other product for usage. I said, "used occasionally neat" because recently, using lavender and tea tree neat has become less popular due to the concern of causing sensitization of the skin. This is a valid concern and should not be overlooked, but there are emergencies in which neat is best.

For instance, late one night, my two young daughters decided to play with the light bulb in their lamp. We were alerted by shrieks of terror. My four year-old had put her wet hand onto the light bulb. Her palm had already formed a blister and she was hysterical. I applied a small amount of lavender to my hand and rubbed it into her hair to calm her. I then poured straight lavender essential oil onto her burn and put a sock over her hand. She promptly fell deeply asleep. In the morning, she took the sock off her hand and was surprised to find she had no pain and no blister. Her wounds had healed overnight. She displayed her hand to me with disbelief and exclaimed, "Look Mommy! Your medicine worked!"

When my kids ask for medicine for their "owies," they are referring to lavender essential oil. They are true believers by way of their life experiences with it.

Aromatherapy Tip: Next time you have a migraine from your job, or your child is not in the mood to "go nighty-night," turn to earth's gift of lavender essential oil, remembering of course, that fragrance oils are not a substitute for essential oils. If you are not getting your beauty sleep, put a small amount of lavender essential oil onto a cotton ball and put it into your pillowcase. Or if your face suddenly breaks out with one big red pimple on the tip of your nose, apply some tea tree essential oil to the affected area.

Aromatherapy for All Seasons

Colder seasons cause dry skin that can become chapped and cracked. The cool weather of fall and winter can be rough on skin. Fall and winter climates force the skin to deal with a lot of harsh environments: strong winds, cold air, indoor heaters, rain, snow, sleet, and an overall lack of a good healthy dose of sunlight.

Cold-Weather Cleansing: Put away foaming and soap cleansers and stock up on crème cleansers. Cleansing crèmes, lotions and milks are very effective cleansers and they do not contain the typical surfactant or detergent ingredients that most cleansing gels contain; these can be too harsh on the skin during the cold months.

Wintertime Toning: Put away your astringents and switch to a toner for fall and winter. The skin needs to be soothed and balanced and not dried out further by an astringent.

Mid-Winter Moisturizing: Choose heavier crèmes in the winter than you would in the summer months. Feel free to use your heavy eye crème around your lips and entire face. If your skin is itching it is because the dry air is causing the moisture in the top layer of your skin to evaporate quickly. You will need to slather those areas with extra moisture until you feel relief. Never be afraid of using pure oils on your skin in the cold months. A bottle of jojoba oil or olive oil is a great thing to have on hand all fall and winter.

Hands and Body: During the cold and flu season, hands should be washed liberally, but be certain to apply a heavy hand crème every time. Shea butter, balms, butters and whipped butters are great body moisturizers in the fall and winter.

Extra Exfoliation: Central heating plays havoc on the sebum our skin normally produces, which makes our skin lose the water that should be retained in the lower dermis. During the winter months there are thousands of dry skin cells ready to be sloughed off the surface, and they become clumped together with oil, which forms what appear to be flakes. Exfoliate the body with sugar or salt scrubs that are full of rich oils or butters. Exfoliate your facial skin with crème-based exfoliates that contain jojoba beads. Exfoliate twice per week to remove dead skin cells.

In-Home Hydrotherapy: One spa treatment can be done in most homes with a simple hot, steamy shower on a daily basis. However, just at the end, switch the water to cold for about fifteen seconds. Repeat the process for two minutes. This hydrotherapy technique will revitalize skin by stimulating the flow of blood through the skin. During cold and flu season, add one to five drops of eucalyptus essential oil or Breathe Green essential oil blend to the corner of the shower and let the steam create a wonderful aromatherapy treatment.

There are dozens of recipes out there teaching how to make traditional body scrubs with oils, salts and sugars. Here is one that's just a little bit outside the box for you.

Solid Shea Butter Sugar Scrub Recipe
6 ounces Melt and Pour Soap Base
4 ounces Shea Butter
11.5 ounces Turbinado Raw Sugar
0.2 ounces Peppermint Essential Oil Blend

Directions: Heat up your Melt and Pour Soap Base (you can use any brand on the market or any of the soap base recipes from my book *How to Make Melt and Pour Soap Base from Scratch*.) Add shea butter and allow it to melt into the hot soap and next, stir in peppermint essential oil. Your product will be poured into soap molds, so once you are ready to pour add turbinado raw sugar to your melted soap, stir and pour quickly into soap molds. Allow your product to cool for 2-4 hours before un-molding.

:: Chapter 6 ::
The Business of Aromatherapy

Aromatherapy can seem like a daunting subject when you are first introduced to it, and the therapeutic value can get lost in the thick textbooks. However, spa treatments have been around since the Roman Empire which was known for bath treatments called *Sanus per aquam*, meaning: health through water. The Romans set up Kur towns around curative waters all over the German countryside. In Germany, holistic medicine includes regular trips to Spa Kur (Cure). Today's international spa holistic body treatments come from the centuries-old German traditional Kur System. The German Kur is based on the use of natural therapies used in spa treatments.

In Germany, a doctor will send their client to a spa village with the right climate, altitude, and treatments to benefit the overall condition of their patient. In America we are lucky to convince our fast-paced culture to slow down for the day. Destination spas can include the climate, altitude, and treatments as part of the curative value of their location.

Holistic wellness can be achieved through a balanced life which includes taking care of oneself physically, mentally, spiritually and emotionally. A holistic approach to wellness includes spa treatments at home or in addition to regular visits to the spa for body therapy. Body therapy treatments address the physical and emotional needs of your client. In essence, you become more than your clients' esthetician or massage therapist; you become their holistic body therapist and address the needs of their mind, body, and soul.

Creating Luxurious Spa Treatments

As your clients' holistic body therapist, you have the opportunity to revive your client's immune system, satisfy their need for human touch and bring deep relaxation to their potentially chaotic world. Holistic body treatments include the use of facials, massage, hydrotherapy, body wraps, hot packs, aromatherapy, herbal therapy, body scrubs, sauna, steam room, thalassotherapy, and baths in order to revitalize, detoxify, and boost the immune system all while relaxing the client.

While some treatments like massage and wrap are best reserved for the spa, many spa-type activities can be done right at home. Not all of your clients will be able to afford regular trips to the spa, but nearly everyone is interested in products they can use at home to pamper and restore their mind and body.

Just remember that your client is in your hands to achieve a personal metamorphosis. Whether your client is spending one hour or an entire day with you, their time is precious. It is your responsibility to do your homework and provide the safest and most effective treatments to every client that walks through your doors.

Choosing Spa Products

First and foremost, the products used for treatment must be addressed. During body treatments, the pores and respiratory system are wide open and absorbing the products used during the treatment. It is vital that, as your clients' advocate and care taker, you go the extra mile to ensure all of the products you use for treatment are good for your client. Not all spa products are of the same quality. Don't fall for the marketing fluff, read your ingredient lists, do your research, and get outside advice on the products you are using.

Once you have found the right product, determining the features for your facility is the next step. Steam rooms, saunas and spa hot tubs are all bonus features of your spa that can make your spa stand out among your competitors. Encourage your clients to use the added features of your spa before their treatment to enhance the aromatherapy benefits of their stay. Warm skin allows for faster absorption of essential oils and opens and prepares the respiratory system for their healing properties. Encourage your clients to come a little early to take advantage of those extra tranquil moments so that when they reach your table they are already on the journey of relaxation.

Spa Treatments

Cellulite treatments are a fabulous example of programs that will cause your client to purchase and use package deals. The use of herbal reduction and/or detox wraps, along with essential oils combined with massage oil in a take-home kit, will offer great results and loyal customers. Choosing the right treatments that will sell your services and your product lines are vital to the financial health of your spa. You want your client to repeatedly come back and you want them to provide the best advertising of all: word of mouth.

Body Polish

A body polish increases the absorption of essential oils via the combination of vigorous massage and exfoliation of the skin. Essential oils can be added to oil or butter-based scrubs at three percent. Simply add 15 drops of a combination of the detoxifying essential oils to one ounce of scrub.

Subtle Aromatherapy

The use of hot aromatherapy towel packs and cold distillate water towels during treatments offers a fabulous finishing touch to the spa experience for your client. A hot towel soaked in herbs and/or essential oils and then placed on the table just before your client lies down is a fabulous vehicle for subtle therapy. A hot towel with a few drops of eucalyptus, lavender, or geranium each, can bring a different subtle aromatherapy experience to any treatment. Eucalyptus would make your stuffy client more comfortable during the treatment by easing congestion; lavender would make an uptight or uncomfortable client relax easier, and geranium would have valuable hormonal properties that could bring your female client into balance during her stay with you.

The options are limitless with cold water packs applied to the face to cool a client after a hot treatment, bath or sauna. Cold teas offer soothing effects while having great antioxidant properties. Brewing a pot of chamomile, rooibos, or green tea and refrigerating it for the day will give a cool treat to your clients during a variety of treatments. Distillate waters are a wonderful option because they can be purchased in bulk and used over several months. There are a wide variety of distillate waters available on the market including: lavender, chamomile, witch hazel, cucumber, rose and orange blossom.

While distillates are aromatic in nature, their aroma is very subtle. Distillates are the perfect choice when a gentle aromatherapy treatment is called for. They have a very delicate and often short shelf life—less than a year for most of them.

Distillates are commonly sold under the terms distillate waters, hydrosols, hydrolates, hydrolats, plant waters and floral waters. Distillates contain all of the plant's material, including the water-soluble components and the essential oil molecules in solution. They are aromatic byproducts collected during the steam distillation of plant material in the extraction of essential oils.

All distillates, like all aromas, smell differently on different people. The chemistry of an individual has been known to make the aroma of orange blossom distillate smell like cat urine on some and like heaven on others.

Scrubs

Full body scrubs remove toxins, increase circulation, rehydrate the skin and release a natural radiance. There are so many ingredient options when it comes to body scrubs. Some of the typical exfoliating ingredients include coffee, walnut shell powder, jojoba beads, and various grades of salt and sugar. Additional ingredients that add to the detoxifying effect of scrubs are mustard, sea kelp, herbs, cayenne pepper, turmeric, and essential oils. There are a handful of companies making foaming scrubs with exfoliants. These are perfect for clients who are concerned about using oily products.

It is realistic and economical for a spa to mix their own special scrubs or buy an unscented natural bulk scrub base to which they add herbs, essential oils and additives for each treatment. This flexibility allows for customized treatments and the also the ability to treat customers with allergies and sensitivities. At my last two spa experiences, both at different locations, I had to change my treatments because they did not have unscented or pure essential oil based body scrubs. Surprisingly, neither large facility had the ability to customize their scrubs to accommodate my allergy to fragrance oils. It is no longer an option to not have fragrance-free options. Many potential consumers are staying away from spas because they can't count on a fragrance oil-free treatment.

A great example of a customized body scrub treatment could be accomplished with a natural bulk butter body scrub base or a bulk salt scrub base with a choice of three different additive packages. One variation could be an immune boosting scrub in which the spa adds mustard powder and laurel leaf essential oil to the base for the treatment. A second option could be a detox scrub in which the spa adds sea kelp and the essential oils of cedarwood (*Cedrus deodora*) and grapefruit. The third option with the same base could be a cellulite scrub in which the spa adds ground coffee beans, cayenne pepper and the essential oils of rosemary, fennel, geranium, juniper, lavender, and bergamot. This would allow three separate treatments using one base with a few bulk ingredients to your back bar.

Wraps

Body wrapping is best done in a true spa setting. Wrapping is a therapeutic body treatment using detoxifying natural ingredients to tighten, tone, and stimulate the body to rid itself of toxins and excess fat. It is also an excellent addition to any weight loss and exercise program. Selecting an herbal reduction detox wrap that uses herbs, minerals, clay, and even coffee to cause lipids to be broken down and released into the lymphatic system will give your clients verifiable results. Since the skin is the largest eliminative organ of our body, a wrap, along with directions to drink a lot of water, can create significant results.

Wraps create a "sealing in" effect that decreases the essential oil's likelihood of becoming volatile and dispersing into the air. This sealed-in warmed area can increase the rate of absorption of the essential oil. Most wraps are created with a cloth material that is soaked in a mixture of water and essential oil or a clay masque combined with essential oils that are then painted onto the body. These then can be applied to the affected area and covered with plastic or Mylar wrap.

The lymphatic system needs to keep moving for optimum health. A body wrap causes the system to kick into gear and release the garbage stored in the body's cells, moving it into the lymphatic stream and expelling it through normal elimination processes by the body. A body wrap made with clays, herbs, minerals and salts that draw toxins out of the body is the optimal choice. As the toxins are drawn out, the soft tissue is compressed and compacted as the skin regains elasticity by being detoxified. This leaves a smoother and firmer muscle base over which the soft tissue lies.

Body wraps are most effective when they are done in a series of two to six wraps at least five days apart from each other. An exercise and healthy eating program will aid in maintaining weight loss. A healthy regimen will promote thorough cleansing, detoxifying, and toning. An herbal body wrap program as a series or in combination with aromatherapy based massage treatments will provide the best results for the client both in appearance and health.

Because of the warming nature of a wrap, essential oils should be added to wrap material at 1% unless the wrap immediately follows a massage that has left a protective oily layer on the skin. To add detoxification to a procedure, simply add five drops of any of the detoxifying essential oils to one ounce of clay or wrap material.

Massage
In Robert Tisserand's book, *Aromatherapy*, he relates a case study of a twenty-nine year old client with heavy cellulite on her thighs, hips, and buttocks. She was treated with massage and the essential oils of rosemary, fennel, geranium, juniper, lavender, bergamot, and chamomile. During a three-week period, the client came in twice per week for aromatherapy-based massage of her problem areas. After three weeks she had only a small patch of cellulite left, which was cured by changing her sitting position at the piano to allow adequate circulation.

Massage with essential oils is also best in a professional spa setting because the rate of absorption of essential oils is increased with massage. Blood flow is increased and the temperature of the skin is raised, allowing for faster intake of essential oils into the blood stream. This was proven by Jäger in 1992 when a blood sample taken five minutes after a massage application of essential oils found linalyl acetate and linalool in the blood stream.

Aromatherapy works best when using synergetic blends of two or more essentials oils. You can choose any two or more of any essential oil to add to fractionated coconut oil. The percentage of essential oil used can range from one to 3% depending on the health of your client. For every one ounce of carrier oil add five drops of essential oil to create a product with 1% essential oils.

Creating detoxifying massage oil is very simple. Fractionated coconut, meadowfoam and jojoba oil are the best oils for massage because they will not leave your sheets smelling musty or rancid. Fractionated coconut has a fabulous slip and good staying power to last for a full body massage. Jojoba oil has the same chemical make-up as the skin's sebum which makes it the perfect oil for all skin types. Jojoba oil is a must have for any facial massage. Fractionated coconut oil is the most affordable option of the three.

For a detoxification treatment, the massage therapist should focus on the areas of the skin most permeable to essential oils. The palms of the hands, soles of the feet, forehead, scalp, behind the ears, inside the wrists and armpits are more permeable than the legs, buttocks, trunk and abdomen. Subcutaneous fat has a poor blood supply which means that essential oils applied to these areas may take longer to be absorbed. Also, remember that mature or dehydrated skin slows the absorption of essential oil. Increased water consumption for up to 26 hours after the detoxification treatment is always recommended.

Essential Oils Commonly Used in Detoxification Treatments

Aromatherapy is an effective spa experience for detoxification of the body.

- Basil is a restorative essential oil, general stimulant, anti-inflammatory, and skin tonic.
- Cedarwood (*Cedrus deodora*) is cleansing, tonic, dries oily or blemished skin, and topically works as a natural astringent which softens skin.
- Cypress increases circulation, and reduces fluid retention and cellulite. It also is an astringent and reduces excess sweating and overly oily complexions.
- Grapefruit reduces fluid retention, tones congested skin, and detoxifies. It is an astringent for oily congested skin, reduces cellulite, increases circulation, and stimulates lymphatic system detoxification.
- Juniper reduces fluid retention, is a diuretic, and has tonic effect. It also increases circulation and reduces fluid retention.
- Lemon balances sebum and is a general tonic and detoxifier. Plus, lemon aids epidermal circulation.
- Orange is a diuretic and general body tonic that reduces water retention while increasing circulation, cell hydration, and general detoxification.
- Rosemary is good for circulation. It reduces cellulite and is a general tonic.

Almost all massage treatments end with moisturizing with either a massage oil or body lotion. At the end of a treatment the body will readily absorb whatever you apply. It is vital that you apply a lotion that isn't full of chemicals. It would be like going for a great run and then smoking a cigarette. It just doesn't make sense to pollute the body with unnecessary cosmetic chemicals after any holistic body treatment. Look for lotions that achieve their properties and body from natural oils and butters and avoid fillers like carbomer and triethanolamine, which are thickeners and fillers that have allowed the cosmetic formulator to use less active ingredients. They create thickness and body instead of allowing the texture of the formula to come from natural oils.

Thalassotherapy

Thalassotherapy is the medicinal use of seawater. It was developed in the seaside towns of Brittany, France in the 19th century. There are trace elements of magnesium, potassium, calcium sulfates and sodium found in seawater.

Treatments include:

- Soaks or scrubs
- Baths or showers in warm sea water
- Sea salts added to soaks
- Marine mud used in baths or wraps
- Algae or seaweed added in wraps
- The inhalation of steamed sea water

The main objective of thalassotherapy is to increase blood circulation by replenishing the mineral content of the body with the minerals from the sea. Vital minerals are depleted from our body due to stress, pollution, and poor diets. Good health, mental wellness, and healthy skin are dependent on the correct balance of sodium, potassium, and fluids in the body.

Different salts from various regions of the world have unique minerals available in them. The mineral content of the Dead Sea is significantly different than ocean water. Most salts from seas or oceans are about 97 to 99% sodium chloride. A study of the concentration of minerals in the Dead Sea salt found it to be 30.4% sodium chloride, 14.4% calcium chloride, 4.4% potassium chloride, and 50.8% magnesium chloride. Brittany Sea salt contains 95% sodium chloride with unique trace minerals. Hawaiian sea salt also has the mineral alaea from volcanic baked red clay added to enrich the salt with iron oxide. These salts, as well as Celtic salt, flake salt, grey salt, Italian salt, and sea salt are all good salts for any thalassotherapy treatment.

:: *Chapter 7* ::
Creating Aromatherapy Bath Products and Soap

Making Aromatherapy Bath Salts

The easiest bath products to make are bath salts and soaks. You can buy pre-mixed bath salts or blend your own using a variety of salts on the market. Once you pick your salt or salts, it is just a matter of determining if your salts can be completely dry or should have a light coating of carrier oil. The key to making a good bath salt is using the skin safety measure of adding an equal measure of carrier oil as essential oil whenever you go over 2% essential oil in your recipe. For 2% and below, you can create an oil-free bath salt safely. For 2.1% and above, it is best to coat the salt with carrier oil.

2% and Under
16 ounces Any Salt
.32 ounces Most Any Essential Oil

2.1 to 5%
16 ounces Any Salt
0.34 Up to 0.8 ounces Most Any Essential Oil
0.34 Up to 0.8 ounces Any Carrier Oil

There are many different salts available on the market, my favorites include:

Atlantic Fine Sea Salts
INCI: *Sodium Chloride*
Sea salts soften the water and can be used for a cleansing, abrasive exfoliate and help draw toxins from the body. People worldwide have used the healing power of salts baths for centuries. The minerals and trace elements deep clean and revitalize the body. Atlantic sea salt is produced using the ancient method of solar evaporation in a region that is free of pollution and has high evaporation rates.

Dead Sea Salts
INCI: *Sodium Chloride*
Dead Sea salt is salt dried from the Dead Sea. Dead Sea salts are available in fine and course grades, which give you a nice variety of visual choices for your bath salts. Dead Sea salts have a high mineral content that has been used for treating and preventing various diseases such as psoriasis, acne, and

rheumatism. Dead Sea salt is beneficial to the skin and the rest of the body, because the skin absorbs salt, vitamins, and other substances into the body.

People come from far and wide to bathe in hot springs, mineral baths, and the Dead Sea because of the unique mineral compositions of each place. In Israel, the Dead Sea attracts visitors because it is the lowest point on the earth and contains a high percentage of natural minerals. In many countries people with conditions labeled "incurable" have reduced their symptoms or completely resolved them after being treated with mineral hydrotherapy

Dendritic Salt
INCI: *Sodium Chloride*
Dendritic salt is a fine-grain salt which has been crystallized to provide more surface area and irregular surfaces. This is desirable in bath salts because the increased surface area helps retain fragrance, requires fewer pigments, and reduces clumping. This natural salt absorbs essential oils twice as efficiently as other salts used in bath mixes. It's specially formulated to prevent caking, add flow-ability, and keep the scent in your salts longer. I recommend using one cup of dendritic salt to every 20 cups of other salts used.

Epsom Salt
INCI: *Magnesium sulfate*
Epsom salt is a chemical compound containing magnesium, sulfur, and oxygen. Medical research indicates that magnesium may reduce inflammation and relieve pain, making it beneficial in the treatment of sore muscles, migraine headaches and fibromyalgia. Soaking in an Epsom Salt bath is one of the most effective means of making the magnesium that your body needs readily available. The best method for making an Epsom Salt soak is to add two cups of Epsom Salt to warm water in the bathtub and soak for 12 to 15 minutes. For a foot bath, add one cup of Epsom Salt to a tub of warm water and soak.

According to the Epsom Salt Council, the magnesium in Epsom salt helps ease stress, improves sleep and concentration, helps muscles and nerves function properly, reduces inflammation to relieve pain and muscle cramps, and improves oxygen use. And the sulfates in Epsom salts help flush toxins, improve absorption of nutrients, and help prevent or ease migraine headaches.

Himalayan Salts
INCI: *Sodium Chloride*
Himalayan salts contain 84 beneficial trace elements and have a unique crystal structure. Pink Himalayan Salt is mined from ancient sea beds inside the Himalayan Mountains. Himalayan salts are completely unrefined, raw, and remain in their natural form. Himalayan salts are pure and free of

contaminants and pollutants. The pink color of the salts comes from the high content of Iron. Himalayan salts are said to contain trace amounts of 84 minerals and elements including potassium, magnesium, calcium, iodine, zinc, and sodium.

These coarse-grain salts make excellent additions to bath salt blends and are used at 100% of the salt portion of a formula. For thousands of years, the salt has been used as a main ingredient in baths, body scrubs, drinks, and foods and has been revered for its unique crystalline beauty and its folk-medicinal properties.

Solar Salt
INCI: *Sodium Chloride*
Solar salt is an extra-coarse white crystalline form of sodium chloride that is produced by the solar evaporation of seawater from the Great Salt Lake. The salt crystals are refined by washing with clean saturated brine to remove surface impurities, then drained of excess moisture, dried and screened to size. The appearance of solar salts is a good enough reason to add them to your recipes to give texture to your product, but they also contain minerals that are unique to the extremely saline Great Salt Lake.

Making Aromatherapy Bath Soaks
Bath soaks often include salts with the addition of other ingredients to enhance the bathing experience. A warm bath can increase the rate of absorption of essential oils. In warm bath water, essential oils penetrate the skin 100 times faster than water does and 10,000 times faster than the ions of sodium and chloride from salt (Römmelt et al 1974, Schilchler 1985). Bathing also involves inhalation of essential oils as well as absorption through the skin.

You can buy ready-made soaks or create your own. To create a detoxifying aromatherapy bath, choose your favorite, unscented salt. A good salt for detoxifying is Dead Sea salt, but any salt will work. Essential oils can be added to the dry salt at 1% by adding five drops of essential oil to every one ounce of salt. If you would like to make a stronger soak you can add up to 15 drops of essential oil to every one ounce of salt, but you must also add 15 drops of a carrier oil to the salts to protect the skin while in the water. Bath soaks generally use 2% or below essential oils because the addition of a carrier oil just makes a soak look like a gloopy mess.

Allantoin
INCI: *Allantoin*
Allantoin is present naturally in comfrey plant and the urine of most mammals. It is a nature-identical, safe, non-toxic chemical compound that is used for its healing, soothing, and anti-irritating properties. It has the ability

to help heal wounds and sores, and it stimulates the growth of healthy tissue. Allantoin is a skin softener and an anti-irritant, which inhibits allergic type responses. In bath soaks it is traditionally used at 1% or less of a recipe.

Aloe Powder
INCI: *Aloe vera barbadensis miller*
Aloe powder is freeze-dried, cryo-dried, or spray-dried aloe powder with deionized water to a single strength equivalency (SSE). Once the aloe powder is reconstituted, the finished product requires preservatives in order to remain stable, which is why using aloe powder in a bath soak is so wonderful. It requires no preservation because the bath soak has a single-use application.

There are many different Aloe Powders available on the market today. I prefer 100 % pure aloe vera that is IASC Certified. The International Aloe Science Council is a third-party verification process that ensures purity of aloe products. The aloe that we use comes from freshly harvested leaves of the *Aloe vera barbadensis miller* variety of aloe. The inner gel (a.k.a. fillet) is carefully removed to minimize disruption of the aloin layer. The resulting gel is processed to remove the pulp and fiber. The gel is then pasteurized to maintain efficacy and concentrated using low temperature evaporation. The gel concentrate is then freeze-dried without the use of matrix, preservatives or any other additives. The finished concentrate allows us to follow an exact formula to reconstitute the aloe to a single strength equivalency (SSE) aloe juice. Because aloe powder is so concentrated, it can be easily used at less than 0.5% in any bath soak recipe.

Bentonite Clay
INCI: *Bentonite*
Bentonite clay is a combination of montmorillonite and volcanic ash. Montmorillonite is a soft phyllosilicate group of minerals found in the Midwestern United States and in Canada. It is highly absorbent clay that pulls oils and toxins from the skin. Bentonite Clay is the best clay to use in a soak, because it increases the rate of detoxification. To ensure that your customers don't detoxify too quickly, I recommend using only one pound or less of bentonite in a 20 to 30 minute soak. There are many who recommend higher concentrations of bentonite clay to bath water, but with the addition of aromatherapy this is not necessary.

To create a relaxing and detoxifying treatment with Bentonite clay soak, add lavender, juniper, cedarwood (*Cedrus deodora*) or cypress essential oils. For example: To 1 lb. bentonite clay add 30 drops lavender + 30 drops cedarwood (*Cedrus deodora*) + 10 drops cypress + 10 drops juniper essential oils and mix.

Bentonite clay is a wonderful example of how injecting lab animals with safe cosmetic ingredients can produce bad scientific data. Bentonite clay is commonly used in cosmetics and some people even consume it, but when it is injected into rats it is fatal for the rat. That data, in the hands of an organization with an agenda, could be used to incorrectly label bentonite clay as "dangerous." Misrepresentation of the safety of cosmetic ingredients has been done many times on perfectly safe cosmetic ingredients in order to promote an organization's cause.

Blue Green Algae
INCI: *Aphanizomenon flos aquae*
Blue green algae powder comes from the Klamath Falls in Oregon. It is the purest, most nutrient intact algae available in the world. It is a wild-harvested, organic-certified, single-celled organism which occurs in the remote area of the Oregon Cascade Mountains. It is highly bio-available and contains a full spectrum of minerals: chlorophyll, B vitamins, beta-carotene, pro vitamin A, lipids, active enzymes, essential amino acids, nucleic acids, DHA, and EPA fatty acids. Because blue green algae powder is so concentrated and dark in color, it can be easily used at less than 0.5% in any bath soak recipe.

Green Clay
INCI: *Montmorillonite*
Green clay is from a subcategory of clay minerals known as illite clay, which often occur intermixed with kaolinite clays. The green color of the clay comes from a combination of iron oxides and decomposed plant matter, mostly kelp seaweed and other algae. The mineral montmorillonite is a component of green clay, as well as other minerals including: dolomite, magnesium, calcium, potassium, manganese, phosphorus, zinc, aluminum, silicon, copper, selenium, and cobalt.

Green clay is regarded as a useful treatment for stimulating the skin and removing impurities from the epidermis. Clay soaks are great because they adsorb impurities from the skin cells, causing dead cells to slough off. Clay tones by stimulating the flow of blood to the epidermis. Green clay produces a slight cooling effect on the skin, constricts follicles, and deep cleanses the epidermis. It is very absorbent and cleansing to the skin sebum.

Green clay is rich in calcium, magnesium, potassium, and sodium. It energizes the connective tissue. It is antiseptic and healing. It gently stimulates and is effective in increasing the lymph flow and circulation, enabling oxygen, and speeding the elimination of wastes. Green clay has a high mineral content. Green Clay can be added to a bath soak from 0.5 to 50% of the recipe.

Goat Milk
INCI: *Goat's Milk Powder*
Goat milk leaves the skin with a hydrated appearance, feeling silky smooth.
Upon absorption, the milk smoothes, firms and softens the skin. Milk has a
long standing in beauty history. Goat milk, in particular, is a natural emollient,
containing vitamins A, B6, B12 and E. It contains three times more beta-casein
than cow's milk. Goat milk can be added to a bath soak from 0.5 to 50% of the
recipe.

Kaolin Clay
INCI: *Kaolin*
Kaolin clay originally came from the Kaoling Hill in Kiangsi Providence in
China. It is a white powder, insoluble in water, and absorbent. It absorbs
oils secreted from the skin and draws out impurities and toxins through
absorption. It is great to add to a soak after insect bites and stings. It is
composed of silica, iron, magnesium, calcium, sodium, zinc and other
minerals. Kaolin clay has an electromagnetic quality and attracts oils and
particles left on the skin. Kaolin clay can be added to a bath soak from 0.5 to
100% of the recipe.

MSM
INCI: *Methylsulfonylmethane*
Methylsulfonylmethane is a naturally occurring nutrient found in plants,
meats, dairy products, fruits, and vegetables. MSM is therefore found in the
normal human diet. It is an odorless, tasteless, white water-soluble, crystalline
solid in its purified form. Your bath soak recipes can incorporate up to 5%
MSM in it.

MSM supplies sulfur to the body which allows it to heal itself. It produces
muscle relaxation and reportedly a whole host of beneficial qualities. It has
been used with great success in eliminating chronic back pain, muscle pain,
and repairing cut, scraped, burned, and damaged skin. We've seen reports
of MSM eliminating wrinkles, brown spots, skin tumors, and spider veins.
MSM is being used for burn victims and for repairing scar tissue. Many people
report relief from allergies after using MSM. Other reports indicate that MSM
will remove parasites from the body and help the body to detoxify itself.

MSM is anti-inflammatory and antimicrobial. MSM feeds the formation of
collagen and elastin while preventing and reducing cross-linking between cells,
which is the primary cause of wrinkles and scar tissue. MSM is a natural sulfur
compound that contributes to healthy skin, hair and nails. MSM has been used
orally and topically to aid skin disorders. When used topically, in the form of a
cream or lotion, sulfur is helpful in treating skin disorders including acne, psoriasis,
eczema, dermatitis, dandruff, scabies, diaper rash and certain fungal infections.

Mustard Powder
INCI: *Sinapis alba*
Mustard has been used for many years by cultures around the world due to its reputation to increase circulation and open pores. It is thought to stimulate sweating, which, in turn, helps the body rid itself of toxins. Mustard soaks are a staple for me during cold and flu season. Because of the aroma of the mustard I recommend using up to 1% mustard powder in your soaks.

Pink Clay
INCI: *Kaolinite*
Pink clay is rich in trace elements and used to detoxify and cleanse the face and body. It is composed of silica, iron, magnesium, calcium, sodium, zinc and other minerals. Because pink clay can easily stain linens I recommend using just a hint of pink clay in your recipes.

Rhassoul Clay
INCI: *Moroccan Lava Clay*
Rhassoul clay's most impressive properties in skin improvement are its capacity of absorption due to its high level of ion exchange. In addition to its oil removal characteristics, rhassoul clay masks certainly have the ability to smooth and improve dry skin. Rhassoul clay has been used for over 12 centuries by populations from North Africa, South Europe, and the Middle East.

Clinical studies have been conducted by two different research laboratories in the United States (International Research Services, Inc.) to evaluate rhassoul clay masks on skin conditions. The study results showed that a single use of our rhassoul clay mask statistically: reduces dryness, reduces flakiness, improves skin clarity, improves skin elasticity and/or firmness, and improves skin texture.

Sea Kelp
INCI: *Ascophyllum nodosum*
Sea Kelp grows deep in the cold sub-tidal waters and it is responsibly harvested, dried and milled following organic standards. It is a yellowish-green colored powder with a fish-like, seaweed odor and flavor. The medicinal part is the stem-like part of the thallus, which is reminiscent of root, leaf or stem-like organs. It grows in the North Atlantic Sea. Sea kelp contains chlorophyll which helps detoxify the skin and body, essential fatty acids which improve skin elasticity, and carbohydrates which stimulate the skin's ability to heal, and vitamin A that normalize skin cells. Sea kelp contains proteins and amino acids which are the building blocks of cells and act as skin conditioners. Because of the strong odor of sea kelp I recommend using less than 1% in a bath soak recipe.

Sodium Bicarbonate
INCI: *Sodium Bicarbonate*
Common Name: Baking Soda
Sodium bicarbonate is better known as baking soda and is used in all kinds of bath soaks, bath bombs, and fizzies. It is a natural alkaline that neutralizes acids and washes away oils and dirt. Its natural pH balance leaves the skin soft, silky and smooth. Sodium bicarbonate often makes up the bulk of a bath soak and up to 95% of a recipe.

Making Aromatherapy Fizzies and Bath Bombs

The chemistry of bath bombs is simple. Do you remember the volcano project you (or your child) did in 4th grade? Well, bath bombs are pretty much the same chemistry concept, minus the smelly vinegar. The foundation of a bath bomb is the combination of sodium bicarbonate ($NaHCO_3$), which is a base, with citric acid ($C_5H_7O_5COOH$), which is a weak acid. Each of the ingredients is unreactive when they are dry and separate from each other. Once they are combined and come in contact with water (H_2O), they create a vigorous reaction. This reaction, of an acid and a base, generates carbon dioxide (CO_2) which builds up and releases as bubbles.

The wonderful byproduct of this whole chemical reaction is the release of therapeutic essential oils into your bath water and the air around you. Bath bombs can also incorporate other beneficial ingredients into the formula that are soothing, moisturizing, or bubbly.

I've had a few people ask why my Kitchen Chemistry videos or in other recipes that I share never include the traditional bath bomb recipes that are all over the internet. There are a million and one bath bomb recipes out there on the market. The reason is simple: I don't like to share recipes that may fail depending on humidity in the air, how much witch hazel you spritz or don't spritz, or whatever other reason traditional bath bomb recipes fail. I prefer no-fail recipes over the ones that have a high failure rate. Bath bombs should be simple, but they are greatly impacted by the moisture in the air and hence temperamental.

At Essential Wholesale we used to have bath bomb machines that were custom built for us. These machines allowed us to make 12 bath bombs per machine at a time. We had four machines in total. The machine applied the right amount of pressure every time. Our recipe weighed out exactly the right amount of witch hazel per batch. And the sealed room, in which we manufactured the bath bombs, had a dehumidifier in it. And still, sometimes batches of bath bombs failed! Failed products are a huge waste of time, supplies, and money. I don't want to waste your time or supplies. And I especially don't want to waste your money.

The other reason I don't share those recipes is that they have already been done. There are dozens, if not hundreds, of websites out there sharing the traditional "one part citric acid, two parts sodium bicarbonate with a spritz of witch hazel" recipes. I'm not bashing the traditional bath bomb or anyone who teaches how to make them. I'm simply sharing that when I evaluated the economics of making bath bombs, my readers and I chose to go the no-fail route to save you time and money. My advice to everyone who makes traditional bath bombs is to invest in a dehumidifier. The investment will increase your profits in the end.

Bath bombs are a wonderful way to use aromatherapy in your bathtub. Here are a few fun and easy bath bomb recipes to get your creative juices flowing. You can choose to use the essential oils or essential oil blends that I used or make up your own.

Fizzing Bath Powder
1 cup Sodium Bicarbonate
1/2 cup Citric Acid
1/4 cup Corn Starch
1 Tbsp. Pink Clay
1/4 cup Dendritic Salt
1 Tbsp. Taming the Wild Child EO Blend (from Essential Wholesale)

Directions: Mix together with gloved hands and package into air tight containers or bags. Really, it is that simple.

Messy Cupcakes Recipe
2 cups Sodium Bicarbonate
1 cup Citric Acid
2 tsp. Lavender 40/42 Essential Oil
Spritz
Witch Hazel USP

Directions: Mix ingredients together with gloved hands and pack into cupcake molds, with or without cupcake liners. If you pack each mold with an even top you will only get a slightly messy cupcake. In order to create a very messy cupcake you must create a packed, rounded top first. Once you are happy with the level of your cupcake, spritz the top heavily with witch hazel. It will start to fizz like crazy, so let it go. If you get too much overflow you can push the sides in when it is just starting to dry and is pliable.

Bubble Bars Recipe
Dry Ingredients
1 cup Sodium Bicarbonate
1 cup Crème of Tartar
2/3 cup Sodium Lauryl Sulfoacetate (SLSA)
1 tsp. Sea Kelp Powder (optional)
Wet Ingredients
1/4 cup Bio-Terge 804
3 Tbsp. Cocamidopropyl Betaine
2 tsp. Breathe Green Essential Oil Blend (from Essential Wholesale)

Directions: First, mix all of the dry ingredients together with a gloved hand, while breaking up any clumps. Then, add all of the wet ingredients and continue mixing until it feels like a sticky dough. You can press this into a mold, or roll the dough into a log and cut it into slices while it is still soft. If you wait too long it will become very hard to cut.

Bubble bars were made popular by LUSH™ in the past decade, but good working recipes on how to make them have been hard to come by. I created this one that is very simple and looks just like the ones make popular by LUSH™. You can add any color of your choice and essential oils to create your own varieties from this recipe.

Ingredient Information: Bio-Terge 804 is a surfactant blend that creates high foam and bubbles. Cocamidopropyl betaine is a mild surfactant. I have added Bio-Terge 804 and cocamidopropyl betaine to the glossary for further information on it.

No Fail Foaming Bath Bombs Recipe
Dry Ingredients
1 cup Citric Acid
2 cups Sodium Bicarbonate
¼ cup of Sodium Lauryl Sulfoacetate (SLSA)
¼ cup Cream of Tartar
Wet Ingredients
½ cup melted Deodorized Cocoa Butter
1 tsp. Laurel Leaf Essential Oil

Directions: Chop up the cocoa butter and melt it in the microwave or on a stove top and set aside. Chopping up the cocoa butter allows it to melt faster due to its high melting point. First, mix all of the dry ingredients with a gloved hand. Then pour in all of your wet ingredients and continue mixing. Press your mixture into a dry soap mold or cupcake tin and transfer it to the freezer for 10 to 20 minutes. Remove from the freezer and unmold. If you are patient, you can skip using the freezer and simply allow these to set up over a 12 to 24 hour period and then unmold.

Ingredient Information: Sodium lauryl sulfoacetate (SLSA) is a unique surfactant that is very mild on the skin. I have added sodium lauryl sulfoacetate to the glossary for further information on it.

Lavender Kaolin Bath Fizzies Recipe
Dry Ingredients
2 cups Sodium Bicarbonate
1 cup Citric Acid
2 Tbsp. Kaolin Clay
Wet Ingredients
1.4 ounces by weight Deodorized Cocoa Butter
1 Tbsp. Lavender Essential Oil

Directions: Chop up deodorized cocoa butter and melt it in the microwave or on a stove top and set aside. Chopping up the cocoa butter allows it to melt faster. Next, mix all of the dry ingredients with a gloved hand. Then pour in all of your wet ingredients and continue mixing. Press your mixture into a dry soap mold or cupcake tin and transfer it to the freezer for 10 to 20 minutes. Remove it from the freezer and unmold. If you are patient, you can skip using the freezer and simply allow these to set up over a 12 to 24 hour period and then unmold.

Detoxifying Bentonite Bath Fizzies Recipe
Dry Ingredients
2 cups Sodium Bicarbonate
1 cup Citric Acid
2 tablespoons Bentonite clay
Wet Ingredients
1.4 ounces Illipe Butter by weight
1 tablespoon of Cleanse Essential Oil Blend (from Essential Wholesale)

Directions: Chop up illipe butter and melt it in the microwave or on a stove top and set aside. Chopping up the illipe butter allows it to melt faster since, like cocoa butter, it has a high melting point. Next, mix all of the dry ingredients with a gloved hand. Then pour in all of your wet ingredients and continue mixing. Press your mixture into a dry soap mold or cupcake tin, and transfer to the freezer for 10 to 20 minutes. Remove from the freezer and unmold. If you are patient, you can skip using the freezer and simply allow these to set up over a 12 to 24 hour period and then unmold.

Chocolate Butter Bath Bombs Recipe
.495 lbs. Citric Acid
.565 lbs. Sodium Bicarbonate
.25 lbs. Natural Cocoa Butter
.01 lbs. Sweet Orange EO

Directions: Chop up cocoa butter and melt it in the microwave or on a stove top and set aside. Chopping the cocoa butter up allows it to melt faster due to its high melting point. Next mix all of the dry ingredients with a gloved hand. Then, pour in all of your wet ingredients and continue mixing. Press your mixture into a dry soap mold or cupcake tin, and transfer to the freezer for 10 to 20 minutes. Remove from the freezer and unmold. If you are patient, you can skip using the freezer and simply allow these to set up over a 12 to 24 hour period and then unmold.

No-Bake Bath Cookies Recipe
Dry Ingredients
2 cups Sodium Bicarbonate
1 cup Citric Acid
1 cup Corn Starch
½ cup Epsom salts
½ cup Kaolin Clay
¼ cup Lactose
¼ cup Turbinado Sugar
Wet Ingredients
2 oz. Cocoa Butter
3 oz. Shea Butter
.5 oz. Spicy Citrus Essential Oil Blend

Directions: Chop up cocoa butter and melt it in the microwave or on a stove top and set aside, but first drop the shea butter into the melted cocoa butter to soften it up too. Next, mix all of the dry ingredients with a gloved hand. Then pour in all of your wet ingredients and continue mixing. Finally, you can either hand-shape your cookies, use a cookie cutter, or use a mold to create your bath cookies. While they are soft and pliable, you can still add extra salt or sugar crystals, herbs, or anything you think will give your cookie a unique look. Let them set up for 12 to 24 hours and your cookies are all done. Just make sure you label them clearly so that no one tries to eat your bath cookies!

This No-Bake Bath Cookie recipe works much better in the tub than traditional bath cookie recipes that use egg and are baked. Baked bath cookies don't fully dissolve in the tub, but these do and they look just like real cookies.

Shower Fizzers Recipe
Dry Ingredients
2 cups Sodium Bicarbonate
1 cup Citric Acid
¼ cup Calcium Sulfate (a.k.a. Plaster of Paris)
Wet Ingredient
2 tsp. Well-Being Essential Oil Blend (from Essential Wholesale)
Spritz
Witch Hazel USP

Directions: Mix ingredients together with gloved hands and pack into soap molds and allow to harden up over one to two hours.

Making Soap with Essential Oils

Cold Processed Soap
In the process of manufacturing cold process soap, essential oils are added before the lye has been consumed, which means it is highly alkaline. Cold process soapmakers try to work around potential problems by choosing essential oils that are resistant to strong alkali or can accommodate the changes that occur in non-resistant scents and colors.

According to Kevin Dunn, in an interview with Robert Tisserand, "Essential oils are complex mixtures of dozens of chemical compounds. A given essential oil may contain some compounds that react with alkali, and others that do not. Lavender oil, for example, contains about 42% linalool (which does not react) and 22% linalyl acetate (which does). In fact, when linalyl acetate reacts with alkali, one of the products is linalool. Thus the scent of a CP soap made with lavender oil will smell less of linalyl acetate and more of linalool than the original essential oil.

"The only way to predict which essential oils will react with alkali is to examine the list of components and note which of them are reactive. Such compounds generally consist of esters, phenols, and acids. There is a practical way, however, for a soapmaker to evaluate essential oil reactivity. Add a few drops of essential oil to 1 mL of the lye solution used for soapmaking (typically 25-50% NaOH). A reaction will be visible and sometimes not. In either case, wait a day or two and then compare the scent of the alkaline EO to that of the original. In some cases, there will be no difference in scent. In those cases where the scent changes, the alkaline scent might not be bad, just different from the original.

"Phenols and acids react directly with alkali to produce odorless salts. Clove oil for example, contains a large proportion of eugenol (a phenol). If you add a few drops of clove oil to lye as described above, the resulting solution is bright yellow and very nearly odorless. Esters, on the other hand, are decomposed by lye into an acid salt (usually odorless) and an alcohol, which is often fragrant. In fact, the alcohol produced is often present as one of the components of the original EO. The scent of such an EO changes as the proportions of its components change, but it remains fragrant.

"Phenols are harder to spot, but the most common fragrant phenols are eugenol (clove, cinnamon leaf), carvacrol (thyme, oregano), thymol (thyme), and vanillin (vanilla). Phenols are actually weak acids. Other fragrant acids typically smell sour, e.g. acetic acid in vinegar."

Hot Processed Soap
Essential Oils do not suffer the impact of the strong alkali that cold process soap is exposed to, because the scent is added as a final phase once the alkali has been consumed. Essential oils can even be added to hot process liquid soap when it is completely done processing and has cooled, because the soap is in liquid form. You should be aware that when essential oils are added to completed hot process liquid soap when it has cooled, some of those essential oils will separate. You will need to give a "shake before use" direction on your label.

Melt and Pour Soap
When using essential oils with low boiling points, it is important to add your essential oils to your melt and pour soap at the lowest possible temperature. Melt and pour soap is still pourable at 130 degrees Fahrenheit, which allows you to choose the optimal temperature to add your essential oils before pouring, based on the boiling point of the essential oil used.

Melt and pour soap is the simplest soap making technique, even if you make it from scratch and don't use an already prepared base.

Note: I am not providing recipes for cold process, hot process and melt and pour soap in this book because I believe that it is important to read a thorough book on how to make each of the forms of soap from scratch, rather than to use a recipe out of context of the process. There are many wonderful books and tutorials on cold and hot process. To learn how to make your own melt and pour soap see my book, *How to Make Melt and Pour Soap Base from Scratch*, for methodology, recipes and troubleshooting information.

Always, always, always include any ingredients on the label that you add to your melt and pour soap base. This means if you add lemon essential oil to scent it, yellow 5 to color it, and poppy seeds as an exfoliant, all of the added ingredients must be included on the product ingredient list.

:: Chapter 8 ::
Building Your Brand

Natural Product Industry is the Place to be

The natural product industry continues to have an incredible opportunity to seize a sizable share of the beauty industry. In 2009, sales of natural and organic personal care products increased by 9.5% and were expected to have double digit increases in both 2010 and 2011. Industry research shows nothing but growth through the year 2013 in the natural and organic personal care market. According to Sundale Research, the natural and organic market is expected to account for 17.4% of the personal care industry by 2013, up from the 5.1% of the industry expected in 2010.

It is never too late to become a natural, organic, green growing company. The opportunity to capture this market with spa treatments and products that will produce results and repeat customers is ripe right now. Despite the economic downturn, sales of natural and organic personal care products are up. Currently 10.5% of natural and organic personal care sales are captured by department stores, spas, salons, and boutiques, leaving 89.5% of this multi-billion dollar industry seeking these products elsewhere. As such, the experts in skin care, spas, and salons have an opportunity to capture a larger segment of the natural and organic personal care industry.

According to the leading researcher Mintel in 2010, "Consumers will not just buy discount brands; they will scrutinize products more, and buy those that they perceive as being good 'value'…there are a growing number of online tools to help people pay attention to virtually everything, ensuring transparency – everything is out in the open in the internet age, and secrecy is no longer acceptable for today's consumers." Mintel says, "One-third of all consumers have never tried organic or natural personal care products, suggesting that there is plenty of room for growth in this market."

Research by Sundale has shown that consumers are willing to pay 20% more for safe, effective "green" cosmetics and toiletries. Even in this economy Mintel research says, "Consumers will look for ways to escape from the tyranny of value…"

The good news is that, in a down economy, smart businesses can still thrive based on wise choices. In recent years, conventional personal care products have had a moderate increase in sales. However, natural and organic personal care sales are booming. The greening of the market place has caused a high demand for natural cosmetics and services. This segment of the industry is dominated by small to moderate-sized companies.

Innovative companies seize opportunities in a down economy and thrive. More millionaires were made during the Great Depression than at any other time in U.S. History. When times are tough it is a crucial to make the right changes in your business model.

Evaluate your services and products to work for the here and now. If you have historically sold a synthetic skin care line and sales are down, that could be an indicator that you are missing the boat. If you are in the skin and hair care industry you are in the right industry. But do you have the right products for *this* time in history?

If the product segment of your business did not increase in 2009 and 2010, then maybe you aren't carrying the products that the market is demanding. Evaluate your services against the marketplace as well. Consumers today are stressed out about money and are short on time. Be creative and mold your company to fit the needs of busy stressed-out consumers instead of expecting them to make the time to use conventional services.

The phrase, "I'm waiting for the economy to improve" is overused. Take control of your own economy and stop waiting. Make progressive steps forward despite the economy. If you are standing still waiting then your company is slipping backwards faster than you can afford.

Delete the phrase "waiting for the economy to change" from your vocabulary. Accept the economy of today and move forward. Don't spend a single day waiting. Spend every day working toward your vision.

Business Advice
Use technology to work smart
The social media frontier is the single most cost-effective means of increasing sales that is available on the market today. If you don't have a blog, newsletter, You Tube channel, e-commerce website, Twitter account, or Facebook page you are losing thousands of contacts per day. Consumers are living their lives out on the internet. They make purchasing decisions, form loyal relationships and spread incredible word-of-mouth advertising on the internet every day.

There is a conversation happening online. Word-of-mouth advertising and many other opportunities abound in the virtual marketplace of social media. More than any other marketing method in the course of history, the arena of social networking gives small business the upper hand over big corporations.

The intimate atmosphere that naturally occurs in social networking creates abundant opportunity to influence untapped markets.

Currently, Facebook has over 800 million active users and more than 50% of them are signed logged every single day. Consumers spend over 700 billion minutes per month on Facebook. In March 2011 Twitter had an average of 460,000 new accounts being singed up per day. In 2011 Twitter had one billion tweets being sent per week. And even this information will be outdated in a minute, because Twitter is constantly growing. In 2007 there were 5000 tweets per day, 300,000 per day in 2008, 2.5 million tweets per day in 2009, there were 35 million tweets per day in 2010 and in the month of March in 2011 there was an average of 200 million tweets per day! Social media is moving that fast, and you simply have to be part of it to keep up with it.

Due to the millions of consumers on Facebook and Twitter each day, it is logical to assume that your customers and potential customers are spending their time there as well. A recent study by GroupM Search found that, "Consumers exposed to a brand's influenced social media and paid search are 2.8 times more likely to search for that brand's products."

Small businesses are no longer slaves of the once most important factor in business, "location, location, location." Whether your business is on Main Street America, in your home, or on Corporate Lane USA the new mantra is "Google, Yahoo or Bing search-ability."

The key to social networking influence is whether search words lead your potential customers to your branded website, blog, social media sites or to your competitor. Small businesses that do not have a strong social networking presence, whether they have traditionally depended on foot traffic or web traffic, will be shuttering their doors due to missed opportunities.

In a room full of small businesses and multi-million dollar corporations, the most common excuse I have heard is, "we don't have the time for social networking." With the culture of consumers changing every single day to the online community at an alarming rate, every company must make the time to follow their customers to the internet.

The excuse that comes in a close second is, "We don't know how to use social networking." There are tutorials and blogs all over the internet that will teach any company the basics of joining the online conversation. Another method is to spend a few days on the sidelines watching some active user's methods.

The fact is that if you haven't joined the online conversation, then you cannot direct the conversation toward your business. The internet is today's Main

Street America. A small business that does not have a blog, newsletter, Facebook page, or twitter account is literally doing business without a storefront sign in today's society. Consumers are readily available for direct one-on-one contact with brands. The story of your product creates value, credibility and furthers consumer hunger for education regarding natural, safe, green, and organic cosmetics. Join the conversation and direct the conversation toward your business.

Get the right people working on the right tasks

If you have a person with extensive web design skills answering phones, you might be wasting a valuable resource, especially if you are paying them extra for their education and skills. Make sure you don't have your high-paid employees doing the mundane tasks that an employee at a lower cost could do. And most importantly, as the owner of your company, don't waste all of your time working *in* your business on mundane tasks that you could hire out, leaving you with no time to work *on* your business.

You are your most valuable salesperson and best cheerleader. It is important that you spend your time working on the things that will help grow your business. The difference between working in your business and working on your business can mean the difference between success and failure. Even if today you are a one person operation, don't disregard this tip—plan your business toward this goal with the things you do today.

Determine your best sellers

Focus on the top 20% of your products and services that bring in 80% of your sales. Phase out the rest unless they are support products for your top sales items. On a spreadsheet, list every single product and service and put the total dollars sold next to each item. Sort them from highest to lowest and then determine which products make up the top 80% of total sales. You will find that they will be your top 20% of products or services.

Cut inventory by moving inventory

As long as you make money on your inventory, whatever the margin, in tough times you may need to lower your expectations on profits. Flat is the new growth and if you are holding out for higher profits then you may be hurting your long-term momentum. Essential Wholesale just cut margins on all essential oils, carrier oils and almost all our cosmetic bases. We have built our business based on six to twelve turns a year on inventory which ensures that you only get the freshest ingredients. We are not a company that will buy two years-worth of inventory just to save twenty cents a pound. We prefer fresh material and, as you already know, we can still stay competitively priced without having to inventory 50 drums of sweet almond oil that will take two years to sell off.

Focus on the money-making aspects of your business first

Don't get busy doing busy work while setting aside the most important tasks of your day. It is easy to choose to do the easiest things and then get around the hard things later, but it's usually the hard things that help you make money. Your daily to-do list should say, "First, do hard things. Second, do the hard thing that makes money first!"

Review your marketing

Take a close look at your company to make sure your company is sending the right message to your customers at the right time. Ensure that your products and services match your message. Evaluate every dollar you spend against how many dollars it returns. Cut the marketing that doesn't have a good return and focus on the marketing that does.

Above all do not repeat the last seven words of a dying company, "We never did it like that before!" Don't stick to what you have done in the past. Focus on new ways of doing business that can open doors and introduce a potential bonanza of loyal customers. Shamelessly advertise business in traditional outlets and social media. Ask for business through newsletters, social media, blogs, and up-selling. Reward loyalty more than you ever have in the past. Don't be afraid to get creative in ways that are not part of the history of your business.

Reduce overhead – trim expenses from multiple sources

Employees are often the number one cost of doing business. Look to see if you can consolidate jobs and eliminate any redundancies. Involve your employees in the solution. Only do this if you want to create a teamwork atmosphere and only if you are really planning to incorporate their input. No one wants to be asked their opinion if you are not going to take it.

Employees: You should only keep A players and B employees that are on the way to being A players, and let everyone else go. This is a painful, but critical piece of advice for any employer. People wonder why Essential Wholesale has such an amazing staff and the truth is that we have practiced this piece of advice for years. We use nothing but the best ingredients in our products and keep no one but the best employees on our team.

Go with your gut and act immediately and decisively. You know when the new person you thought was perfect is just not right. Waiting 3 more months for them to change is only going to put you 6 months behind and cost you thousands in wages and training dollars. You should know within 2 weeks, at the most, whether or not that new hire is right. And if you have older employees that have been with you since your company started that have not been able to grow and change with your company as it has grown and changed,

111

then you really need to consider making them available to the market again. If they have shown no desire to change their knowledge base to become an asset of the company again, then stop wasting your time and money and hire up.

Communication Phones, Cells, and Faxes: Faxes should be streamlined. EFax is free up to a certain number of faxes per month and nominal fee after that. Cell Phones could replace a land line altogether.

Leases: Try to renegotiate any long term leases you have, including your building rent, equipment, or technology leases. No vendor wants you to fail and is almost always willing to defer or change your terms temporarily to help you stay in business. They lose if you don't succeed.

Reduce COGS: Most CEOs and owners focus on improving their bottom line by doing one of three things and neglect to look at all three. Successful businesses look at all three all the time.

- Increase sales (1%)
- Decrease cost of goods (1%)
- Increase price of goods sold (1%)

If you did all 3 you have moved 3% to your bottom line. Choose to make it 0.5%, 2%, 5%, or whatever changes you wish, but the idea is to work on many fronts simultaneously. All of these are changes are increases that are small enough to not impact the buyer and big enough to impact the bottom line for your company when done together.

- **Example of Increased Sales:** If you sold $1,000 worth of product per month, then you would need to increase sales by $10 (1%), $20 (2%), or $50 (5%), and that isn't very much at all. Anyone can increase their sales by $10, $20, or $50 in a month.
- **Example of Decreased Cost of Goods:** If you currently buy lavender 40/42 from Essential Wholesale you could decrease your cost of goods by buying in larger volumes. Forecast your sales and chose the size that will work for you. Increasing volume from one ounce to two ounces saves 14.5%; one ounce to four ounces saves 28.9%; one ounce to eight ounces saves 43.3%; one ounce to sixteen ounces saves 50.2%; one ounce to thirty-two ounces saves 57.5%; one ounce to twenty-five pounds saves 64.2% on cost of goods sold per ounce.
- **Example of Increased Price of Goods Sold:** If you sell a bar of soap for $5 currently, then increasing the price by:
    - 1% would make the price $5.05
    - 2% would be $5.10
    - 5% would make that same bar $5.25

All of these are price increases that are small enough to not impact the buyer and big enough to impact the bottom line for your company. Buy in bulk to reduce your COGS (Costs of Goods Sold). Take advantage of any term deductions like the "1% Net 15" or the "2% Net 10" options that many suppliers offer if you have terms.

Evaluate current expenses: Stop spending money on things that don't add a single dollar to your bottom line. Changing the packaging, printing new catalogs just to change a picture or two, upgrading your website, and buying new shoes may all look good and give you a better image, but they will not immediately change your bottom line in a positive way. During economic downturns, you need to mitigate any new expense unless it is something you can sell for a profit immediately.

Fire Bad Customers: I bet if you were to look at your customers you will find that 20 to 30% of your customers do 70 to 80% of your volume. And that the bottom 80% of your customers account for only 20% of your total sales. You may even have one or two customers who do 10% or more by themselves. And you will likely find that the problematic or high maintenance customers tend to be in the bottom 80%. They are never satisfied.

You have to be willing to fire customers, too. When you have exhausted all your resources and have jumped through every single hoop imaginable and the customer is still never happy, then that is a good sign that they never will be no matter what you do, and they probably treat everyone else with contempt as well. It could be time for you to invite that unhappy customer to find a new supplier since you "do not seem to be able to meet their needs anymore." As painful as this breakup could be, it will free you up to concentrate on serving the needs of the majority of your customers.

Trust me, you will sleep easier when you know your customers are happy and if you are anything like us, you go to great lengths to do right by your customers in ALL situations. As a company, we don't believe the customer is ALWAYS right (we are all only human), but we do believe the customer should ALWAYS be treated right.

Give Your Business Regular Check-ups

You have to keep constant tabs on your business and go with your gut. One prime example for me happened in my family life. I kept noticing that Keegan's eyes had an occasional yellow hue. His color would return just in time to stop me from calling the doctor. Then at one doctor appointment I mentioned it, but since he showed no yellowing at the time we decided to wait and see, but a nagging feeling told me something wasn't right.

Finally one day I glanced over at Keegan and was stunned by the shade of yellow in his eyes. I called the doctor's office and got an appointment. His doctor wasn't in, but I was able to get him in that day to see another one. I wanted to get him in there while his eyes were actually yellow.

We had never met the doctor that we saw that day. She thought Keegan looked completely healthy and turned to Keegan and said, "We will do some blood work, but I think your mom is over-reacting and nothing will show up." I was stunned. I wondered if this doctor was a mother herself or had somehow missed the reality of a mother's instincts.

I didn't say anything, because I only cared that his liver was going to be tested. I even held my tongue when the doctor called back a few hours later to confirm that indeed there was something wrong with his liver. Thankfully it was only Gilbert's syndrome, which does absolutely no harm other than cause occasional jaundice.

That incident reminded me that when something isn't quite right with our children, our maternal instinct is very accurate. That same instinct is very powerful in the spirit of the entrepreneur. Trust your instinct. If it feels like something isn't quite right with your business, then take a step back and investigate it. Even if you can't quite put your finger on what it is, don't brush away the instinctual alarm that is sounding.

Give your business a regular and thorough exam; don't be afraid to seek outside help in the form of mentors or seek business guidance from other members in your industry through organizations like Indie Beauty Business. You will never regret spending time working *on* your business not only *in* it.

What We Learned Along the Way

Ever since our Christmas craft project turned into a business, people often ask me, "When is the best time to start a new company or launch a new product line?" My answer is always the same, "Right now!" It does not matter what time of year it is, what time of your life you are in, the current state of the economy, or who you are. The time that you are thinking of starting a business is the time to get started. The following 10 points are lessons we learned from starting our own company and supporting thousands of start-up companies through Essential Wholesale.

1. Make a mess and clean it up later.

Don't keep getting ready to get ready…Get started! If you keep sharpening your pencils and filing papers in your files, then all you will have is an organized office. Too many "would-be" entrepreneurs are stuck in the planning phase and need to just jump in. You can't grow and learn without the mistakes and lessons of actually doing the dirty work. Yes, there is a place for planning, but eventually enough is enough. Don't get stuck in the paralysis of analysis. Make a mess and clean it up later when the money starts rolling in.

2. Use your passions to pick a product line.
If you love lavender, purple, or pure products then use your passion to choose your product line. But remember to keep it simple. Start with a minimum number of products. Your focus and your financial commitment should not be too broad. Don't let all your money get gobbled up in getting started. You will need your capital later. Put as much focus as possible into marketing a few great products and not tons of average products. And trust your gut when you start having customers tell you that you need to add this or that product to your line; it could be another distraction.

3. Choose to be the Muscle or the Brain.
A key decision in your business model should be to decide whether to be the Muscle or the Brain of your organization. Focus on your gifts and talents. Some people are born marketers. Some are born to create. Others are super human and can do both. Find what you do best and do it. If your only option is to do it all, then by all means do it all. But be smart.

When I first started making my own soaps and cosmetics I personally made every drop of product that we sold. I couldn't even imagine a day when another set of hands would be involved in the process. Dennis had to pry me away from being involved on every level of every product, but once I started to let go it got easier with time. Had I not changed, and had Dennis not gently eased me into change, we never would have grown past what I personally could physically make each day. I also would have burned out years ago. Dennis and I have changed our roles in the business depending on the season in our family's life, the stage of our business, and what was needed at the time to take our business to the next level.

There are four routes to choose from as you find the right balance of Muscle and Brain.

Muscle^2 ≥ Brain - In this scenario you do it all, including product manufacturing, labeling, marketing, filling, selling, and social media, all while running the day-to- day operations of your business. It can be done. This is the heavy blood, sweat and tears version but the cost is sanity, time and balance.

Muscle ≥ Brain - In this scenario you chose to use pre-manufactured Bulk Bases which cuts down significantly on your manufacturing burden, but you continue to do the labeling, marketing, filling, selling, and social media all while running the day to day operations of your business. With manufacturing off your plate this frees up a significant amount of time allowing for more balance in your life. If you want to get out there and sell then you need to be content to buy finished unscented base products that you can simply scent, repackage, slap a label on and call it good.

Muscle ≤ Brain² - In this scenario you chose to contract-manufacture your products. There is a larger capital investment up front but you have bought back a large portion of your time. You no longer manufacture, fill or label your product. Your time is spent focusing on marketing, selling, social media along with running and growing your business. You have the ability to grow your business far beyond your capacity in the Muscle2 ≥ Brain because you don't have to worry about keeping up with your growth.

Muscle ≤ Brain - In this scenario you choose to use the Essential Wholesale Private Label Selector. This means that you don't have a large capital investment needed to get started, but you still free yourself from all of the manufacturing, filling, and labeling your product. This point and click method of Essential Wholesale's Private Label Selector allows you to sit back and wait for your small run finished product to arrive to your doorstep. That way you can focus purely on bringing your product to market.

4. Don't undersell your product.
Think ahead when setting your price point. Remember that eventually you will have employees and other expenses. This is one of the most common mistakes of home businesses. Eventually you can't do it all, but you are stuck because you did not establish a large enough margin in your price point to hire help, pay yourself and grow. The choice will be either to stay small and do it all yourself, or grow and increase your price point which may result in the loss of some of your customers. It is a terrible position to be in.

The first step in setting the retail price of your product is to determine your costs to produce it, including paying yourself, overhead costs and material costs. From there determine the gross profit that you would like to make and work backwards. Then check your price against what the market will bear. Instead of selling your product at $3.99 to compete with Wal-Mart, you should set it at $5.99 so that you have room to grow and to offer your larger customers extra pricing incentives. Business is all about thinking ahead. You can always lower your price, but it is very hard to raise it.

There are two industry standards for pricing merchandise, including keystone and discount. Keystone pricing is using a 50/50 formula in which the retail price is double the wholesale price. Discount pricing uses a 60/40 formula. In this formula the retail price = the wholesale price multiplied by 1.667.

A high-end spa selling mass merchandiser products with low price points does not really convey the exclusive message you want to convey if your business means to reach teens and men. Men and teens will not spend excessive amounts of money on their skin. The price point of the teen care and men care products you chose to use for your business should be just slightly lower than your skin care products for women. If you have the miracle product for acne, you may be able to charge a bit more because moms will spend the extra money to help their teen look better.

If your price point puts you in the upper-end marketplace, don't promote to the local drug store just because they saw you at a trade show and wanted your product. They will require you to discount your product so low that it will only result in losses for you and frustration for them. Keep focused on who you are trying to reach and understand where they shop, what they buy and what motivates them to buy. If you do have a Wal-Mart knocking on your door, but you don't have a product that will meet their price point, then you should consider developing a new product that can.

5. Make a good first impression.
First impressions will make or break you. Product packaging followed by product aroma is your first impression. Your product description and marketing will cause the customer to sample the goods. While you think the product itself is the most important part, in reality, to the consumer, it is not as high on the consumer's list. You must have a good product to keep them coming back. Getting them to pick it up in the first place is all about the marketing.

Proper packaging for aromatherapy, organically preserved, and naturally preserved products, is more important to the formulator than how pretty the package looks. The needs of natural, organic, or aromatherapy-based products are different from other personal care products. Products containing water that are organically and naturally preserved must be packaged so that neither air, light, nor fingers come in contact with the product. This tip will help you identify the difference between a natural organic look-alike and the real thing.

Invest in good packaging from your internet site design, to your brochures and Point of Purchase (POP) displays, right down to your product packaging and labels. Don't skimp on the cheapest bottle or label out there. This industry is saturated with "the best thing since sliced bread" products, and the ones that get noticed are those that grab the attention of the consumer. If you need help then contact a graphic designer that has experience with personal care products. Make sure you check out their portfolio and if they don't have the type or quality of work you want for your products, then don't hire them.

6. Know your product inside and out.

You need to be able to compare and contrast your product for the average consumer and the well-educated buyers alike. Translate to the consumer what makes you so passionate about your product. Keep it honest but enthusiastic. If you don't really believe in your product, no one else will either.

I am a registered and certified aromatherapist, so people who insist on telling me that their product - which smells like a synthetic watermelon - is made with only pure essential oils quickly lose their credibility with me. Watermelons don't produce an essential oil.

If you don't know what's in your product because you buy a bulk base, ask questions. They should be willing to disclose information and they must provide you with the complete ingredient list. Then learn all about those ingredients. Your customers will appreciate your knowledge, and it will make the difference between you and the other guys. Do not try fitting your square peg into a round hole.

7. Know who your market is.

Often people waste time marketing to the wrong consumer for their product line. Know who your product will appeal to. Meet the needs of your consumer group, and success will follow. Differentiating whether your market is tweens (10 to 12 year olds), teens (13 to 19 year olds), or men makes a huge difference in the choice of products you pick for your business. Teens, young adults, and men have typically been under-served. However, this segment of the market is now among the shoppers of natural and organic products.

From the cosmetic formulator's viewpoint, teen and men's care products are developed with different objectives in mind than your typical skin care line. Men's care products are designed around the unique skin care needs, aroma preferences, special issues surrounding facial hair and results expected from the product. Teen products are developed with all the issues surrounding blemished skin including changing hormones, antibacterial needs and reduction of breakouts. The focus becomes creating active products that will produce specific results related to hormonal skin.

Fully understanding the mind of a cosmetic formulator can help you choose the right products for your business. There are often three major issues that a formulator must work around when in the development including: price of the finished product, aroma and therapeutic value. Packaging, marketing and message also are important to the formulator but are secondary to price point, aroma and results. When formulating for teens and men it is important to produce fast results, appealing aromas, and visually attractive packaging.

Another overlooked but growing segment of the population is of ethnic descent which makes it important to carry products that address the specific needs of ethnic men. Shaving products that address the common issue of ingrown hairs, razor bumps, and keloids will benefit from the increased growth of the ethic segment of the market. Traditionally, African-Americans have been the focus of ethnic products, but there is a large and growing under-served segment of the market that includes Asian, Hispanic, Middle Eastern, and Mediterranean descent. Thick coarse hair is a common trait among many of these ethnic groups and can be addressed with the right personal care products.

The younger and older populations cannot be overlooked either. Anti-aging products are becoming more popular with this rapidly aging population of America, and they have the highest level of disposable income. Marketing to men 55 years and older with services and product offerings will help capture a piece of this lucrative market. Empty-nesters are the fastest growing segment of the market and yet only have a handful of products to choose from. The teen category is also expected to continue growing with a younger generation that cares more about grooming and personal care than ever before. Your skin care business will benefit greatly by capturing these growing markets.

Most importantly, once you know who your market is, be true to your market.
If your marketing campaign is based on aromatherapy and you use synthetic fragrance chemicals to scent, your end product is contrary to your mission statement. Aromatherapy treatments should not contain any level of synthetic fragrance chemicals. An aromatherapy treatment should only be done with essential oils. Aromatherapy benefits cannot be achieved with fragrance chemicals. Synthetic fragrance chemicals are not the same as natural made aromas. If you have a fruity aromatherapy product make sure that the aroma is coming from orange, lemon, bergamot, lime, litsea, tangerine, mandarin, blood orange, pink grapefruit, white grapefruit, or another citrus that produces essential oils.

Aromatherapists are regularly asked for aromatherapy blends with scents such as passion fruit, banana, coconut, kiwi and strawberry. By definition, aromatherapy is treatment with the scented liquid that comes naturally from essential oils. However, the only fruits that produce essential oils are citrus fruits. All other fruit scents are made with fragrance chemicals and have no aromatherapy value at all. Only natural plant materials have these therapeutic properties and effects of essential oils.

If your market loves strawberry bubble gum, tooty-fruity, or sugar plum and other fun fragrances, just know that they can only be created synthetically and the aromatherapy marketing would be misleading. Thus the fragrance oil market is the right choice for you, and that is okay; both markets have a huge audience.

Just keep in mind that consumers are insulted by companies claiming to use aromatherapy while using synthetic fragrance oils that are contrary to their marketing and mission statement. Make it easy for your customers and align your scenting practices with the message of your company. Whether you are a fragrance or essential oil user, the goal is to be true to yourself and to your customers.

8. Keep your goal in front of you.
If you are creating your own business so that you can be home with your family, keep that in mind. Put photos of your kids and the vacation you want to take with them on your desk and refrigerator. Visual re-enforcement will help you through those long days and nights. And there will be days, lots of them, where you wonder why in the world you are going to all this trouble. Just remember what motivates you during those times and the little things will fade.

9. Find a mentor or someone you can count on for sound advice.
Your mentor should not be your best buddy but someone with experience in business development and more. Your local Small Business Administration (SBA) will generally have a SCORE department made up of retired business people that are looking for someone to mentor. Trust me, your family and friends just might think you are nuts starting up a company, but don't let that discourage you.

Other company owners know and understand what drives you. Don't seek advice from your non-supportive best friend, otherwise you might just lose your dream altogether. Your mentor needs to be someone who isn't afraid to offend you and who will point out where you are going wrong.

10. Follow the leader.
There are so many success stories in this industry and there is room for many more. A person like Donna Maria Coles Johnson of the Indie Beauty Network is just one of the exciting stories in the beauty industry. If you see the growing trend toward the mineral make-up industry, or the success of those in the 5 billion-dollar organic products industry, follow them. Don't see competition as a negative; see it as a positive because you can always learn from them. It also means that you are positioning yourself in a hot marketplace.

Trends in natural products will come and go, but ethical responsibility and sustainability will always trump price in the natural industry. According to

Mintel's latest report on green living, "the environment remains a concern for the majority of Americans. More than one-third (35%) of survey respondents say they would pay more for 'environmentally friendly' products."

At the core of the natural products industry is a desire to protect the earth, use non-toxic products and support companies with ethical business practices. Chasing ingredient trends will lead nowhere if the core of the corporation isn't in alignment with the cornerstone of the natural industry. Brands, big and small, that do not undercut another brand to sell themselves will find consumer loyalty. Like never before, a brand's ability to speak to consumers honestly and forthrightly will supersede those that only *talk at* their market without *listening to* their market.

Top Ten Things I Love about Being an Indie Business

As I mentioned, you have to keep your goal in front of you, and part of that is knowing exactly why you want to be an Indie (independent) small business owner. I know my "why." Do you know yours?

1. **Foundation Building** - We get to build something really amazing that reaches out and touches people's lives in different ways every day. I am humbled by the responsibility, and I am honored to have built a company alongside my husband that supports thousands of businesses. I feel blessed for having the perfect partnership that allows us to succeed as a team in tandem with thousands of businesses.

2. **Freedom** - I have the freedom to work the hours I want to. I can work while my kids are at school and after they go to bed. I have the freedom to be available for chaperoning every one of my kids' field trips, and I can be a cabin mom when they go to camp. I have the freedom to dash out to a cina-meeting with my husband if we want to. (Cina-meeting definition: "business meeting" with my partner held while watching a movie at the theatre in the middle of a work day.) I have the freedom to sneak a kiss to my "boss" at work.

3. **Passion** - I get to focus on what I am passionate about and I get to share it with the world. I love aromatherapy, writing, research, tinkering in the lab, making cosmetics, watching people learn, and my family. I get to live inside the bubble of my passions every day. I can make whatever my creative mind comes up with or my awesome team dreams up. It has left me with good skin and my whole family always smells good—at least that is what everyone at the checkout stand, bank, drive thru, school, and physician's office says when we approach.

4. **Sharing** - We have the financial ability to support missions, charities and organizations that we believe in. We get to experience the joy of giving. And I get to watch my husband be giddy like a school kid in the act of giving.

5. **Training Up Our Kids** - We can teach our children that they can fail, get back up again, fail, keep going, take a misstep, start all over again, and eventually succeed. We can live by example and model the full spectrum of business ownership before their eyes. And our income will support their dreams.

6. **Watching Other People Succeed** - We get to be part of the success of other people's businesses. We've had the opportunities over and over again to watch dreams become a reality. We've watched businesses grow even beyond their expectations. I feel like a proud momma seeing the success of other people's businesses.

7. **Employees** - We get to employ some amazing people. We have had three Essential Wholesale weddings and one Essential Wholesale baby. We have watched as our employees have grown up before our very eyes. We have been family for many. We have been through stress, tough times, good times, parties, friendships, good-byes, laughter, arguments, lots of good food, and teamwork with some of the greatest people in the Portland metropolitan area.

8. **Control** - Business ownership gives us the ability to take new steps, enact change, and react to things out of our control. We have the responsibility of making the final call and the freedom to do what we think is right.

9. **We've Made Our Parents Proud** - Our poor families stood by as we struggled financially to get our business off the ground. When we worked around the clock for next to nothing pay, they wondered—mostly quietly—why we didn't just go get real jobs. But now they get to see the vision that we had come to fruition. My parents bit their nails for the first thirty-ish years of my life and now get to sit back and let their nails grow long. I can't take back the grey hair I gave them, but I can give them all the free products they will ever need.

10. **Community of Entrepreneurs** - We get to be part of an amazing community of entrepreneurs. We share the highs and lows of business ownership with friends that we have made in the course of this great endeavor. We get to support one another, promote each other and be the cheerleader when one of us is heavily burdened. Technology has

made the community of entrepreneurs as close as neighbors. I won't be surprised someday if Donna Maria sends me a 'direct message' through Twitter to borrow a cup of sugar. But I would be surprised if she used it to bake instead of making a body scrub out of it.

:: Chapter 9 ::
Navigating Industry Regulations

An Essential Oil Bias

As a certified and registered aromatherapist, I am admittedly biased toward essential oils over fragrance oils. I am also allergic to fragrance oils. I was forced to live a fragrance-free life long before it was popular. Once I found aromatherapy it opened up a whole new world to me. Having admitted all that up front let me share the debate from the view of an aromatherapist.

The differences between essential and fragrance oils can best be described by comparing a real orange to a piece of orange candy. The real orange has health benefits for the body and comes directly from nature. The orange's color, shape, flavor, scent, taste and vitamins, as well as the psychological and physiological benefits, all come directly from nature. It was designed to nourish our body as well as provide vitamin C for health benefits. On the other hand, a piece of orange candy gets its sweetness from refined sugar and its shape from gums. It is artificially flavored and colored, has no health benefits whatsoever, and can actually be bad for our bodies.

In that example an essential oil is the orange, and fragrance oil is the piece of orange candy. The body gains nothing of value from fragrance oil because this man-made substance was only created to duplicate a natural aroma and not the properties. Whereas the essential oil is a function and byproduct of a plant created to protect, heal and pollinate life and is far more beneficial. The hormonal, antimicrobial, antibacterial, and antiviral properties of a plant are captured in the essential oil and enable the human body to use the plants vital energy to benefit itself.

Some plants produce a variety of essential oils from different parts of the plant. For instance, the citrus family produces neroli (*Citrus aurantium*) from orange blossoms, sweet orange (*Citrus sinensis*) from the zest, and petitgrain (*Citrus aurantium*) from the leaves. Although all of these essential oils come from the same plant family, only sweet orange from the zest smells like an orange.

The Great Debate

The dispute between fragrance oils and essential oils has been going on since 1868 with the invention of coumarin, the first synthetic fragrance. From there the trend toward synthetic fragrances took hold, making synthetic scenting economical and aromas consistent. Still today, the positive side of fragrance oils over essential oils is the consistency, cost and variety of non-plant based aromas.

The debate inside the industry was originally fueled by legitimate concerns regarding the authenticity of some brand's natural or organic claims. However, the backlash of lawsuits and outright brand-to-brand attacks has left the consumers with a lack of confidence in the natural industry. In the case of many safe ingredients "the baby has been thrown out with the bath water" thanks to misleading information from watch groups. This trend has the potential to erode consumer confidence even further in the natural industry. In order to gain consumer confidence, common ground within the natural industry must be found.

In 2010, beauty products trended toward organic ingredients, revisiting attributes like authenticity, provenance, and local production. We must respect that there is a place for natural, naturally derived, and synthetic because— and here is the rub in the natural industry—you ,simply cannot make every personal care item out of ingredients picked directly from the earth.

The most heated debates in the industry are centered on surfactants, emulsifiers and preservatives. While there is a place in the marketplace for the ultra-natural brands that avoid all three categories, there are not enough consumers willing to do without traditional personal care items. There is a large base of consumers who desire natural products, but not at the price of beauty or high prices at the checkout stand.

This is where the fluency of common sense must prevail in the natural industry. Many already agree that ingredients like cetearyl alcohol, cetyl alcohol, decyl glucoside, phenoxyethanol, and - even on some lists - sodium lauryl sulfate have a place in the natural industry. Expect claims like "free from" and "sustainable" to appear on products that simultaneously contain synthetic actives like peptides, hyaluronic acid, ceramides, or collagen. The vital function of ingredients that act as surfactants, emulsifiers, and preservatives simply cannot be achieved using natural substances in all cases.

Synthetic fragrances are cheaper and always smell consistent because they are lab created. Nature does not always produce the exact same scent with each and every harvest of plant material. Essential oils can vary due to environmental differences from year to year and with the varying countries of origin for plant material.

The unfortunate side of a synthetic fragrance is that the manufactured scent does not contain the therapeutic properties of their counterparts, whole-plant based essential oils. Thus, the true power and purpose of aromatherapy is lost.

For example, one drop of peppermint fragrance oil does not contain the same natural pharmacy that one drop of the essential oil has. The synthetic version only attempts to duplicate the aroma and not the properties transferred from the plant material itself.

Synthetic fragrances have had several other negative issues come to light over the past few years. These include a high rate of allergic reactions, as well as the controversy surrounding the undisclosed aroma chemicals and preservatives in every fragrance oil. Many people have chosen to work with fragrance oils because they are intimidated by the powerful properties of essential oils, only to find even fragrance oils often contain minute amounts of essential oils.

The Fragrance Exception

By law, even when a label says "essential oils" or a product is sold as an "essential oil," it is not a guarantee that the product does not contain synthetic fragrance chemicals. This practice is perfectly legal and runs rampant in our industry. In fact, you can claim you use "essential oils" even if you use fragrance oils, reconstitutes, adulterated oils, perfume compounds, aromas, synthetic fragrance ingredients, or diluted essential oils. It is legal to claim that a product only uses essential oils, when in fact there are added synthetics in the product. The practice of using fragrance oils and labeling them essential oils is even more common in blends that are being sold as essential oil blends.

According to the rules set in place by the FDA, all ingredients must be listed in order of predominance on a cosmetic ingredient list EXCEPT ingredients added to give a product an odor. Because of this loop hole the word "fragrance" or "parfum" may represent many hundreds of ingredients in one product. The term "fragrance" is defined by the FDA as "any natural or synthetic substance or substances used solely to impart an odor to a cosmetic product."

If a "fragrance" is added to mask or cover up the odor of other ingredients it is not required to be added to the label. Therefore, a product that contains fragrance chemicals can be labeled "unscented" or "fragrance free." This means that if an ingredient in a product gives it an undesired scent, then the manufacturer can add fragrance oils to mask the smell and never disclose them at all. Prior to my aromatherapy and cosmetic education I had always wondered why I still had allergic reactions, ranging from eczema to asthma, to products bearing the label "unscented" or "fragrance free."

The fragrance exception allows formulators to not only maintain a consistent product scent, but even preservatives can be hidden behind the "fragrance" title. A preservative with the trade name Naticide has been given the coveted INCI name of "fragrance," hence allowing unscrupulous manufacturers to call their product "preservative free."

How do I know this? A sales representative called me to sell us what he termed "the greatest new preservative that wouldn't have to be claimed or disclosed on an ingredient list." I asked for a full ingredient list and was denied it because with the "fragrance" INCI name, it is granted the trade secret protection. I asked the sales person to have someone from the lab call me so I could ask technical questions and clarify the safety of the preservative. Believe it or not, no one called me back.

Any host of undesirable preservatives could be hidden within this preservative system. They could be good, bad, or ugly, but with the INCI name of "fragrance" we will never know. One company calls Naticide "manuka oil" in their ingredient list, but I have a bottle of Naticide sitting right here on my desk, and it is undoubtedly not manuka oil as it does not remotely smell or feel the same as manuka oil.

According to the Naticide manufacturer the trade name is "Naticide," the type of ingredient is a "preservative," the functionality is "preservative, broad spectrum (gram+/-, yeast, and fungi), and ideal for preservative free formulations." Its INCI name is parfum a.k.a. fragrance. How can an ingredient be called a preservative, used as a preservative, with the functionality of a preservative and yet be marketed as ideal for preservative free formulations? It can't.

When you buy essential oils or aromatherapy products be sure to do your own research. Many salespeople have been taught that their "aromatherapy-based products are totally natural and scented solely on essential oils, but you need to do your own research. So many spa lines are full of chemicals, fragrance oils and fluffery. You are responsible to your client for their health and wellness. If you are attempting to do aromatherapy with synthetic fragrance chemicals, you are doing more harm than good to the industry. As a therapist you should abide by the physician's creed of "first, do no harm."

An Educated Nose

The best way to know the difference between adulterated and unadulterated essential oils, so that even a poorly labeled product will not sneak past you, is to educate your nose by smelling pure unadulterated essential oils next to fragrance oils. Once you smell the difference it is unlikely that you will ever be misled again. Nothing man-made smells as pure and natural as the essential oil or distillate water that comes from true plant material.

Thanks to the blurred line between what is technically allowed and what is actually true, contaminated and adulterated essential oils are widespread in the market place. It is a common belief that if the FDA allows the ingredients of any fragrance component to all fall under the heading "parfum" or "fragrance" then there is no reason to inform the consumer. Manufacturers and consumers of cosmetics are being tricked into believing that they are using pure essential oils, when in fact they are being sold adulterated goods.

If a company is selling a product that they claim is an essential oil, but they cannot produce a Material Safety Data Sheet (MSDS), Certificate of Analysis (C of A) and tell you the botanical name and country of origin, you should look elsewhere. You cannot rely solely on labels, websites or a claim that something is pure and unadulterated. Absolutely every opinion can be backed up by real facts or "facts." The simple truth is that you can find research to back up any stance you want to take on any given subject. I can find an argument online or in a chat room to back up or discredit any opinion I hold.

Truly the only safeguard against false claims is an educated nose, asking a lot of questions, and knowing exactly what plants do produce essential oils and from what part of the plant do those oils come. For instance, you can get an essential oil out of the leaves of a strawberry plant, but it won't smell like strawberry at all. It would smell herbaceous and green and not sweet and fruity. If you are being sold "strawberry essential oil," ask questions. Request the botanical name of each ingredient and the country of origin.

Sensitive and Allergy-Prone Skin

As an aromatherapist, I'm often asked if fragrance oils are safer to use than essential oils because of the potential property effects of essential oils, and my answer is always a resounding "No". Fragrance oils are made up of a long list of various chemicals, often including essential oils with little regard for the natural qualities that make these oils so precious.

There are said to be anywhere from 2,000 to 5,000 raw fragrance components used to formulate fragrance oils. I didn't count the list, but feel free to go to the site yourself to see a full list of raw fragrance ingredients, and decide for yourself what is acceptable to you. You will find a combination of natural and purely synthetic ingredients on the list of raw fragrance components. (To learn more look in the Resource Guide in the back of the book: The Scientific Committee on Cosmetic Products and Non-Food Products Intended for Consumers)

It is important to know that synthetic fragrances work differently on the human body than natural essential oils do. According to many reputable allergy specialists, lab-created fragrances or "essential oils" misbranded as pure, unadulterated plant essences are the most common cause of cosmetic-related allergic reactions, but current laws do not require the full disclosure of the synthetic chemicals making up the fragrance oil

For instance, the formula for green tea fragrance oil contains the chemical compounds in citrus essential oils that cause photosensitization. In addition, it contains nutmeg and cinnamon essential oils. Cinnamon essential oil renders the skin hypersensitive to the sun and is photosensitizing. The combination of these two items can be irritating. But since fragrance oil ingredients are not fully disclosed, the consumer may be unaware of any potential issues. The crafter using this fragrance oil would not be aware of the presence of cinnamon in the blend when creating their products, and may even think that this synthetic fragrance is safer than a natural one.

Skin allergies are very common, but allergies can impact any area of the body. A skin allergy reaction can appear in the form of a rash, welt or hives. These inflammations of the skin may be in isolated patches or in general areas. In order to have an allergic reaction you simply need to have been exposed at least one time to a substance, at which time your body identifies it as a foreign invader. The next time you are exposed to that substance, your body sends out the troops to protect itself, and suddenly you have an allergic reaction. Your body has an exaggerated immune response. The same substance will cause absolutely no reaction in non-allergic people because the body sees the substance as harmless, because it is if you aren't allergic to it. Many times an allergic reaction shows up on the skin whether it was caused by topical exposure or not.

For those who suffer from allergies, there is a tendency to label a cosmetic ingredient or a cosmetic in general as "bad," because of their allergy. I know, because I've had my moments as an allergy sufferer in which I want to assume all products that have allergy triggers are bad. But it simply isn't true. The bad guy in my body really is my immune system and not the allergen.

An allergy is the body's immune system rejection of a substance. It is caused when the immune system sees a substance as a foreign invader. In reaction to the foreign invasion of allergens, the body sends T-cells—a group of white blood cells—out to fight. In skin allergic reactions, this causes redness and irritation. Your risk of developing an allergy to cosmetics isn't necessarily related to the natural or chemical formulation of a cosmetic, but instead it is related to your parents' allergy history.

I am one-quarter Irish and suffer from both sensitive skin and allergy-prone skin. People with red hair, or who have Celtic, Irish, British, or Scottish heritage often suffer from sensitive skin, which is characterized by very thin, fragile and pink colored skins. Sensitive skin is often mistaken for allergy-prone skin. In sensitive skin the blood vessels and nerve endings are closer to the surface of the skin, which causes it to get irritated and redden easily from external or internal irritants. Not only can topical application of a cosmetic cause sensitive skin to redden, but so can eating spicy food, consuming caffeine or alcohol, taking niacin (vitamin B3), exposing the skin to sun, or using tobacco.

Sensitive skin is much more likely to develop reactions and allergies to cosmetics and essential oils. However, many reactions for people with sensitive skin may not be associated with true allergies. I can attest to this phenomenon. In reaction to some cosmetic ingredients or internal stimulus, my skin just gets a little reddened, while my reaction to others is a rash, welts or hives. It takes special attention to the details of foods and cosmetic ingredients to isolate what is causing simply red, irritated skin versus what is causing a true allergy. Either way, anyone with sensitive skin knows that whether it is a true allergy or simply a reaction from sensitive skin, it is desirable to avoid the cause of the reaction in the future.

Fragrances are a common source of allergic reaction in cosmetics. A commonly unknown cause of allergic reaction to "fragrance-free" cosmetics is actually fragrance chemicals. This is one loophole in the cosmetic law that I would love to see closed. It is perfectly legal to call your product fragrance-free and not label it with the term fragrance if, and only if, the fragrance was added to mask the aroma of another chemical in the formulation.

"The ingredient or mixture of ingredients acting as a masking agent, i.e., covering the undesirable off-odor of a product without adding a discernible odor to it, may be declared by their individual name(s) or as "fragrance" (in lieu of a better designation). A masking agent present in a product at an insignificant level may be considered an incidental ingredient under § 701.3(1) (2)(iii) in which case it need not be declared on the label."

Source: FDA Labeling Manual.

I don't believe in the term "hypoallergenic" when it comes to cosmetics. It is an oxymoron because there are absolutely no substances on earth that can be guaranteed to not cause an allergic reaction for some people. Hypoallergenic really means that it is less likely to cause an allergic reaction. For the same reason there no essential oils that cannot cause an allergic reaction in someone. I am allergic to fragrance oils, but I am not allergic to essential oils. I have known people who are allergic to certain essential oils but not fragrance.

For this very reason, you should never claim to manufacture anything hypoallergenic. You can avoid formulating with common allergens, but you simply cannot formulate hypoallergenic for all consumers. Again, there simply is nothing on earth, whether man-made or natural that is guaranteed to be hypoallergenic.

Allergies have become such a hot topic that the European Union has created labeling laws to respond to them. The Seventh Amendment to the European Union Cosmetics Act—amongst other things—placed a labeling obligation on final cosmetic products containing any of the 26 identified allergens present at 0.01% in products rinsed off the skin, or 0.001% in leave-on products. This was required by March 2005, but the following was added to Annex III, Part I requiring that:

- "The presence of the substance must be indicated in the list of ingredients referred to in Article 6(1)(g) when its concentration exceeds: — 0.001% in leave-on products — 0.01% in rinse-off products" for products sold in the European Union. This means that essential oils, naturally or adulterated, that contain the following components must disclose said component on the ingredient list if in the given formula the concentration exceeds 0.0001% in leave-on products and 0.01% in rinse of products.
    - Amyl cinnamal
    - Benzyl alcohol
    - Cinnamyl alcohol
    - Citral
    - Eugenol
    - Hydroxy-Citronellal
    - Isoeugenol
    - Amylcin namyl alcohol
    - Benzyl salicylate
    - Cinnamal
    - Coumarin
    - Geraniol
    - Hydroxy-methylpentylcyclohexenecarboxaldehyde
    - Anisyl alcohol
    - Benzyl cinnamate
    - Farnesol
    - 2-(4-tert-Butylbenzyl) propionaldehyde
    - linalool
    - Benzyl benzoate
    - Citronellol
    - Hexyl cinnam-aldehyde
    - d-Limonene
    - Methyl heptin carbonate
    - 3-Methyl-4-(2,6,6-trimethyl-2-cyclohexen-1-yl)-3-buten-2-one
    - Oak moss extract, and/or Treemoss extract

Fragrance-Free Policies and Regulations

And then there is the city of Portland, Oregon which adopted a new Fragrance-Free Policy, imposing on all their employees, contractors, product vendors and visitors a blanket fragrance-free ban. I thought it was a joke at first, but sadly it is not. The policy was passed by the City Council on February 23, 2010.

The policy means that all employees, contractors, vendors, and visitors of Portland City buildings must be free of fragrances. While digging for it, I found this policy that was passed in 2004. I can't find the current new law and have to assume that it is broader than the one below. I have emailed the City of Portland requesting a copy of the current law. In a nutshell it was created to ensure a workplace free of airborne irritants, and so the Bureau of Emergency Communications (BOEC) is designated as a fragrance-free zone. This means that all "employees, contractors, product vendors, other city bureau employees and visitors to BOEC are subject to the following rules:

3.1.1 Perfumes, after-shaves, and any other scented products are prohibited.

3.1.2 Clothing or personal items carrying detectable fragrances are prohibited.

3.1.3 Magazines and catalogs containing fragrance samples must have the samples removed.

3.1.4 Gifts, flowers, candles and other items which are scented are prohibited.

3.2 BOEC employees wearing scented products will be asked to wash off the scent or change their clothing.

3.2.1 If an employee is unable to remove the scent at work, they will be sent home to bathe or change.
1. Employees sent home may use their lunch/breaks or vacation time to cover their time away from work.

3.2.2 Employees wearing scented products to work will be counseled and the documentation of that counseling will be placed in the supervisor's file under the employee's name.

3.2.3 Once counseled, future violations will result in discipline up to and including termination.

3.3 Contractors, product vendors, other city bureau employees or visitors wearing a scented product or scented clothing will not be allowed on BOEC-controlled premises and will be asked to leave.

3.3.1 A BOEC supervisor may make exceptions if the offender is performing emergency repairs on critical equipment, however, every precaution will be taken to protect employees working within the operations area.

3.3.2 Violations by other city employees will be documented and immediately referred to their own bureau supervisors.

3.3.3 Documentation of repeat offenders or of any confrontations from contractors, product vendors, other city bureau employees or visitors will be forwarded to the appropriate manager for follow up and may result in that person being banned from BOEC.

3.4 Visitors and contractors in areas under BOEC control but outside of the Operations floor, will be advised of the Fragrance Free policy and asked to comply."

In My Opinion (IMO)

This is going too far. People who are allergic to peanuts cannot honestly petition for peanuts to be banned worldwide. But they do have the right to have it disclosed to them if a product they consume or use contains or has been processed near peanuts.

Again, keep in mind that I have terrible allergies and asthma, but I do not support government policies like this one. At our company we ask our employees not to wear synthetic perfume and cologne in the workplace because they cause asthma and headaches for three of our employees. We have an abnormally large population of chemically sensitive people who work for us because our business specializes in natural, organic and aromatherapy based products. None of my employees need a policy in place to respect the health issues of their co-workers. The use of essential oils in any form or fashion is encouraged.

I don't need the city to impose a policy in order to function as an asthmatic with allergies to chemical fragrances. If someone is wearing a perfume or cologne that bothers me I simply move further away from them. This policy doesn't only restrict the use of synthetic perfumes and colognes. It also restricts natural ones. It would restrict the essential oil blend that I use to aid my asthma. I certainly hope I don't have any business to take care of within any City of Portland buildings.

Before you say it, I'll say it: "What's next, a flatulence-free zone?" Let me tell you, it's been asked, and there already is one. The southern African nation of Malawi has a new fart-free zone which states, "Any person who vitiates the atmosphere in any place so as to make it noxious to the public to the health of persons in general dwelling or carrying on business in the neighborhood or passing along a public way shall be guilty of a misdemeanor."

Voluntary Industry Standards

IFRA Standards
The International Fragrance Association (IFRA) is the official worldwide representative body of the fragrance industry to insure safety of fragrance materials, including essential oils. IFRA has their own Code of Practice which applies to the manufacture and handling of all fragrance materials. IFRA requires that all member companies follow the IFRA Code of Practice. IFRA makes annual Amendments to the Code, as needed based on new scientific developments. These contain either new usage restrictions or revisions of existing usage restrictions.

According to IFRA Standards
"The IFRA Standards form the basis for the globally accepted and recognized risk management system for the safe use of fragrance ingredients and are part of the IFRA Code of Practice. This is the self-regulating system of the industry, based on risk assessments carried out by an independent Expert Panel.

The Expert Panel is made up of renowned independent experts from the fields such as dermatology, toxicology, pathology and environmental sciences. Their role is to evaluate the data on a fragrance to see if it supports the current use level, to make sure that there is no risk for the consumer. In cases where the safety assessment does not support the current use, the Panel instructs IFRA to issue a Standard either restricting or banning a material.

The Standards amount to 174 substances which have been either banned or restricted in their use in fragrance products. All members of IFRA are required, as a condition of membership, to observe the IFRA Code of Practice. The fragrance industry spends approximately $8 million (annually) in joint research on the safety of fragrances, and much more at the individual company level.

IFRA provides information on the exposure situation (usage concentration, variety of use, volume of use), chemical composition as well as the olfactory profile and olfactory potential (importance) of a fragrance ingredient to the Research Institute for Fragrance Materials (RIFM), the scientific arm of IFRA. RIFM then prepares comprehensive dossiers on the materials including all available safety data and, if necessary, initiates and organizes any missing safety studies on the fragrance ingredient.

The Standards are established according to the following process:

1. IFRA provides information on the exposure situation (usage concentration, variety of use, volume of use), chemical composition as well as the olfactory profile and olfactory potential (importance) of a fragrance ingredient to RIFM;

2. RIFM prepares a comprehensive dossier on the material including all available safety data and, if necessary, initiates and organizes any missing safety studies on the fragrance ingredient;

3. The RIFM Panel of independent experts, evaluates the data to see if it supports the current use level, to make sure that there is no risk/danger for the consumer; if the safety assessment does not support the current use, the Panel instructs IFRA to issue a Standard*;

4. IFRA prepares a Standard in accordance with the Panel's instructions and conclusions;

5. The draft Standard is consulted with the IFRA membership and stakeholders for a period of about a month, to ensure that IFRA/RIFM are aware of all data on the material and to provide holders of additional data that might alter the outcome of the Panel's risk assessment with the opportunity to share those with IFRA/RIFM;

6. If no additional information is received via the Consultation phase, the final Standard is published in a notification procedure as part of an "Amendment to the IFRA Code of Practice".

* The final decision on the content of the Standard is solely in the hands of the Expert Panel, not IFRA or RIFM."

IFRA Compliance Program
"The IFRA Compliance Program focuses on the safety of fragranced consumer products by ensuring that the IFRA Code of Practice is fully applied and adhered to. It involves the analysis of a variety of consumer products for the presence of fragrance ingredients regulated by IFRA Standards.

Each year, IFRA selects the segment in each category on a rotating basis. Ten countries where IFRA is linked to Fragrance Associations (through direct membership or through a regional association of IFRA) are selected every year by a random computer program operated by a supporting external laboratory which also operates as a third party administrator.

For the initial cycles of the program the top leading 15 products for each segment in each country, are identified based on their ranking of the preceding year. This selection process will be modified in future to include lower ranking and more local products.

After elimination of the products common to several country rankings and likely to contain identical fragrances, 15, 15 and 20 products according to the breakdown below are selected at random by a computer program also operated by the third party administrator:

- 15 in one segment of the fine fragrance category (e.g. Eau de Toilette, Perfume)
- 15 in one segment of the cosmetics and toiletries category (e.g. shampoo, deodorant)
- 20 in one of two segments of the household and detergents category (e.g. air freshener, fabric conditioner, washing powder).

These products are sampled from each related market and channeled to the external laboratory in charge of the analysis of the products.

The products are analyzed by a third party administrator, eurofins Consumer Product Testing GmbH in Hamburg, Germany. The product analysis is defined in specific procedures and is coordinated by the third party administrator in order to eliminate any conflict of interest.

The third party administrator is well accredited and scientifically recognized and follows internal procedures to ensure confidentiality and impartiality in each step of the program" Source IFRA (11/2011)
                    -This information is reprinted with permission from IFRA

National Association of Holistic Aromatherapists Code of Ethics

1.1 Demonstrate commitment to provide the highest quality aromatherapy service to those who seek their professional service

1.2 Conduct myself in a professional and ethical manner in relation to my clients, fellow aromatherapists and colleagues and the general public so as to comply with the highest standards of moral behavior and integrity and to uphold the dignity and status of my profession under all circumstances.

1.3 Share professional knowledge, research, and experiences with fellow aromatherapists and colleagues to support the advancement of aromatherapy.

1.4 Provide services within the scope of scope and in accordance with holistic principles and render professional services for no other purposes than the total well being of the client.

1.5 Educate clients in the quality and availability of true aromatherapy products and services.

1.6 Refrain from engaging in any sexual conduct or sexual activities involving clients.

1.7 Recognize that my primary obligation is always to the client and agree to practice Aromatherapy to the best of my ability for my client's benefit. My client's comfort, welfare and health must always have priority.

1.8 Provide clients with informed consent/disclosure statement and information that includes training, certification, scope of practice, payment structure, benefits, limitations and expectations of both the practitioner and client.

1.9 Endeavor to serve the best interests of my clients at all times by providing the highest quality of service and I shall undertake continuing education and improve upon my Aromatherapy skills and professional standards whenever possible.

1.10 Provide services within the scope and the limits of my training. I will not employ techniques for which I have not had adequate training and shall represent my education, training, qualifications and abilities honestly. I shall acknowledge the limitations of my skills and when necessary, refer clients to the appropriate qualified professionals.

1.11 Not diagnose, prescribe or provide any service, which requires a license to practice unless specifically licensed to do.

1.12 Maintain client confidentiality and not divulge to anyone the findings I acquire during consultation, or in the course of professional recommendations, without my clients consent except when required by law.

1.13 Support other Consultants at all time and shall never criticize, condemn or otherwise denigrate other Consultants in the presence of a client or other lay persons.

1.14 Respect the rights of other healthcare professionals and aromatherapists and will cooperate with all health care professionals in a friendly and professional manner.

1.15 Where another Consultant refers a client to me, I shall return such clients to the original Consultant when the specified recommendation is completed. I will not denigrate another Consultants recommendations.

1.16 Not make false claims regarding the potential benefits of Aromatherapy and shall actively participate in educating the public regarding the actual benefits of True Aromatherapy.

1.17 Not give guarantees regarding the results of any recommendations, nor exploit a client for financial gain through inferences or misrepresentation of any sort.

1.18 Practice honesty in advertising, promote my services ethically and in good taste, and practice and or advertise only those skills for which I have received adequate training or certification.

1.19 Maintain my premises in a hygienic condition, and ensure that my premises offer my Clients sufficient privacy.

1.20 Maintain complete records of each Client, including specific details of my recommendations.

1.21 Refrain from the use of any mind-altering drugs, alcohol, or intoxicants prior to or during a professional Aromatherapy consultation or while representing the National Association for Holistic Aromatherapy.

1.22 Dress in a professional manner, proper dress being defined as the attire suitable and consistent with accepted professional practice.

1.23 Represent a united front to the public and refrain from criticism of colleagues either in writing or verbally before clients or the general public.

1.24 Shall, upon being found to have transgressed any of the By-laws of the National Association for Holistic Aromatherapy and/or this Code of Ethics voluntarily surrender and return my membership certificate to the Association.

NAHA Scope of Practice – Policy Statement

The scope of practice for Aromatherapists and their knowledge in this field of expertise is one of the most important issues for both client and practitioner. It is also an area in which the National Association for Holistic Aromatherapy (NAHA) supports its members and the public through information and guidelines to educate and share our knowledge in the safety and benefits of essential oils and hydrosols. NAHA and its members are dedicated to the advancement of Aromatherapy as a unique healing modality and to the recognition of Professional Aromatherapists as qualified practitioners.

NAHA Policy Statement: Raindrop therapy

One of the fastest growing new areas for aromatherapy is the Spa industry. Here essential oils and hydrosols are used primarily for esthetic, detoxification, massage and relaxation 'treatments.' As interest in the use of aromatics increases in this field the need for in-depth training in Aromatherapy for Spa practitioners also becomes imperative. Clients seeking treatments should consider the scope of practice to be expected from a Spa and/or Spa treatments and should carefully decide at what point health concerns require expertise available only from a professional Aromatherapist or other qualified health practitioner. In particular there is concern regarding cure-based treatments such as Raindrop therapy.

Cure based treatments are those that claim to cure diagnosed medical conditions including structural, spinal, or skeletal problem i.e. scoliosis, as is the case with Raindrop Therapy. Any practitioner claiming to cure a diagnosed medical condition or making diagnosis without referring the client to a medical or qualified health practitioner may be practicing medicine without a license. Raindrop therapy is no longer allowed in the country of Norway, as the claims to cure scoliosis etc. are unsubstantiated.

Due to the wide variation in skin sensitivity, essential oil quality, and reaction to topical absorption, it is virtually impossible to gauge exactly how an individual may respond to undiluted application of some of the oils specifically used in Raindrop therapy. Certain of these essential oils can cause dermal reactions ranging from mild to severe and for this reason professional Aromatherapists most often prepare custom blends for their clients to accommodate individual needs. Adequate education in the chemistry, therapeutic attributes, contra-indications and appropriate use of essential oils and other aromatics is absolutely necessary both to maximize the potential health benefits and to prevent any inappropriate effects or actions. Make sure your practitioner is properly educated.

NAHA has created detailed standards for education of qualified Aromatherapists. These educational guidelines require a minimum of 200 hours of specific aromatherapy education including anatomy and physiology relevant to the effects of aromatherapy in the body and basic pathology allowing a practitioner to know when referral to other qualified practitioners is necessary or appropriate. Full details of the NAHA education requirements and a list of qualified schools may be found at www.naha.org where you can click on "education."

NAHA also offers a database of qualified Aromatherapy practitioners and educational establishments as a resource for the public and our members. Source NAHA (11/2011)
            -This information is reprinted with permission from NAHA.

AIA Safety Statement

The AIA is committed to ensuring public safety by providing reliable and current information through public education, qualified practitioner members, recognized schools and the AIA Research Committee.

Promotion of the safe use of aromatherapy, as described in the supporting links below, is the keystone of the AIA organization. Proper assessment of the individual client, high quality essential oils, dosage, dilution, duration, storage of essential oils, and the level of education of the individual selling and/or administering the essential oils are all paramount to the safe practice of aromatherapy. Consulting with a qualified aromatherapist for oil selection, best application methods and concentration levels will ensure safe and effective outcomes.

Aromatherapy in professional practice requires aromatherapists to maintain an incomparable level of safe practice for both the client and the aromatherapist. Safety in the use of essential oils and client care is foremost and fundamental to all AIA aromatherapy education programs. AIA Aromatherapists are required to comply with health and safety issues legally, as prescribed by law, professionally, in personal behavior accepting the AIA's Standards of Practice and ethically adhering to the AIA's Code of the Ethics in practice. These Aromatherapy Standards of Practice guidelines identify the scope of care and reflect professional norms that are inherent in the practice of clinical aromatherapy.

Clinical Member Aromatherapists (CMAIA) are required to maintain a valid First Aid/CPR/AED certificate, possess practitioner liability insurance and obtain 20 hours of Continuing Professional Development training annually, protecting both the client and the aromatherapist within a structure of responsibility.

AIA Standards of Practice, by Laraine K. Pounds, RN, MSN, Adopted by the AIA Membership on October 19, 2007

We are entering a new era in health care where the public is informed regarding choices in health care and the availability of alternative and complementary health care modalities. There is an increasing expectation for mainstream health care providers, such as physicians, nurses, health administrators, and educators to be knowledgeable regarding the existence, availability and benefits of alternative and complementary healthcare modalities.

For the clinical aromatherapy community to grow as a profession and take its place with more-established complementary care modalities, it has the obligation to identify and establish standards of care and practice. Professional standards of practice reflect the current knowledge base and practice in any given field and imply accountability. Standards are dynamic, and subject to evaluation and subsequent change through time as practice norms evolve.

The following Aromatherapy Standards of Practice are stated to identify the scope of care and reflect professional norms that are inherent in the practice of clinical aromatherapy. This is in contrast to the use of essential oils by individuals for home and family use or as a hobby.

Definitions:
Qualified aromatherapist – one who has completed a recognized training in aromatherapy at the minimum level of 200 educational contact hours (such as approved by the National Association of Holistic Aromatherapy or the Alliance of International Aromatherapists) or has been recognized through a standardized exam, such as provided by the Aromatherapy Registration Council

Interdisciplinary cooperation – collaboration by a collective of health care providers in response to a client's health care needs

Standard I: Theory and Practice

The qualified aromatherapist understands and applies appropriate, scientifically sound theory as a basis for essential oil use. The art and science of

Aromatherapy is characterized by the application of relevant information that provides the basis for a skilled use of essential oils and subsequent evaluation of the outcomes.

The Aromatherapy Registration Council (ARC) has categorized the scope of aromatherapy education based on historical input by leading schools in aromatherapy. For example, the knowledge base includes, but not limited to:

[1] Basic Concepts of Aromatherapy - essential oils, sources, history, client assessment;
[2] Scientific Principles - botany, extraction, chemistry, anatomy and physiology
[3] Administration - therapeutics, safety, delivery methods, contraindications, blending
[4] Professional Issues – documentation, quality control, ethics

This standard also applies to those engaged in fragrance blending or product development as these activities are predicated on the basic concepts relating to essential oils, chemistry, and blending.

As a member of the Alliance of International Aromatherapists, I shall:

1. conduct myself in a professional and ethical manner in relation to my clients, health professionals, and the general public.
2. recognize that the public has the right to share in decisions pertaining to their health care. I shall educate and guide clients toward this goal and actively encourage them to take responsibility for their care and well-being.
3. represent my education and qualifications honestly in advertising and practice and acknowledge the limitations of my skills, as indicated.
4. provide the highest quality of aromatherapy products available.
5. provide services within the scope and the limits of my training and to refer to appropriate qualified professionals as indicated.
6. maintain professional confidentiality except when failure to take action could constitute a danger to others.
7. refrain from guaranteeing a specific wellness outcome, acknowledging that aromatic extracts support self-healing and that holistic health outcomes are influenced by many factors.
8. visibly display a copy of the AIA Code of Ethics for the benefit of employees and the public.
9. avoid discrimination against individuals on the basis of race, creed, religion, gender, age and national origin.
10. appreciate the importance of thoroughness in the performance of duty, compassion with clients, and the significance of the tasks I perform.

11. respect the law and avoid dishonest, unethical, or illegal practices.
12. refuse primary responsibility for health care for any client. Individuals who are licensed or otherwise authorized to provide primary health care are excluded.

Standard IX: Research

The qualified aromatherapist contributes to the continuing development of knowledge of clinical aromatherapy through data collection, research activities and documentation of findings. Source AIA (11/2011)

-This information is reprinted with permission from AIA

The Personal Care Products Council Consumer Commitment Code

Preamble

Cosmetic products are the safest products regulated by the U.S. Food and Drug Administration (FDA), a fact that has been recognized by a number of FDA Commissioners over the last several decades.

To further strengthen industry safeguards for consumers, the Personal Care Products Council has instituted a Consumer Commitment Code for the cosmetic industry. This incorporates and strengthens some practices already in place for most companies, such as the current reporting of manufacturing establishments; and it includes new practices such as a Safety Information Summary Program that makes information relevant to cosmetic product and ingredient safety readily available to the FDA upon request.

The Council's Board of Directors unanimously supports the principles and practices embodied in this Code. It will formally take effect for all Council members on January 1, 2007. Throughout 2006, the Council will commit substantial resources to educating its members on the practices embodied in the Code and gaining their commitments to the Code. The Council will also reach out to many related trade associations and other organizations to encourage broad recognition of the Code by 2007.

During this time, we will continue to work closely with the Food and Drug Administration to provide as much information regarding cosmetic safety as the agency needs to evaluate the safety of the products. In providing FDA with access to this information we seek to provide consumers with the continued confidence that the proper steps are being taken by government and industry to assure the continued safety of all cosmetic products, and to allow consumers to make fully informed choices when purchasing cosmetic products.

The Personal Care Products Council Consumer Commitment Code

The following principles constitute the Personal Care Products Council Consumer Commitment Code:

1. A company should market cosmetic products only after ensuring that every ingredient and finished product has been substantiated for safety. The decision that an ingredient has been substantiated for safety may be based on a finding by the Cosmetic Ingredient Review Expert Panel that such ingredient is safe for the use intended by the company or on other appropriate data and information.

2. When marketing a cosmetic product containing an ingredient that exceeds limits on concentration or product type established by the Cosmetic Ingredient Review Expert Panel, a company should possess information sufficient to substantiate the safety of the ingredient for its intended use in such product and be willing to make that information available for inspection by the Food and Drug Administration.

3. When marketing a cosmetic product containing an ingredient for which the Cosmetic Ingredient Review Expert Panel has found insufficient data to determine safety, a company should possess information sufficient to substantiate the safety of the ingredient for its intended use in such product and be willing to make that information available for inspection by the Food and Drug Administration.

4. A company should participate in the applicable parts of the FDA Voluntary Cosmetic Reporting Program set forth in 21 CFR Parts 710 and 720 for products marketed in the United States, and file timely reports regarding its manufacturing establishments and ingredient usage.

5. Although adverse events that are both serious and unexpected are extremely rare for cosmetic products, a company should notify the Food and Drug Administration of any known serious and unexpected adverse event as a result of the use of any of its cosmetic products marketed and used in the United States. "Serious" and "Unexpected" are defined in accordance with FDA's definition for such experiences related to drugs in 21 CFR 314.80(a). Information related to other product experiences as described in the Council's Safety Information Summary Program should be maintained in the safety information summary described in Paragraph 6 below. Such information should be made available for inspection by FDA under the conditions specified in that program.

6. A company should maintain a safety information summary of ingredient and product safety information and data regarding its cosmetic products marketed in the United States as specified in the Council's Safety Information Summary Program Guideline, and make any information in that safety information summary available for inspection by FDA under the conditions specified in that program.

The Code should not be construed as a legal standard. All companies have an independent obligation to ascertain that their cosmetic products comply with all current laws and regulations.

The Council's Safety Information Summary Program Guideline

The Program:

The purpose of the program is to provide a means for the U.S. Food and Drug Administration (FDA) to access proprietary information on cosmetic, toiletry, and fragrance formulations. In order to assure the availability of necessary information, companies should compile the following information on each individual formulation they market in the U.S. (except that formulations that change only by color may have a single compilation for all), and should make those compilations (Safety Information Summaries) available to FDA for inspection when requested as described below.

Safety Information Summary Contents:

- An identification code for each product using the formulation so that individual products can be related to the relevant formulation.

- The semi-quantitative formula for the formulation, using INCI nomenclature to identify the raw materials and providing their concentrations in ranges of >50%, 50 to >25%, 25 to >10%, 10 to >5%, 5 to >1%, 1 to >0.1% and 0.1% or less.

- Raw material specifications, particularly considering limitations for possible impurities such as microbial flora, heavy metals, etc., and reference to the methods used to determine the specifications (or general discussions of the methods if they are not published).

- Finished product specifications, including limitations on microbial content, and reference to the methods used to determine the specifications (or general discussions of the methods if they are not published).

- A summary of the manufacturing process, which may be represented by a simple flow chart.

- A statement that the product has been manufactured under the good manufacturing principles as outlined in the Council's Quality Assurance Guidelines.

- A statement that the product's safety has been substantiated in accordance with the principles of the Council's Safety Testing Guidelines, and a summary of the elements that are the basis of the safety assessment, with appropriate citations.

- A computation of the incidence of adverse health effects in the United States (e.g., number per 100,000 or million units distributed) that have been medically confirmed as caused by the product in question. Minor, transient health effects need not be included in this computation.

Safety Information Summary Availability:

All of a company's relevant safety information summaries may be kept in one central location, in multiple locations, or may be a part of a database or databases from which a safety information summary can be readily assembled. Request for a particular safety information summary should be made by written request by the FDA District Director stating the basis for the request. The request should be made to the CEO, General Counsel or other official designated by the company to receive such requests. The request should specify the information the FDA is relying on to question the safety of the product, and must be based on a legitimate and specific safety concern or question related to a product, or ingredient in a product, manufactured by that company. The company should provide the safety information summary for inspection at a mutually agreed location within a reasonable time after receiving the request. Source PCPC (11/2011)

-This information is reprinted with permission from PCPC

:: Chapter 10 ::
Do Not Pass Go Without
Collecting Safety Information

What's What

Testing is an essential part of the aromatherapy industry. It keeps everyone honest by revealing whether an essential oil has been extended or adulterated. There are many common marketing terms for "grade" of essential oils including therapeutic grade, aroma therapeutic grade, perfume grade, massage grade, pure grades 1,2,3, and so forth. This is where the marketing department comes in, because most of these "grades" or "standards" are trademarked by the company selling that particular grade of essential oil.

This marketing ploy creates a dependence on that supplier for the "grade" that is perceived to only be available from them. The perception is true, because the grade was randomly set by the supplier and cannot be followed by another supplier. There is no regulatory agency that defines, monitors, or enforces these marketing "grades" and "standards." There is little to no difference in the chemical make-up of essential oils sold with these various marketing ploys.

A true standard that can be followed all the way back to the crop of plant material is the term certified organic. If an essential oil is listed as certified organic then it means that the plant material used was cultivated and processed according to the National Organic Program (NOP) standards as defined by the USDA. You should be able to trace the certifying agency back an agency, like the Oregon Tilth which works directly with growers and manufacturers to assure that the NOP standards are being met by all parties using the USDA label. Agencies like Oregon Tilth monitor the farm production and address issues when guidelines are being overlooked or ignored.

No matter what you hear about grades and standards, the reality is that there are only two legitimate standards that are certified in aromatherapy: Food Chemical Codex (FCC) and certified organic. You will see other terms such as "non-sprayed," "cultivated without chemicals," or "wild-crafted" as well, but these are not certified terms. And then you see the purely marketing term "therapeutic" grade and various scales of "grades" of essential oils both from the marketing department. Essential oil chemical make-up is related more about where a plant grew, and the climate of a given year, than a random and uncertified grade placed on it by a supplier.

There are also terms used in the food and drug industry that, when also seen in the world of essential oils, are often misused. For example, an essential oil should never be labeled United States Pharmacopeia (USP) grade or National Formulary (NF). These standards are regulated by The United States Pharmacopeia, which is a non-governmental, not-for-profit public health organization that sets standards for all prescriptions, Over-the-Counter (OTC) medicines, and other health care products manufactured or sold in the United States.

By Federal law, all prescription and OTC medicines available in the United States must meet USP "pharmaceutical grade" standards. However, essential oils are not allowed to be sold as OTC drugs. If a company makes claims that put essential oils into the category of healing, curing or remedying, by definition, that company is creating an OTC drug.

In my early years as an aromatherapist, I longed for the day when essential oils would become part of traditional medicine, or at least be considered as over the counter drugs. After years in the cosmetic industry, I am grateful that aromatherapy remains an alternative treatment available to everyone. I have been through the process of manufacturing an OTC sunscreen and learned that the cost, paperwork, and regulation of making essential oils into OTC drugs would put the majority of aromatherapists out of work.

FCC is one of the few US Pharmacopeia terms that can be used in essential oils. The Food Chemicals Codex (FCC) is an internationally recognized standard for testing the purity and identity of food, food ingredients, food additives and food processing aids. The FCC standard is more commonly found as a standard in aromatherapy because many essential oils are used by the food and flavor industry. Once an essential oil is given the FCC rating it tends to remain with the product even when it leaves the food industry and enters the aromatherapy market.

Forms of Essential Oil Adulteration
Essential Oil Dupes are essential oils sometimes adulterated by creating oil from other, less expensive, oils that smell like it. An example would be using palmarosa mixed with rosewood and selling it as rose.

Stretching is the practice of extending an expensive essential oil with a less expensive essential oil. An example would be stretching neroli by adding petigrain.

Chemical Constituent Stretching is the practice of adding a chemical constituent that naturally occurs in the essential oil to it in order to stretch it. An example of this practice is adding the chemical constituent linalyl acetate to lavender essential oil to stretch it further.

Using Fragrance Chemicals involves creating synthetic fragrance oil and selling it as an essential oil. For instance, creating chamomile fragrance oil and selling it as Roman chamomile essential oil.

Country Blending is the practice of using a cheap version of an essential oil from one country and blending with an expensive version of the same essential oil from another country. For instance: mixing inexpensive Chinese lavender with an expensive French lavender and then selling it as French lavender.

Carrier Oil Extending is the use of cheap carrier oil mixed with an expensive essential oil and then not disclosing the carrier oil on the label.

Alcohol Extension is the practice of extending an essential oil with alcohol and then not disclosing it on the label.

Purity Tests for Essential Oils
Your nose is the least expensive testing tool available. However, it takes years of practice and experience to develop a well-trained nose.

Gas Chromatography (GC) is an analytical technique used to separate components. The test is run by vaporizing a sample and then separating the constituents by their solubility. The test results look like a graph filled with peaks and valleys.

Mass Spectrometry (MS) is an instrumental analytical technique used to concretely identify components. The mass spectrometer shatters molecules. Each fragment has a different mass associated with it, which gives the fingerprint of that molecule.

Flame Ionization Detector (FID) is a device that gives the quantity of each component. It is the only test that gives the actual percentage of components in an essential oil.

Specific Gravity tells the ratio of the weight of an essential oil to the weight of an equal volume of water measured at a specific temperature.

Optical Rotation is a test that tells the rotation of the plane of polarized light by transmission through an optically active substance.

Refractive Index is measured with a refractometer. It is a measure of the bending of parallel rays of light of a given frequency when passed from a less dense medium into a denser medium.

Contraindications and Safety Warnings

You will find that contraindications are one of the most debated topics in the aromatherapy world. Some believe in erring on the side of caution while others throw caution to the wind. Historically many properties and contraindications given for essential oils are from herbal use and oral use, but the information is still very important.

International Fragrance Association Safety Warnings
IFRA Banned Sensitizers: costus root, elecampane, verbena, fig leaf, peru balsam.

IFRA Severely Restricted Oils: calamus oil (*Acorus calamus*), *Backhousia citriodora*, lemongrass, *Litsea cubeba*, melissa.

IFRA Restricted Oils: cinnamon bark, cassia, oakmoss extracts, treemoss extracts, fennel, opoponax, styrax, verbena absolute, pinaceae extracts, Peru balsam, and tagetes.

IFRA listed Phototoxic/sensitizers: bergamot, orange, lemon, grapefruit, lime, tangerine, mandarin, blood orange, rue, fig leaf absolute, tagetes, angelica root, celery, clove bud, pimento, cornmint, peppermint, cassia, savory, clove leaf, thyme, folded orange.

IFRA Severe Irritants: garlic, massoia, horseradish, mustard.

IFRA Neurotoxicants: hyssop, camphor, cedar leaf, tansy.

IFRA Hepatotoxicants: pennyroyal, buchu, spearmint, catnip, peppermint, cornmint, aniseed, star anise.

IFRA Teratogens: savin (*Juniperus sabina*), Spanish lavender (*Salvia lavandulifolia*)

IFRA Methyl Salicylate Toxicity Causing: wintergreen, sweet birch.

Most aromatherapists will agree on the following Contraindications.
Internal Use of Essential Oils: No matter what internet idea you read, essential oils should never be taken internally; many are highly toxic, and some can be fatal if consumed. Internal consumption of essential oils is always contraindicated.

Contact Dermatitis: Many safe essential oils can cause a form of contact dermatitis in some people with sensitive skins including: ajowan, allspice, sweet basil, black pepper, borneol-type thyme, cajeput, caraway, Virginian cedarwood, cinnamon leaf, clove bud, cornmint, eucalyptus, garlic, ginger, lemon, parsley, peppermint, pine needle (Scotch and longleaf), white thyme, and turmeric.

Sensitization: Contact sensitization is a hot topic regarding essential oils and cosmetics in general. Sensitization is an allergic reaction that can occur when the body's immune system reacts against a particular chemical constituent of an essential oil. Severe reactions may be avoided by doing a 24-hour patch-test on individuals with sensitive skins before use of any oil known to cause sensitization. Some essential oils are more apt than others to cause contact sensitization. These include: ylang ylang, cassia, cinnamon bark, costus root, bergamot, fig leaf, elecampane, verbena, aniseed, clove stem and clove bud. other essential oils known to cause sensitization in some people include: French basil, bay laurel, benzoin, cade, cananga, Virginian cedarwood, chamomile, citronella, garlic, geranium, ginger, hops, jasmine, lemon, lemongrasss, lemon balm, *litsea cuba*, lovage, mastic, mint, orange, peru balsam, pine (Scotch and longleaf), styrax, tea tree, white thyme, tolu balsam, turmeric, turpentine, valerian, vanilla, violet, and yarrow.

Photosensitivity: Some essential oils render the skin hypersensitive to the sun, causing skin reactions in the presence of ultraviolet light. This is called phototoxicity or photosensitivity. Photosensitizing essential oils include: angelica root and seed, caraway, cassia, cinnamon bark, lime, bitter orange, bergamot, lemon, cumin, lovage, lemon verbena, melissa, rue, and ginger.

Phototoxic oils: (generally citrus oils) including angelica root, cumin, ginger, bergamot, lemon, lime, lovage, mandarin, orange, tagetes, and verbena.

High Blood Pressure: Some essential oils are generally avoided for those with high blood pressure (hypertension), but honestly, the evidence is shaky, especially with aromatic massage proving to actually lower blood pressure. To be extra cautious avoid hyssop, rosemary, sage (*Salvia officinalis*), and thyme.

Low Blood Pressure: Avoid clary sage (*Salvia sclarea*), lavender, lemon, marjoram, melissa, and ylang ylang.

Cancer: Clients with cancer should be always treated with great caution. It is extremely important to communicate that essential oils will soothe, comfort, and aid the patient but not cure them. Avoid anise, basil, fennel, laurel, myrtle, nutmeg, and star anise.

Epilepsy: Avoid white camphor, sweet fennel, hyssop, peppermint, rosemary, all types of sage and tea tree.

Diabetes: Avoid angelica.

Glaucoma: Avoid lemongrass, melissa, and litsea.

Kidney Disease: Avoid Indian Dill, juniper, parsley leaf/seed, and black pepper.

Cardiac Disease: Avoid nutmeg.

Liver Disease: Avoid Indian dill, parsley leaf/seed, or oils containing menthol.

Acute Respiratory: Avoid garlic, onion, and sage (*Salvia officinalis*).

When using homeopathic treatments: Avoid black pepper, camphor, eucalyptus, peppermint, and rosemary.

Pregnancy: The use of essential oils during pregnancy remains a contentious subject debated by many in the industry. From aromatherapist to aromatherapist you may get varying answers when it comes to prenatal aromatherapy. Some believe that essential oils should be completely avoided during the first trimester. Others believe they should be avoided all together, and then there are others that don't avoid them at all.

I am asked about aromatherapy in pregnancy most commonly by those who become pregnant while running their own soap, aromatherapy, spa, or personal care product line. However, I worked as an aromatherapist through two of my three pregnancies. I handled, blended and manufactured using essential oils on a daily basis with no ill-effects on my pregnancy or babies. I also used aromatherapy for massage, and baths to treat my stress, body aches, fatigue, morning sickness and labor successfully. To confidently use aromatherapy in pregnancy, it is vital to understand the root of aromatherapy warnings and contraindications.

The History of Aromatherapy Warnings for Pregnancy

The fears surrounding aromatherapy in pregnancy are found in historical cases in which essential oils were misused purposefully or accidentally. All cases of adverse reactions in pregnancy are related to women drinking large doses of essential oils. Any responsible aromatherapist would never suggest that essential oils should be consumed. Essential oils, no matter what the circumstances are, should never be taken orally.

There has *never* been a reported case of a woman or baby being harmed by topical or inhalation therapy used during pregnancy or labor. Aromatherapists all warn their clients away from pennyroyal essential oil due to a case in the USA in which a woman drank a large dose of pennyroyal in order to induce an abortion that proved fatal to her (Gold and Cates, 1980). One out of four cases in which pregnant women accidently drank camphor oil instead of castor oil resulted in the death of the baby (Weiss and Catalano, 1976).

Another reported case in which pennyroyal and parsley seed were taken in large doses caused hepatotoxicity which resulted in the death of the baby. There are two other cases in which women consumed the same large doses of pennyroyal (100 to 200 times the recommended topical application) in which both the mothers and the babies survived unharmed. It is cases like this that give essential oils their warnings and contraindications.

A large number of midwives and nurses worldwide have become Certified and/or Registered Aromatherapists over the past ten years. Aromatherapy in the labor and delivery room has been a common practice in England since 1987. After 22 years of regular use of aromatherapy by midwives and nurses in England, one would think that if topical and inhalation usage of essential oils was dangerous during pregnancy then there would be a case reported, but there have been none.

The most recent case of a pregnant woman consuming essential oils resulted in a midwife losing her job and license, but no harm came to the mother or baby. The Daily Mail reported that in North Wales, midwife Sandra Hughes, who was trained in aromatherapy, mixed some sweet almond oil with two drops of lavender and one drop of lime in a plastic cup and left it by her patient's bedside. Her intention was for it to be massaged onto the patient, but while Sandra was out of the room, there was a mix-up and the patient drank the blend. The mother and baby were monitored but suffered no ill effects. Communication and proper application of essential oils is vital.

In reality, essential oils have been safely used by pregnant women for thousands of years. Most perfumes on the market use essentials oils, or components of essential oils, combined with synthetic fragrance chemicals. Yet we never see a warning on perfume bottles to avoid use during pregnancy. Chemical components of essential oils have historically been used in the production of fragrance oils and have caused no ill effects during pregnancy. For instance, nutmeg essential oil is one of the ingredients used to make green tea fragrance oil. Below you will find nutmeg on the "essential oils to avoid during the first trimester" list, however, it is a component of a common fragrance oil that pregnant women use every day all over the world with no ill effects.

According to Martin Watt, "There are NO essential oils that, used externally, are proven as harmful to a developing foetus. The vast majority of oils you have listed are common food additives. This is all stuff from the aromatherapy novel writers."

Be aware that during pregnancy a woman has a heightened sense of smell. Always use half-doses of essential oils for pregnant women. The highest percentage of essential oil in aromatherapy products for pregnant women is 2%. Be completely in tune with what essential oils she finds repulsive or dislikes during pregnancy. I have found that most pregnant women in the first trimester of pregnancy find essential oils that are highly hormonal to be distasteful. My theory is that her body is warning her away from essential oils with properties that it does not need at a given time. I have also found that women crave and adore highly hormonal essential oils when they have PMS or are going through menopause. It is as if her nose is leading her to oils that she needs at given times in her life.

There is no documentation on whether or not essential oils pass through the placenta, but because they have low molecular weights and are negatively charged molecules it is feasible to assume that they do. The placenta acts a barrier to positively charged molecules but negatively charged molecules do cross the placenta (Maickel and Snodgrass 1973) which makes choosing the right essential oils used during pregnancy vital. For instance, savin and Spanish sage (*Salvia lavandulifolia*) could be extremely detrimental during pregnancy. They are not common essential oils used in aromatherapy. However, they are a good example of why precaution is used by aromatherapists.

Savin (*Juniperus savina*) and Spanish sage (*Salvia lavandulifolia*) essential oils contain the compound sabinyl acetate which has been proven to have a teratogenic effect (ability to interfere with normal embryonic development) in laboratory animals (Guba 2002).

Many essential oils are believed to have emmenagogic actions (cause uterine contractions believed to induce menstrual cycle) and are believed to be dangerous to use during pregnancy. However, many aromatherapists believe that emmenagogic actions are not enough to affect a stable pregnancy. The controversy lies in the history of a pregnant woman. If a woman has had miscarriages in the past, it is always best to err on the side of caution and avoid emmenagogic essential oils.

The safest essential oils to use in pregnancy are the citrus essential oils which include bergamot, lemon, lime, sweet orange, mandarin, grapefruit, and tangerine. They all have such low molecular weights that they disperse into the air shortly after application. There are no contraindications, no safety data, and no warnings that are related in any way to pregnancy.

Occasionally you might find them on a list of essential oils to avoid during pregnancy, but that is only when the aromatherapist has taken every essential oil with a warning and included them in their "avoid during pregnancy" list.

The only warning for all citrus essential oils is that they may be phototoxic, which means that they may increase the risk of sunburn when used undiluted. But since you won't be using any essential oil over 2% on a pregnant woman, you are well within safety limits.

I highly recommend the use of grapefruit essential oil for massage throughout pregnancy. It is the only citrus essential oil that is not phototoxic, so you even avoid that warning. It uplifts the spirit, eases the mind, helps with water retention, has an astringent property that leaves the skin feeling great, and is generally known as safe in all cases. If you were to add one essential oil for pregnancy massage, grapefruit is the safest, most universally liked essential oil on the market.

Common Essential Oil Warning for Pregnancy

Emmenagogic essential oils: basil, carrot seed, blue and roman chamomile, sweet fennel, clary sage (*Salvia sclarea*), juniper berry, lavender, sweet marjoram, myrrh, rose, rosemary, peppermint.

Safe throughout pregnancy: bergamot, lemon, lime, sweet orange, mandarin, grapefruit, and tangerine.

Avoid in first trimester: palmarosa, sweet fennel, peppermint, carrot seed, nutmeg, bay, anise, cinnamon, sage (*Salvia officinalis*) myrrh, juniper, lovage, roman and blue chamomile, cajuput, peppermint, melissa, marjoram, rose otto, rosemary, clary sage (*Salvia sclarea*), vetiver, basil, oregano, black pepper, sandalwood.

Essential oils to avoid completely during pregnancy: savin, Spanish sage (*Salvia lavandulifolia*), angelica, calamus, buchu, wormwood, davana, mugwort, mustard, wild basil, calamint, wormseed, brown and blue and white camphor, horseradish, blue cypress, turmeric, bitter fennel, Bulgarian geranium, wintermint, star anise, cade oil, latana, Spanish lavender, bog myrtle, dog basil, Brazilian sassafras, parsley seed, lavender cotton, sassafras, tansy, thuja, dill, yarrow, tarragon, caraway, camphor, broad-leaved peppermint, hyssop, pennyroyal, spearmint, rosemary, tagette.

It is critically important to know the difference between various essential oils. For instance, clary sage (*Salvia sclarea*) is very helpful in the last stages of labor, yet Sage (*Salvia officinalis*) is contraindicated for pregnancy. Aromatherapists use Latin nomenclature to identify essential oils for that very reason. For instance, clary sage is *Salvia sclarea* and *Salvia officinalis* is sage. When buying essential oils, always cross check them by using their Latin nomenclature in combination with their common name. This will ensure consistency and safety above all. Using both names to identify and crosscheck your essential oil choices is the best practice to protect your business.

157

Do you need an MSDS?

A very common question that many in the aromatherapy, cosmetic, soap industry ask is, "Should I collect a Material Safety Data Sheet (MSDS) or not?" The best way to answer that question is to give you a thorough understanding of what the MSDS is designed to do.

The purpose of an MSDS is to inform you of proper handling of a material, first aid treatment, accident response protocol, effect on human health, chemicals with which it can adversely react, as well as the chemical make-up and physical properties prior to usage. The MSDS is often used by employers, employees, emergency responders, freight forwarders, soapmakers, and home crafters. Sometimes you may find an MSDS formatted differently by some manufacturers, but they all contain the exact same information required by law. Once you get the hang of reading MSDS you won't even notice the differences.

The MSDS is a single document prepared by the manufacturer that contains all the information about the chemical make-up, use, storage, handling, emergency procedures, and the potential health effects related to a hazardous material. MSDS was originally intended for hazardous materials only in order to comply with Federal regulations. However, many materials with no hazards now have an MSDS simply for product liability purposes alone.

Today an ingredient that has an MSDS is not necessarily a hazardous material, nor may it cause health effects. Much of the information from the MSDS information is misused to make an ingredient look bad in personal care items. This is the practice of organizations like the Environmental Working Group and their database Skin Deep. The fact is that an MSDS sheet is simply giving information about the safe handling of the ingredient at full concentration, which does not translate to normal cosmetic usage, since you never use any ingredient at 100% concentration in any cosmetic formula.

A perfect example of how the MSDS does not translate to the finished product is with lye. The MSDS shows that it causes eye, skin, digestive, and respiratory burns. However, in the finished product it causes no ill effect to the consumer. Unfortunately, those with regulatory agendas misuse the MSDS information to create propaganda against many ingredients that are perfectly safe in the finished product.

All MSDS information is required to contain the same uniform categories of information including chemical identity, health hazard data, manufacturer information, precautions for safe handling and use, hazardous ingredients, exposure controls/personal protection, physical/chemical properties as well as fire and explosion hazard data. When new regulatory information or health effects information becomes available, the MSDS must be updated.

Many are concerned that the MSDS is hard to interpret. That is because the original purpose of an MSDS was for industrial hygienists, chemical engineers, and safety professionals who were trained to read them. The MSDS has become more widely used but the language was never changed to laymen terms.

If you are manufacturing with raw materials, you should get a copy of the MSDS for your knowledge and records. The most important parts to read include the name of the material, hazards, safe handling, storage requirements, and emergency procedures. Store the MSDS in a file that will be easy to access if emergency responders such as Occupational Safety and Health Administration (OSHA), fire fighters, hazardous material crews, emergency medical technicians and emergency room personnel need them.

If you have employees, you are required by law to maintain readily accessible MSDS for any hazardous materials "known to be present" in the workplace. The MSDS is designed for employees who will occupationally come in contact with hazardous materials. The OSHA Hazard Communication Standard requires that safety training on proper handling of materials be conducted and all hazardous materials be labeled appropriately. If you have contractors on the premises you must inform them of the potential hazards. The MSDS is designed to help employers and employees protect themselves from hazardous chemical exposures and to teach them to handle material safely. Not only is it important to follow all those steps, but it is critical to log and document it all.

Are you left wondering if you need to collect MSDS sheets or not? The answer is simple. Do any of the ingredients you use have a hazardous rating above zero? Do you use lye? Do you have employees? If the answer to any one of these questions is yes, you must collect an MSDS for ingredients you use with a hazard rating above zero.

The National Fire Protection Association (NFPA) believes that the MSDS and labeling of material with the NFPA hazard diamond are relevant for anything flammable. The NFPA hazard diamond uses a standard system for identification of hazardous of materials for emergency response. You don't really want your emergency responder to have to read the whole sheet; the NFPA hazard diamond on the material will tell them everything they need to know in a glance.

My Top 12 Aromatherapy Safety Rules
History and safety testing have given us useful aromatherapy data. For review of this chapter, please study the following twelve rules that I think are the most important when it comes to using essential oils safely.

Rule #1 - **Never consume** essential oils. Even if you read a book by an aromatherapist from a country that uses essential oils internally, they should never be consumed. The practice of consuming essential oils is dangerous and was designed to be done under the care of an aromatherapist trained in that form of therapy. In addition, studies have shown that topical aromatherapy is more effective than internal aromatherapy methods.

Rule #2 - Always dilute your essential oils before applying them to the skin. There are a very small handful of exceptions to this rule including lavender and tea tree which can be occasionally applied neat, or directly, to the skin. In different aromatherapy books there may be recommendations of essential oils over 3% in massage oils but it simply isn't necessary. Less is more in the world of essential oils. There is no need to overdose and it is always better to be safe than sorry.

Essential oils are incredibly potent and need to be dispersed into a carrier before applying them to the skin. You wouldn't wrap your body in 30 lbs. of plant material so don't apply that much or more directly onto your skin. Typically, essential oils are diluted into products at 1 to 3% - sometimes less and sometimes more, but that is the general rule of thumb. Some essential oils have an intense aroma and price tag combination that allows for their use as low as 0.1% Take jasmine, blue chamomile and neroli for example.

Raindrop therapy is a good example of how undiluted and too high of concentrations of essential oils can be dangerous. This method of applying essential oils is the practice of dripping pure undiluted essential oils directly onto the skin which has many adverse effects. People have had burns, skin irritation, and intense detoxification effects that could have been avoided if this dangerous practice was no longer taught. The human body does not need to detoxify at such a rapid rate, and the skin should not come in direct contact with undiluted essential oils. The practice of raindrop therapy has become such a big problem as a multi-level marketing ploy that NAHA has set up a reporting site to document burns and adverse reactions caused by the spread of this dangerous misinformation.

Rule #3 - Keep all essential oils out of the reach of children; they are notorious for putting everything in their mouths. Compared to adults, essential oils should be used in half the dosage rate for children for topical application. They are not miniature adults, and their bodies were not designed to process the same ratio of essential oils on their skin. I have safely used aromatherapy on all three of my children since 1998.

I heard of a case of a woman who read that tangerine essential oil would help with hyperactivity in children. She decided to put undiluted tangerine essential oil directly on the palms of her child's hands. Thankfully, tangerine is a safe enough essential oil and the child suffered no serious ill effect. But she had decided to try it on a day that the child had a big test to take at school, and the high concentration of tangerine oil knocked the child out for the entire day and he slept through his test, lunch, dinner…and into the next morning.

Rule #4 - Stay with the tried and true essential oils. Avoid ones that are not the common essential oils used historically in aromatherapy. Unless you understand the chemistry, it is best to stick with the commonly used essential oils. A trained aromatherapist can read the chemical composition of an essential oil profile and make an educated decision about the safety of an essential oil. But without that training you would not know whether you should avoid or use essential oils based on their chemical composition of aldehydes, esthers, ketones, phenols, and monoterpene hydrocarbons.

Rule #5 - Know which essential oils to avoid or use with caution. Avoid them even if you like the way they smell or the properties that you read about them. Essential oils to be avoided altogether include: unrectified bitter almond, basil *ct. methyl chavicol*, birch, boldo leaf, blue cypress, bitter fennel, bog myrtle, buchu, unrectified cade, calamint, calamus, (brown, blue or yellow) camphor, cassia, cinnamon bark, costus, davana, dog basil, elecampane, fig leaf, horseradish, jaborandi, lantana, *melaleuca bracteata*, mustard, mugwort, parsley seed, pennyroyal, rue, dalmatian sage, santolina, sassafras, savin, tansy, tarragon, tea absolute, thuja, tonka bean, verbena, wintergreen, wormseed, and wormwood.

Essential oils that should be used with caution or at very low dosages include: yarrow, dill, tarragon, caraway, white camphor, hyssop, spearmint, rosemary *ct. verbenone*, and tagette.

Essential oils that should be heavily diluted due to potential skin irritation include: cassia, cinnamon bark, cinnamon leaf, cumin, lemongrass, oregano, clove stem, clove bud, clove leaf, wild thyme, and red thyme.

Rule #6 - Always wear protective gear while handling essential oils. Remember that essential oils are very concentrated and should not be applied directly to the skin. If you wear gloves while handling essential oils you lessen the chance of spilling undiluted essential oils directly onto your hands. Even if it doesn't hurt at the moment, it could hurt later. A good example is how peppermint essential oil spilled directly onto your hands might not hurt at the moment, but later when you touch your eye, it will burn like crazy.

Rule #7 – Work in a well-ventilated area. Remember that essential oils can enter the body through inhalation. Some essential oils can cause euphoria, sleepiness or can be extremely stimulating. In a closed space with poor circulation the essential oils can become overwhelming.

Rule #8 - Use extra caution when using essential oils on children and the elderly. The dosages should be at least half that of what you would use for a healthy adult. And essential oils are toxic to cats so never ever use essential oils on them.

Rule #9 - Use common sense. Essential oils are safe when used in moderation. Many substances on earth are toxic when used in the extreme. Too much water can lead to water poisoning, and carrots, tomatoes, saffron, and mustard will all cause illness when consumed in excess.

Rule #10 - To safeguard your business, do not make healing claims about your products. That would transform your cosmetic into a drug. The rules and regulations for drugs are completely different, and aromatherapy does not qualify on any monograph for approved over-the-counter drugs.

Rule #11 – Always use the botanical name for essential oils when ordering. I never make an aromatherapy decision without reviewing the botanical name. The botanical name tells the genus and species of the plant and includes information about the variety, cultivar, chemotype, and hybrid when needed. Often these details are the difference between an essential oil being safe for use or not.

Rule #12 – Check contraindications of an essential oil before using it. You don't want to be making a sleepy time bath with essential oils that are contraindicated for insomnia like peppermint, basil, lemon verbena, cornmint, or rosemary.

:: Chapter 11 ::
Cosmetics, Drugs, and Soaps... Oh My!

Drugs, Aromatherapy and Cosmetics

There is a fine line between drugs, aromatherapy and cosmetics. It is important that as aromatherapy and cosmetic companies we clearly stay on our side of the line and not walk the tightrope between the two definitions. Our job as cosmetic companies is to cleanse and to promote beauty. We have plenty to do inside our own world without tinkering with the drug definitions.

There are some that claim, "If you can't pronounce it, it can't be good for you." This statement was made by the Environmental Working Group and placed on a banner at Natural Products Expo. It should take the award as the most uninformed, illogical statement ever made by a political action group. It simply proves they have no business attempting to be experts in the field of cosmetics and personal care like they attempt to be with their fatally flawed Skin Deep Database.

International standardization to ensure consumer safety worldwide means that we can't just put everything into basic English. It means that some words in cosmetic labeling will be difficult to pronounce; I still can't say *Butyrospermum parkii*, but Shea Butter is as safe as ingredients come. Whether you can pronounce the INCI term or not, the use of INCI nomenclature is the law. **NOTE:** All *italics* that follow were added by me as examples and not official FDA comments. All quotes are from the FDA.

What is a Cosmetic?

A cosmetic is defined in the Federal Food, Drug, Cosmetic Act, Section 201 (i) as being:

"Articles intended to be rubbed (*serums, moisturizers, etc.*), poured (*bubble baths, oils, etc.*), sprinkled (*body powders, bath powders, etc.*), or spray on (*body deodorant, perfumes, body mists, etc.*), introduced or otherwise applied to the human body or any part thereof for cleansing (*cleansers, exfoliants, etc.*), beautifying (*exfoliants, moisturizers, makeup, etc.*), promoting attractiveness (*makeup, perfumes, deodorants, etc.*) or altering the appearance (*cleansers, exfoliants, serums, moisturizers, makeup, etc.*)"

Cosmetics: are not as regulated as drugs. They do not require pre-clearance by FDA, and GMP is not required. Cosmetics have simple labeling regulations, and voluntary adverse effects reporting. You cannot make any claims other than cosmetic usage even if it is accurate or nature's wonder "drug." The Cosmetic Legality Principle does not require pre-market approval or notification of products or ingredients, clearance of products safety, or substantiation of product performance claims (*moisturizing, cleansing, deodorizing, etc.*). Mandatory establishment or product registration is currently voluntary.

Cosmetics exclude soap, but if your soap claims to be "cleansing, beautifying or moisturizing," it is a cosmetic and must be labeled appropriately. This means you are required to include a full International Nomenclature of Cosmetic Ingredients (INCI) ingredient list on every bar of soap and follow all cosmetic regulations ONLY if you make claims that go above and beyond cleansing, beautifying, or moisturizing. The Manufacturer is responsible for making cosmetics safe and they must not be adulterated or misbranded.

Adulterated is defined as harmful or injurious to user under customary conditions of use such as microbiology, unapproved color additive, chemical contaminant or prohibited ingredient.

Misbranded is defined as when labeling is false or misleading; Package does not exhibit labeling information required by statute or regulation; Packaging not in compliance with 1970 Poison Prevention Packaging Act (PPPA). All cosmetic ingredient lists must use INCI (International Nomenclature of Cosmetic Ingredients) names for all cosmetic ingredients in a finished product. The use of trade or common names is not allowed on cosmetic ingredient lists.

What is a Drug?
A Drug is defined in Federal Food, Drug, Cosmetic Act, Section 201 (g) as being:

"Articles intended for use in the diagnosis, cure (*anti-wrinkle, antibacterial, anti-fungal, anti-acne etc.*), mitigation (*pain reliever, headache reducer, muscle relaxant, etc.*), treatment (*acne treatment, fungal treatment, wrinkle cures, psoriasis and eczema, anti-cancer treatments, etc.*) or prevention (*anti-scar, wrinkle cure, cancer prevention, anti-perspirant, etc.*), of disease. Articles (*other than food*) intended to affect the structure (*wrinkles, perspiration, scars, etc.*) or any function (*cell regeneration, collagen formation, etc.*) of the body."

Drugs: are highly regulated and require pre-clearance by FDA, and GMP is required. Drugs have highly regulated labeling laws (i.e. Drug Facts). They require reporting of all and any adverse effects known, and they can make proven, specific, and tested claims that follow the monographs requirements.

In the Drug Legality Principle, a product meets the definition of drug if it complies with ALL requirements for drugs (even if it also meets the definition of cosmetic). All cosmetics that meet the definition of a drug have to be registered and regulated by the FDA. A product is considered a drug if it makes claims such as being a sunscreen, antibacterial soap, anti-dandruff shampoo, anti-acne, anti-wrinkle, antiperspirant, etc.

"The FDA interprets the term "soap" to apply only when:

- The bulk of the nonvolatile matter in the product consists of an alkali salt of fatty acids and the product's detergent properties are due to the alkali-fatty acid compounds, and
- The product is labeled, sold, and represented solely as soap [21 CFR 701.20]." FDA

What is Soap?
It is very common to find melt and pour soap, as well as true soaps, improperly labeled and containing drug claims. However, most melt and pour soaps do not meet the first standard, because the bulk of the product is not alkali salt and fatty acids.

"If a product intended to cleanse the human body does not meet all the criteria for soap, as listed above, it is either a cosmetic or a drug. For example, if a product consists of detergents or primarily of alkali salts of fatty acids and is intended not only for cleansing but also for other cosmetic uses, such as beautifying or moisturizing, it is regulated as a cosmetic."

Melt and pour soaps consist of detergents and, according to the FDA's definition, they are a cosmetic and not soap. Detergents are essentially de-fatting agents which allows them to remove fats, lipids, dirt, make-up, and debris from the surface of the skin. Detergents aren't bad; they just aren't soap by definition. You are required to include a full International Nomenclature of Cosmetic Ingredients (INCI) ingredient list on every bar of melt and pour soap, and you must follow all cosmetic regulations.

Your Products Intended Use Can Make Your Cosmetic a Drug
Example #1: Product's Intended Use: Drug - A product with any of the following intended uses is a drug: antiperspirant/deodorant (*stops perspirations*), dandruff shampoo (*treats dandruff*), sunscreen/suntan preparation (*prevents sunburn*), fluoride toothpaste (*prevents cavities*), and skin protectants (*helps heal cuts*).

Example #2: Product's Intended Use: Cosmetic - A product with any of the following intended uses is a cosmetic: deodorant (*cover up odor*), shampoo (*cleanse hair*), suntan preparations (*moisturized while tanning*), toothpastes (*cleans teeth or freshens breath*), skin protectants (*moisturize skin*). Notice that both the ingredients and the intended use of the product make a difference in whether it is considered a drug or a cosmetic.

Three Types of Claims that Can Cause Your Cosmetic to be a Drug

1. *Claims that suggest physiological change* - For instance, if you say "younger looking" rather than "younger" you are a cosmetic. If you say "removes" or "prevents" wrinkles, rather than "covers" your product is a drug.
2. *Claims that sound scientific* - For instance, if you claim that your soaps are "Compounded in our laboratory under the most sterile conditions," or "If blemishes persist, see a doctor," your products is a drug.
3. *Claims that appear in an applicable OTC monograph* - Sunscreen products, hormone products, acne, eczema, psoriasis, skin bleaching, etc. Even implied claims by known effects of ingredients. For example, with skin bleaching products, the presence of many ingredients automatically make your product a drug. Remember that even if a cosmetic has a drug action, it must qualify as a drug first and then a cosmetic.

If an ingredient has a monograph it automatically makes a product a drug with the intended use as described in the monograph. The FDA has published monographs for OTC ingredients stating what ingredients can be used and their intended use. Using those ingredients in a product makes your cosmetic a drug—no ifs, ands, or buts about it. Remember, if you use an ingredient with a monograph, that product then meets the definition of a drug, and it must comply with ALL requirements for drugs (even if it also meets the definition of cosmetic).

Are You Transforming Your Cosmetic Into a Drug?
The trick is this, it doesn't matter whether the claim is true or not, it's whether the claim transforms the cosmetic into a drug. You might know that your aromatherapy helps lighten hyper-pigmentation, your ointment helps cure eczema, your serum irons out wrinkles, but as soon as you state or imply that fact on your label, in your literature, in any print advertisement, on your website, or anywhere, you are placing your product into the drug category. Therefore, you must follow all drug regulations and present your product to the FDA before it hits the market. You will also need to present case studies to the FDA to back up your claim. For more information on this, go to The Center for Drug Evaluation and Research (CDER) homepage.

Watch Your Advertising Claims

1. *Environmental Claims*: Claiming something is recyclable, even if true in your area, might not be true in other areas. For example, Polyethylene caps on your containers. There are only a few recycling outlets in the entire USA that recycle PE.
2. *Made in America (or the USA Flag)*: Though your product might be made in the USA, the FTC/FDA requires that all the ingredients originate and remain in the States, too.
3. *Claiming to be an FDA approved product or an FDA approved facility*
4. *Organic Claims*: If you are an organic certified entity, you will be notified of what you can place on your labels. If you are not then you can state "X-percent organic content" on the back of your packaging, but you can't state "organic" on the principal display panel. The verbiage must clearly state it is not certified.
5. *Natural Claims*: involves almost no regulation, however, integrity is recommended.
6. *Product Claims Based on Ingredients*: You can't advertise the effects of a known ingredient. All test studies must be done on the product itself.
7. *Unsubstantiated endorsements* (*such as Celebrity Infomercials*): Again, though a personal claim could be true, it might not necessarily be true for the average person.
8. *Disclaimers like "results may vary" or "not typical for the average consumer"*: It is currently being noted that these disclaimers are not read, but rather the claims are just being heard. Therefore, disclaimers will probably go by the wayside.
9. *Using the term "cosmeceuticals"*: A product can be a drug, cosmetic or a combination of both following the rules of both standards. But the term "cosmeceutical" has no meaning under the law.
10. *Mimicking*: Just because you see another company making claims does not mean you should. If the FDA looks into your claim, you can't use another company's bad judgment as an excuse for your choices. And you don't know if the other company is actually complying with the law since much of it is behind the scenes, with the exception of "drug facts" on the label.

Voluntary Registration with the FDA

Currently registration of your cosmetics on a Federal level is not required. However, there is a voluntary program in place with the FDA. In 2011, several state draft bills popped up all around the country with language that required any business that was not registered with the FDA to register with that state. As of the writing of this book none of that state bills passed in 2011, however Florida already requires that you register with the Florida FDA. I believe that very soon this voluntary program will either be Federally required, or so many states will be requiring that you register with them that if you aren't registered with the FDA then this program will become mandatory or less of a headache than doing it state to state.

Lisa Rodgers, co-founder of Personal Care Truth, had the opportunity to interview Don Havery with the FDA Office of Cosmetics and Colors in regards to the FDA Voluntary Cosmetic Registration Program (VCRP). She gave me permission to share her interview here to help make you familiar with the program in advance.

Lisa: What is your role in regards to the VCRP?

Don: I am the administrator of the Voluntary Cosmetic Registration Program (VCRP) program. I am responsible for daily operation; answering questions, troubleshooting the program when issues come up, and making changes to the program that improve its operation.

Lisa: What is the VCRP?

Don: The VCRP is an FDA program that collects information on cosmetic manufacturing establishments (facilities) and cosmetic products and their ingredients that are in commercial distribution in the U.S. The program has been in operation since 1973. In 2005 the program was modified to allow submission of information electronically over the internet which has made participation in the VCRP much easier.

Lisa: Why should a manufacturer register with the VCRP?

Don: The VCRP helps FDA in its mission to protect consumers. It also helps cosmetic manufacturers and distributors make informed decisions about ingredient use in their products. For example, if it is determined that a cosmetic ingredient presently being used is harmful and should be removed from product use, FDA can notify the manufacturers and distributors of affected products. Since the VCRP is the only source of information about what products are on the market, firms that do not participate in the program won't receive that information directly.

Information from the VCRP database also assists the Cosmetic Ingredient Review (CIR) Expert Panel in determining its priorities for ingredient safety review. The CIR is an industry-funded panel of scientific experts that regularly assesses the safety of cosmetic ingredients. Since cosmetic manufacturers are responsible for assuring that their products and the ingredients in them are safe, participating in the VCRP is one way of supporting the safety review process since VCRP data is used to by the CIR safety review program (See http://www.cir-safety.org).

Lisa: How many manufacturers are presently registered?
Don: We currently have 1,168 firms that have filed 38,450 active products in the VCRP.

Lisa: How does the FDA handle communicating to the companies registered in the VCRP?
Don: Since 2005 when the electronic program was initiated, FDA communicates with VCRP participants primarily via email. More than 99 percent of current VCRP participants do so using the electronic program. For those firms that participate using paper forms, FDA communicates with them using traditional mail or by telephone.

Lisa: Can a company register online?
Don: Yes, online is the easiest and fastest way to participate in the VCRP program and there is no cost to participate.

Lisa: How is the manufacturer's information used?
Don: The VCRP data provides FDA with information on what products are currently on the market, what ingredients are used in them, and how frequently specific cosmetic ingredients are used. The data is also used to support the CIR safety review program. (See earlier answer.)

Lisa: Do you have anything else to add to why a company should register?
Don: Both the FDA and cosmetic manufacturers have a common interest in assuring that cosmetics are safe for their intended use by consumers. Since FDA does not have premarket approval authority for cosmetic products or their ingredients (with the exception of color additives), the VCRP is FDA's primary source of information on what cosmetic ingredients are being used, and what products are on the market. The more firms that participate in the VCRP program, the more information FDA has, and the better able FDA is able to assure that cosmetics on the market are safe for the U.S. consumer.

Industry Self-Regulation and Standards

The Cosmetic Ingredient Review Expert Panel (CIR) is the very best resource for information on the safety of cosmetic ingredients. The mission statement of the CIR is:

"The Cosmetic Ingredient Review thoroughly reviews and assesses the safety of ingredients used in cosmetics in an open, unbiased, and expert manner, and publishes the results in the peer-reviewed scientific literature."

The Cosmetic Ingredient Review was established in 1976 by the industry trade association, now known as the Personal Care Products Council with the full support of the FDA and the Consumer Federation of America (CFA). Many have been critical of the FDA but the CFA by definition looks out for the safety of consumers. The CIR panel is the most qualified organization to make determinations on the safety of cosmetic ingredients. The CIR makes scientific findings that are based on fact and not an agenda. According to the CIR website the CIR procedures are:

- "CIR staff members conduct extensive literature searches, compile data, and prepare draft reports on high-priority ingredients. They organize the literature into several categories: chemistry (including physical properties and manufacture), use (cosmetic and non-cosmetic), general biology (with absorption, distribution, metabolism, and excretion data), and animal toxicology (acute, short-term, subchronic, and chronic studies, as well as dermal irritation and sensitization data). The staff also prepares a clinical assessment of the ingredients that may include epidemiologic studies, along with classic repeated insult patch tests. In vitro test data are also gathered and incorporated into the review. At each stage of the process, CIR seeks the input of all interested parties during a formal 60-day comment period.
- If the open scientific literature contains insufficient information, the Expert Panel will call on industry or other interested parties to provide unpublished data or to undertake specific studies. After multiple opportunities for public comment and open, public discussion, a final safety assessment is issued.
- The Panel may make one of four basic decisions regarding an ingredient:
- Safe ingredients — Ingredients safe in the practices of use (product categories) and concentrations of use for each product category as documented in the safety assessment.
- Unsafe ingredients — These are ingredients with specific adverse effects that make them unsuitable for use in cosmetics.
  - Safe ingredients, with qualifications — The Panel may reach the conclusion that an ingredient can be used safely, but only under certain conditions. Qualifications frequently relate to maximum concentration, but may also address rinse-off versus leave-on uses and other restrictions.
  - Ingredients for which the data are insufficient — if the Panel reaches an "insufficient data" conclusion, it does not state whether the ingredient is safe or unsafe. The Panel is, however, describing a situation in which the available data do not support safety. The specific data that would allow the Panel to complete its assessment always are identified." Source CIR website.

Personal Care Truth co-founder Lisa Rodgers interviewed F. Alan Andersen Ph.D., with the Cosmetic Ingredient Review (CIR). She gave me permission to share her interview here.

Q: Who is the Cosmetic Ingredient Review?

A: The CIR program was created 35 years ago by the cosmetics industry with the support of the FDA and the Consumer Federation of America. CIR's singular mission is to thoroughly review and assesses the safety of ingredients used in cosmetics in an open, unbiased, and expert manner, and to publish the results in the open, peer-reviewed scientific literature.

Oversight of the program is provided by a steering committee comprised of 3 industry representatives (the President of the Personal Care Products Council, the Executive VP for Science at the Council, and the Chair of the Council's CIR Science and Support Committee) and 4 public representatives (Consumer Federation of America, Society of Toxicology, American Academy of Dermatology, and the Chair, CIR Expert Panel).

CIR's procedures call for an initial review of available published and unpublished scientific data relevant for assessing the safety of a cosmetic ingredient or family of cosmetic ingredients. That review is offered for public comment. A draft report is then considered by the CIR Expert Panel. If additional data are needed, an insufficient data announcement describes the required information and interested parties are given time to provide the data. The Expert Panel then issues a tentative safety assessment for public comment. Comments are evaluated and a final safety assessment is prepared.

Recognizing that additional data may later become available, CIR re-reviews every ingredient when the new data become available, but no less than every 15 years. This ensures that CIR's determinations are current.

Q: How long have you been employed by the CIR, and what is your role?

A: I've been the Director of the CIR since 1993 and I'm responsible for the day-to-day operation of the review process and the long-range planning to identify future priorities. Prior to joining CIR, I spent 22 years at the U.S. Food and Drug Administration – moving to FDA directly after receiving my PhD in Biophysics from Penn State.

Q: Do you care about cosmetic safety?

A: Yes! The CIR program offers a unique opportunity to assess the safety of ingredients used in cosmetics and the ex-FDAer in me just loves that we have that capability.

Q: Is there a specific process when testing the safety of an ingredient, before it is made available on the market?

A: No, there isn't a one-size-fits-all approach to establish safety - nor should there be.

For example, some ingredients simply cannot penetrate the outer layer of the skin (the keratinized stratum corneum) and as long as such an ingredient is not inhaled, ingested, or otherwise enter the body; all we have to do is establish that the ingredient will not damage the surface of the skin.

For ingredients that may penetrate the skin, well, we need to know rather a lot more! Where do these ingredients go once they are in the body? Does the body process (metabolize) them? What is produced (metabolites) as a result of processing? Can the ingredient or its metabolites cause damage to genetic material, affect endocrine processes, or cause other adverse health effects? Special concern always exists for any ingredient with regard to the potential to cause cancer, effects on fetal development or reproductive toxicity.

And while natural ingredients are widely used and consumers appear to be comfortable with their safety, ingredients derived from plants often are the most problematic to assess. This is primarily because we don't always know which of the chemicals in the plant are in the plant extract used in the cosmetics. And some of what can be found in plants can be dangerous. Think poison ivy. And even when a concern is not obvious, we need to be vigilant as in the case of aloe-derived ingredients. There is no question that aloe-derived ingredients are widely used and can be used safely, but only if the limits on potentially hazardous anthraquinones that we established are adhered to. We try to leave no stone unturned, so to speak.

Q: How many cosmetic ingredients are on the market?
A: There are around 6000 ingredients currently reported to be used in cosmetics, based on the U.S. FDA's Voluntary Cosmetic Registration Program.

Q: How many cosmetic ingredients haven't been tested for safety?
A: Under the provisions of the Food, Drug, and Cosmetic Act, each company that sells a cosmetic product is required to substantiate the safety of ingredients in that product. With the ongoing movement away from testing safety using animals, more and more will be done without animal testing.

Q: Perhaps a better question would be: How many cosmetic ingredients haven't been assessed for safety?
A: Before I talk about what CIR has done, note that the FDA has reviewed many ingredients used in cosmetics. FDA has evaluated the safety of ingredients used as food additives, color additives, pharmaceuticals, and even medical devices. Additionally, the Research Institute for Fragrance Materials has completed safety assessments of many ingredients used as fragrances.

CIR has completed safety assessments of over 2300 cosmetic ingredients, focusing on the ingredients most widely used in cosmetics. So, formal safety assessments are in place for the ingredients used in most products, but our work continues so that we may address all ingredients used in all products.

Q: What causes an ingredient to be placed on a list of high priority for review?
A: We look at the uses of an ingredient as reported to FDA's Voluntary Cosmetic Registration Program. Our thinking is that the more widely an ingredient is used, the more people will be exposed, and the more important it is to assess its safety. Independent of the use data, we look for information suggesting that the ingredient is a possible hazard. Such information includes the FDA's program to collect information on adverse reactions to cosmetics, monitoring the scientific literature, etc. While such information usually does not establish that a hazard exists, it can suggest that possibility and signal a higher priority for us to do a complete evaluation.

Q: Who makes up the CIR panel?
A: The CIR Expert Panel has 9 scientist and physician members with expertise matched to the approaches for evaluating safety I described earlier.

The Panel Chair is Wilma F. Bergfeld, M.D., F.A.C.P. Dr. Bergfeld is the Head of Clinical Research and Dermatopathology at the Cleveland Clinic Foundation. She is the founding president of the Women's Dermatological Society and is a past-president of the American Academy of Dermatology.

There are two teams that independently review the scientific data on each ingredient.
One team leader is Donald V. Belsito, M.D. Dr. Belsito is the Leonard C. Harber Professor of Clinical Dermatology at Columbia University Medical Center. He is a past-president of the American Contact Dermatitis Society. (Cheryl Boxmeyer)

On this team are:
Curtis D. Klaassen, Ph.D., Professor of Pharmacology and Toxicology, School of Medicine, University of Kansas Medical Center. Dr. Klaassen is a past-president of the Society of Toxicology.

Paul W. Snyder, D.V.M., Ph.D., Professor of Toxicologic Pathology and Director, Veterinary Clinical Immunology and Histopathology Laboratories, School of Veterinary Medicine, Department of Comparative Pathobiology at Purdue University. Dr. Snyder also has an adjunct faculty appointment in the Indiana University School of Medicine.

Daniel C. Liebler, Ph.D., Professor of Biochemistry, Pharmacology and Biomedical Informatics, Vanderbilt University School of Medicine. Dr. Liebler is also the Director, Ayers Institute for Precancer Detection and Diagnosis.

The other team leader is James G. Marks, Jr., M.D., Professor of Medicine,

Chairman of the Division of Dermatology, Pennsylvania State University College of Medicine. Dr. Marks is a past-president of the American Contact Dermatitis Society.

On his team are:
Ronald A. Hill, Ph.D., Associate Professor of Medicinal Chemistry, College of Pharmacy, University of Louisiana at Monroe. Dr. Hill is the author of the chapter on hormone-related disorders–nonsteroidal therapies in Textbook of Organic Medicinal and Pharmaceutical Chemistry.

Ronald C. Shank, Ph.D., Professor and Chair, Dept. of Community and Environmental Medicine, University of California, Irvine. Dr. Shank is also the Director of UCI's Environmental Toxicology Program.

Thomas J. Slaga, Ph.D., Department of Pharmacology, University of Texas Health Science Center, Interim Director, San Antonio Cancer Institute. Dr. Slaga is the founder and editor-in-chief of Molecular Carcinogenesis.

Three non-voting liaison members also serve on the CIR Expert Panel.

Rachel Weintraub, Esq., Senior Counsel, Consumer Federation of America

Halyna Breslawec, Executive VP for Science, Personal Care Products Council

Linda Katz, M.D., M.P.H., Director, Office of Cosmetics and Colors and Chief Medical Officer, FDA's Center for Food Safety and Applied Nutrition

Q: Does the CIR publish its findings of its safety assessments?
A: CIR posts its findings on the CIR website, where it also posts draft reports for public review and comments. Publishing CIR's safety assessments is a core part of the CIR mission. We submit our reports for publication in the peer-reviewed International Journal of Toxicology. Three supplemental issues of the IJT appear each year to ensure wide dissemination of the findings of the CIR Expert Panel. There is an additional benefit to this approach in that industry usually does not have to perform additional animal testing when such data already are captured in CIR safety assessments.

The Side Effect of Fluctuating Standards and One-upmanship

Consumers are seeking natural, organic, green, and true aromatherapy products. However, consumers are confused because of constant bickering among the chief natural companies, certifiers, and resources. The natural industry itself is causing consumers to doubt the reliability of natural products.

According to Mintel, a leading market research company, "In the US, some 42% of consumers indicate they don't know what to believe as to whether natural and organic personal care products actually are natural or organic." The debate over who really is natural within the industry, with one organization bad mouthing another, is creating the opposite effect on the natural industry than desired.

Marketing departments are requiring cosmetic chemists to formulate based on a variety of lists, standards, and variations of misinformation on the internet. The dizzying pace with which one organization declares itself the authority on natural and organic, while another undercuts them to reach the top even makes a natural cosmetic formulator's head spin.

Mintel Beauty Innovation predicted a new consumer standard they coined as "Nu Natural." According to Mintel, it "is a new vision of natural that is less focused on certification and more focused on results, efficiency and safety."

One of the most damaging trends caused by industry one-upmanship was the empowering of the Campaign for Safe Cosmetics and the Environmental Working Group. We have allowed them to use industry backbiting against us in the minds of consumers and in State and Federal government. The very organizations that many believed would support small, natural and organic businesses are the masterminds behind devastating State legislation and many attempts at Federal laws that would do more damage to the aromatherapy, perfuming, natural cosmetics and small businesses than to the big cosmetic companies.

Unfortunately, a lack of science prevails in the efforts of the Campaign for Safe Cosmetics and Environmental Working Group to change the cosmetic laws on Federal, State, County and City levels. The results have been costly in California, where nonsensical lawsuits abound after the passing of Proposition 65 and business killers in Florida where home businesses were literally required to leave the cosmetic industry altogether.

Cosmetics in California

"A company is required to report if all of the following conditions are met:
- It has a total of at least $1 million of cosmetic product sales both within and outside of California (according to previous year tax records)
- It is the manufacturer, packer, and/or distributor named on the label of a product which contains an ingredient known or suspected by an authoritative body cited in the Act to cause cancer or reproductive harm;
- That product meets the U.S. Food and Drug Administration's (U.S. FDA's) definition of a cosmetic (see FDA definition of a cosmetic or cosmetic/drug. Soap and OTC drugs with no cosmetic claim are exempt) and

- That product was sold in California on or after January 1, 2007."
  Ingredient and Incidental Ingredients Defined Products that contain an ingredient on the list must file excluding trace contaminates or incidental ingredients.
  Ingredients are defined as: "According to 21 CFR § 700.3 (e), an ingredient is defined as 'any single chemical entity or mixture used as a component in the manufacture of a cosmetic product.'"
  Incidental Ingredients are defined as: "FDA regulation, 21 CFR § 701.3 (l), states that 'The provisions of this section do not require the declaration of incidental ingredients that are present in a cosmetic at insignificant levels and that have no technical or functional effect in the cosmetic. For the purpose of this paragraph, incidental ingredients are:"
- "Substances that are added to a cosmetic during the processing of such cosmetic but are removed from the cosmetic in accordance with good manufacturing practices before it is packaged in its finished form." [Example: Filter aid.]
- "Substances that are added to a cosmetic during processing for their technical or functional effect in the processing, are converted to substances the same as constituents of declared ingredients, and do not significantly increase the concentration of those constituents." [Example: Sodium hydroxide added to a sodium stearate and stearic acid-containing cosmetic.] ver. 4_14_09 1
- "Substances that are added to a cosmetic during the processing of such cosmetic for their technical and functional effect in the processing but are present in the finished cosmetic at insignificant levels and do not have any technical or functional effect in that cosmetic." [Example: Defoaming agent.]
- "Substances that have no technical or functional effect in the cosmetic but are present by reason of having been incorporated into the cosmetic as an ingredient of another cosmetic ingredient.'"

California created a list containing 783 chemicals that require reporting, however the majority of those are not, have never been, and never will be used in cosmetics or personal care products. Rather than reading through the entire 783 chemical in search of the ones that have ever or could potentially be used in cosmetics I have listed them below.

Common Cosmetic Ingredients:
BHA
Black 2 (also called Carbon Black)
Cocamide DEA
Methyl Alcohol (denaturant in SD Alcohol 1, 3-A, 30)
Retinol
Retinyl Esters (most common are Acetate and Palmitate)
Titanium Dioxide

Less commonly used ingredients:
Acetaldehyde (used in fragrances)
4-amino-2-nitrophenol (used in hair dyes)
Prycatechol
Dibutyl Phthalate
Ethyl Acrylate
Glycol (ethylene glycol)
Formaldehyde (only as anhydrous gas)
Lead Acetate
Spironlactone
Sulindac
Talc that contains asbestiform fibers
Toluene

Chemicals used in fragrances and flavors that may trigger reporting include:
Acetaldehyde
Naphthalene
Benzene, 1,2-dimethoxy-4-(2-propenyl)-[MethylEugenol]
Benzene, ethenyl- [Styrene]
Pyridine
1,3-Benzodioxole
2-Propenoic acid, ethyl ester [Ethyl acrylate]
Estragole, added as such
Phenol, (1,1-dimethylethyl)-4-methoxy- [BHA]
Sulfuric acid, diethyl ester
Sulfuric acid, dimethyl ester
Isoprene
Cinnamyl anthranilate
Dihydrosafrole
Ethylbenzene
Di(2-ethylhexyl)phthalate
trans,trans-2,4-Hexadienal (cis/trans mix)
Quinoline
o-Phenyl phenol
Wood creosote
Ethylene glycol

Regarding the California law, David Steinberg wrote, "Instead of carefully reviewing existing lists of chemicals published by various organizations, California included all of them without considering the fact that the vast majority of these chemicals have never been used in cosmetics and may or may not cause cancer or reproductive toxicity. Those directed to come up with the list of ingredients simply aggregated a large list, which is likely to scare consumers. In fact, California has relied on a study by the Environmental Working Group stating that 54 cosmetic products contain ingredient that the CIR has deemed as unsafe."

He went on to say, "How much money will be wasted to locate these 'unsafe' products? California should save its money; these 54 products are not sold in the United States, much less in California. As an aside, California is in such a poor fiscal position that the office administering this program has mandated closing for three Fridays each month until 2010 - yet it is willing to bleed precious dollars on something of zero value. There is nothing in this law that will make cosmetics safe. Cosmetics are already required by federal law to be safe but California is attempting to make them safer than safe, which makes little sense."

How to Report in California
Go to http://www.cdph.ca.gov/programs/cosmetics/documents/reportinginstructions.pdf

Home-based Cosmetics Banned in Florida
In 2010 Florida passed its own state-level Drug, Cosmetic, and Household Products that are on the state level. What is relevant in the Florida law is section 449.01 Permits which says, "Prior to operating, a permit is required for each person and establishment that intents to operate as: (r) A cosmetic manufacturer."

According to the Florida statute, a "manufacturer" is defined as: A person who prepares, derives, manufactures, or produces a cosmetic. To "repackage" is defined as: Repacking or otherwise changing the container, wrapper, or labeling to further the distribution of the cosmetic. A "repackager" is a person who repackages. Anyone meeting the definition of a manufacturer or is a repackager is subject to the Florida regulations and permitting for cosmetics.

They also include in the definition of a "cosmetic" an article (ingredient) that is intended to be used in cosmetics. Translation: If you sell supplies for cosmetics, make cosmetics, are a vendor of cosmetics, or make soap that has cosmetics claims in the state of Florida, then the cosmetic regulations and permitting apply to you. The State of Florida requires a permit for each person and establishment that intends to operate as a cosmetic manufacturer or repackager within the state. But, if the person uses a private label company, only labels, or changes the labeling of a cosmetic, but does not open the sealed container that comes from a manufacturer outside of the State of Florida then a permit is not required.

Here is the big kicker for small businesses: An establishment that is a place of residence may not receive a permit and may not operate as a cosmetic manufacturer or repackager. That means that all the soapmakers who make soaps that do more than strictly clean, all aromatherapists that make cosmetic products (remember, federally, you already can't make OTC drugs), all small cosmetic home businesses may not operate within the State of Florida. But the real kick in the pants for those small businesses is that if you move out of Florida you could sell your products back into the state without a permit.

And there isn't a way around it within the state because they added: A county or municipality may not issue an occupational license for a cosmetic manufacturer or repackager unless they already have a permit from the state.

If you qualify to be a manufacturer then the current fee is a biennial fee (every two years) of $800. There is an additional fee of $150 for initial applications which require a site inspection and a $100 fee to change the address on file on a permit, which is required to be filed prior to the actual change of address. The permit must be posted in a conspicuous place on the license premises.

Product registration is also required by Florida. Any person who manufactures, packages, repackages, labels, or relabels a drug or cosmetic in the state of Florida must register that product with the Department of Business and Professional Regulation. If you used the private label loophole to skip the permit requirements you are still required to register your relabeled products with the State of Florida with a $20 per product registration fee that is only good for two years. In two years you will need to do it all again. Thankfully there is an Identical Product Certification form that allows you to register products that are identical except for name, size, color, or scents, and that certification only requires one registration.

If your existing registration is no more than 12 months old then each registration for new products is $20. If you have less than 12 months left, then the cost is $10 for any new product registration.

If you make it that far, you then must wait for approval of your label prior to selling your product, and your product must be registered with the State of Florida before you can sell any products.

The State of Florida then gives you a Certificate of Free Sale, which certifies that your cosmetics are registered with the department and can, be legally be manufactured and sold in the state. If you haven't quite paid enough yet there is an additional $25 fee for the Certificate of Free Sale document. If you order additional copies at the same time they are only $2 for additional copies each. Each Certificate of Free Sale can list up to 30 products. And if you need a notarized copy there is an extra $10 fee per notarized Certificate of Free Sale.

The State of Florida also has the right to inspect, monitor, investigate and enforce any registered manufacturer. The State has the right to issue a warning letter, require that you fix issues, stop the sale of any adulterated or misbranded products, to seize products and issue fines as they see fit.

Here is the entire Florida Statue, Chapter 499, Drug, Cosmetic and Household Products
http://www.leg.state.fl.us/statutes/index.cfm?App_mode=Display_StatuteandURL=0400-0499/0499/0499.html

:: Chapter 12 ::
Good Manufacturing Practices and You

Current Good Manufacturing Practice (GMP) guidelines are important for any size cosmetic or soap business to be familiar with. When proper cleanliness is not maintained, your product can be deemed adulterated or misbranded, and you will be prohibited to sell it.

Following GMP is not required for cosmetic products, but the practices are worth knowing and working towards. No matter how much product you sell or how small your company is, now is a good time to implement as many GMP practices into your business as possible.

Early on in our business, my husband Dennis insisted that we become GMP compliant. I knew it was the right thing to do, but when I looked at all the GMP guidelines I was overwhelmed. Nevertheless, piece by piece, we adopted GMP as normal and made it a habit. If I had attempted to tackle the entire project all at once, I would have thrown my hands up in surrender. We were growing fast, and I was making all of the products myself. Dennis believed it was better to start the habits early, so bad habits wouldn't inhibit our growth. He was right. We were just a tiny micro-business when we started following GMP rules, but he believed that we had to "do business like the big boys" in order to grow.

In this chapter I will address GMP guidelines in bite-size chunks. How do you eat an elephant? That's right: one bite at a time. The entire GMP guidelines can be found on the FDA website. The following GMP Guidelines and Inspection Checklist are provided by the FDA. I have provided helpful hints throughout the FDA guidelines from what we learned while growing our home business into a fully GMP compliant business. Later we discovered that being GMP compliant made becoming a Certified Organic Processor and Handler much easier to accomplish.

The following cosmetic establishment instructions, excerpted from FDA's Inspection Operations Manual, may serve as guidelines for effective self-inspection. Take advantage of the fact that the FDA publishes their Inspection Operations Manual by putting on your white gloves to "inspect" your facility. All quotes are from the FDA's website, and non-quotes are my tips to help you make your facility GMP compliant. The boxes correspond to the FDA excerpts.

Guidelines

1. "Building and Facilities. Check whether:

a. Buildings used in the manufacture or storage of cosmetics are of suitable size, design and construction to permit unobstructed placement of equipment, orderly storage of materials, sanitary operation, and proper cleaning and maintenance."

> **Building Suitability Tips:** You may need to designate one part of your kitchen or house as "manufacturing space only" and guard that space with your life. This is not required as long as the space, whether temporary or permanent, is always clean before you begin production.

b. "Floors, walls and ceilings are constructed of smooth, easily cleanable surfaces and are kept clean and in good repair."

> **Counters, Walls, Ceilings, and Floors Tips:** This does not mean you have to remodel your entire kitchen, but your designated area needs to have surfaces that are easy to wipe off.

Counters: Stainless steel, laminate, corian, and staron are all nonporous, smooth surfaces suitable for keeping clean and in good repair. Tiles with grout, wood, and other porous materials are not ideal for this area.

Walls and Ceilings: 4x8 sheets of Fiberglass Reinforced Panel (FRP) are FDA accepted sanitary wall liners. FRP panels are available at Home Depot for approximately $32 per panel.

Floors: Vinyl floors are best for cleaning up. Also having a clean kitchen is okay to as long as the product cannot be adulterated by its surroundings.

c. "Fixtures, ducts and pipes are installed in such a manner that drip or condensate does not contaminate cosmetic materials, utensils, cosmetic contact surfaces of equipment, or finished products in bulk."

> **Fixtures, Ducts, and Pipes Tips:** This may seem obvious, but look up while you are in the midst of a hot cook. Check out all the surfaces the steam reaches. Every surface should be cleaned religiously and be painted with a washable paint if the surface is porous. If it is a painted surface, it must not flake or hold moisture. An example of a good washable paint is Gliddon Evermore super washable flat latex paint for highly washable surfaces. Most brands have a paint that is designed to create an easy to wash off surface. You can also prime or seal any porous surface prior to painting.

d. "Lighting and ventilation are sufficient for the intended operation and comfort of personnel."

> **Lighting and Ventilation Tips:** Be certain that you can clearly see what you are doing. Make sure all areas are well illuminated so you can see whether or not you're working in a clean area. If you are using powders, minerals, lye, or essential oils, you should make sure the area is ventilated as well.

e. "Water supply, washing and toilet facilities, floor drainage and sewage system are adequate for sanitary operation and cleaning of facilities, equipment and utensils, as well as to satisfy employee needs and facilitate personal cleanliness."

> **Water Systems Tips:** When we moved into our second building, we discovered that the walk-through we did with our landlord was not completely accurate. It wasn't until we brought in a plumber to install a three-hole sink that we discovered the plumbing and drainage from the building wasn't sufficient to add the all-important water source. The year and a half that we spent in that building presented many challenges. The landlord simply did not know it wouldn't be possible. So if you are moving into a building, and it needs any work including ventilation, electricity, plumbing, or any other important modification, make sure you bring in an expert before signing a lease for the space.
>
> Having a clean, safe, and well lit facility is an important step in the manufacturing of cosmetics. The best way to avoid a recall is to go above and beyond in the care of your work space. A peanut butter recall and hand sanitizer recall were both related to cleanliness.

2. "**Equipment.** Check whether:

a. Equipment and utensils used in processing, holding, transferring and filling are of appropriate design, material and workmanship to prevent corrosion, buildup of material, or adulteration with lubricants, dirt or sanitizing agent."

> **Appropriate Designs Tips:** Even when you have the right equipment, if it isn't properly maintained, you are wasting your money. It is vital to use the right equipment, maintain it, clean it, and log it all. Creating logs not only gives you a bird's eye view of your own systems but also provides a record of your compliance with GMP regarding equipment.
>
> Depending on what is being manufactured, the right equipment for one company might not be the right equipment for another. In

> general, stainless steel is best for most equipment. The key to cleaning equipment and not transferring contamination from one batch to another is to use non porous materials. Once you invest in the right equipment then maintain it, log it, maintain it, log it, maintain it, and log it!

b. "Utensils, transfer piping and cosmetic contact surfaces of equipment are well-maintained and clean and are sanitized at appropriate intervals."

> **Maintenance Tips:** The key to proper maintenance, cleaning, and sanitizing is to keep a log of all activities. It might all seem redundant, but the extra step of keeping a log is worth it. There is a difference between cleaning and sanitizing. At Essential Wholesale we wash all of our utensils with hot water and soap, rinse, sanitize, and dry. Then, before we put that same utensil into use, we sanitize it again with denatured alcohol. We sanitize right before use in case any contaminate is transferred onto the surface—even if we just finished washing it. It might be overkill but I'd rather be "over the top clean" than contaminate a product.

c. "Cleaned and sanitized portable equipment and utensils are stored and located, and cosmetic contact surfaces of equipment are covered, in a manner that protects them from splash, dust or other contamination."

> **Storage and Locations Tips:** If you are operating out of your home, make sure you have a dedicated area that is not mixed with personal items. Depending on the size of your equipment, there are many options for storage. Just make sure there is no cross-contamination caused by splash, dust or any other possible contamination. Treat your equipment and utensils like precious treasures.

3. "Personnel. Check whether:

a. The personnel supervising or performing the manufacture or control of cosmetics has the education, training and/or experience to perform the assigned functions."

> **Education and Training Tips:** Create Standard Operating Procedures (SOP) so that no one can ever say, "I wasn't told that," or "Oops I forgot that step." SOPs are a standardized set of instructions that you create for every aspect of QC, manufacturing, filling, labeling, logging, packaging, shipping, and any other step your product goes through from the time the ingredients arrive to the moment the finished

product is shipped out of your building. No step is too mundane to include in your SOPs. You cannot purchase a set of SOPs to fit your situation. You must create your own SOP that best suit the needs of your company.

The SOP should be a written document including all the instructions with detailed steps and processes that are simple enough for a 5th grader to follow - with the same results you would get yourself. The steps should be without any variation or change. In this way, you will always get the same results whether you make it yourself or someone follows your SOP to complete the task.

Every employee should be thoroughly trained on your SOP, and their training should be documented. If your SOPs are updated or changed, your employees should be retrained and that training documented. The purpose of the SOP is not to make the job harder, but to make it easier and standardized. Imagine that someday you could go on vacation and your company would run without you. The SOPs get you one step closer to that dream.

b. "Persons coming into direct contact with cosmetic materials, finished products in bulk or cosmetic contact surfaces, to the extent necessary to prevent adulteration of cosmetic products, wear appropriate outer garments, gloves, hair restraints etc., and maintain adequate personal cleanliness."

Appropriate Garments Tips: There is nothing sexier than a hairnet and pair of gloves! Get over feeling silly and make a habit of wearing them. It is the easiest step of all. You can buy them at Costco or Cash and Carry. They are inexpensive and simple. Gloves and hairnets have become so commonplace to me that, when I recently visited a large food manufacturing facility and witnessed an employee touching the food in process without gloves, I nearly fainted. Germs live on our hands and are easily transferred to products. I have read that there are 50,000 bacteria per square inch of skin that are harmless on your skin…But are you willing to gamble that they are harmless to your product? I'm not!

c. "Consumption of food or drink, or use of tobacco is restricted to appropriately designated areas."

Food Tips: If you are in your kitchen this is hard to adhere to but you have to make it a habit to protect the area you work in from cross contamination of food. Pretend that zone, or the time period in which you use the area, is a sanctuary and guard it.

4. "Raw Materials. Check whether:

a. Raw materials and primary packaging materials are stored and handled in a manner which prevents their mix-up, contamination with microorganisms or other chemicals, or decomposition from exposure to excessive heat, cold, sunlight or moisture."

Raw Materials and Primary Packaging Tips: Make sure you store all ingredients and finished products at the proper temperature for that particular product. Not all things should be stored in the refrigerator. Have you ever noticed the condensation in your mayonnaise jar? The same thing can happen to your ingredients or cosmetics. That is why mayonnaise contains EDTA, but your raw ingredients don't have an added preservative in them.

Sometimes we get calls regarding clouding of oils that consumers stored in their fridge. Clouding of carrier oils is caused by condensation that has fallen into the oil. Besides clouding your oil the condensation can grow mold and then contaminate your product. Condensation can also be caused by storing products in the sunlight. For instance, if you are extracting St. John's Wort in oil, and the sunlight is needed to get the red color, make sure you open it every evening and wipe off the condensation. Nothing else has any reason to be in the sun.

Find a room that you can maintain a steady room temperature to store all ingredients. The garage is a very poor choice. One day in a warm area can be equal to approximately 4 days of the product's life and excessive heat accelerates the effect. For instance, 40 degrees Celsius (104 degrees Fahrenheit) is commonly used for accelerated shelf life testing and you don't want to be accelerating your shelf life while you are storing your products. If you use the fridge do not use the door panels. It is best to have a dedicated fridge that won't be opened and closed a zillion times per day.

Don't store your food items with your supplies. Every incoming ingredient should be logged, quality controlled, and marked with a label. At Essential Wholesale we micro test every single incoming ingredient we bring in for resale or manufacturing. It might be too big of a step right now for you to test every incoming ingredient, but you can rest assured that every ingredient and every product has been micro tested at Essential Wholesale before it ever reaches your door. A finished product from Essential Wholesale represents many micro tests as each ingredient is micro tested prior to use, and the finished product is micro tested prior to sale.

> We had an incident that was caused by natural aloe juice that contaminated and destroyed a well-preserved product that had previously passed all challenge tests. Our private label customer had insisted on using their own aloe juice instead of ours. We were already in the practice of micro testing all of our incoming ingredients, so we were shocked when the finished product we had made with the customer's juice failed the micro test. This was several years ago and we were not in the practice of micro testing a customer's incoming ingredients, but everything changed from that day forward. We had to throw away five gallons of very expensive product that had been scented with $235 worth of *Jasmine Absolute*! Trust me when I say we learned a hard lesson and never manufactured with a single untested ingredient again!

b. "Containers of materials are closed, and bagged or boxed materials are stored off the floor."

> **Containers and Storage Tips:** Storing on the floor is a common food and cosmetic violation and it is simple to avoid with low shelving or even cut a pallet to fit the area. Don't just roll a bag up and assume it is closed. Clip it, change packaging, and put it in bins from Home Depot. You need to protect your ingredients from the moisture in the air, the dust floating everywhere, and critters that want to check out what you have in there.

c. "Containers of materials are labeled with respect to identity, lot identification and control status."

> **Log and Label Tip:** Do this as the ingredients come in and keep a log. Document it, log it, document it, and log it. Am I starting to sound like a broken record yet? Logs can be paperless by creating an Excel spreadsheet that includes all of your logs in one place.

d. "Materials are sampled and tested or examined in conformance with procedures assuring the absence of contamination with filth, microorganisms, or other extraneous substances, to the extent necessary to prevent adulteration of finished products. Pay particular attention to materials of animal or vegetable origin and those used in the manufacture of cosmetics by cold processing methods with respect to contamination with filth or microorganisms."

> **Sampling and Testing Tip:** Visual inspection can work for some of these parameters. Otherwise, depend on your supply source or add

micro testing of your incoming ingredients to the steps that you usually take. If you buy from Essential Wholesale you can count on us having all the QC and micro testing documents on every ingredient. With a lot number we can find every detail about an ingredient from when it arrived, when it was micro tested, when it passed, visual inspection, aroma, and many other variations along with a sample of the lot. We take QC seriously on all incoming ingredients, outgoing ingredients, and finished products.

e. "Materials not meeting acceptance specifications are properly identified and controlled to prevent their use in cosmetics."

Failing Specifications Tip: Everything that does not pass your QC process must be destroyed or returned. If you have to destroy or return a product or ingredient, you must log it. Document it all. This will keep you GMP compliant, and your tax preparer can log it as a business loss.

5. "**Production.** Check whether manufacturing and control have been established and that written instructions, i.e. formulations, processing, transfer, and filling instructions, in-process control methods etc. are being maintained. Determine whether such procedures require that:"

Production Tip: Document, Document, Document! Log it, Log it, and Log it! Create SOPs, train your employees on SOPs, and implement SOPs! Your formulas should include methodology that spell out your SOPs for that product and include every step from incoming raw ingredient QC; to storage of raw ingredients, to manufacturing, methodology, filling, labeling, packing, and shipping. The Standard Operating Procedure must be clearly written, followed, and documented consistently.

a. "The equipment for processing, transfer and filling the utensils and the containers for holding raw and bulk materials are clean, in good repair and in sanitary condition."

Condition of Equipment Tip: GMP for Equipment should follow all stages of your product development. That means the equipment for manufacturing—the equipment you use to transfer and fill—is as clean as the containers which hold the raw materials.

b. "Only approved materials are used."

> **Only Approved Materials Tip:** Use your QC Log for incoming materials to keep track of materials you approved and materials that fail QC. Every ingredient or product that fails QC must be added to a Destruction Log that keeps records of what happens to the materials that fail QC. Indicate which materials were rejected and sent back to the supplier or destroyed.

c. "Samples are taken, as appropriate, during and/or after processing, transfer or filling for testing for adequacy of mixing or other forms of processing, absence of hazardous microorganisms or chemical contaminants, and compliance with any other acceptance specification."

> **Samples Tips:** You should take a sample of every incoming and outgoing product that you QC and retain the sample. We retain all of our samples for 3 years. You must also retain all testing documents and QC logs. When you buy an ingredient or finished product from Essential Wholesale, put the Lot # into your incoming records, and that will tie your records to our records to complete the chain of QC Logs. We have records on every raw ingredient and finished product we sell, and they meet every one of the standards listed above for our company and yours.

d. "Weighing and measuring of raw materials is checked by a second person, and containers holding the materials are properly identified."

> **Weighing and Measuring Tips:** For a one-man show, this is a huge hurdle. We are working towards having this changed or waived for small businesses in our legislative efforts. One idea that might work for your small company is to pre-measure, label, and store your ingredients when you have another person with you that can check your measurements. For instance, if you receive 50 pounds of shea butter, but you only use 10 pounds of shea butter per batch of product, have a friend or family member present to check measurements and break down the shea butter into five 10 pound packages. Label, log, and store the shea for future batches. Do the same with as many ingredients as possible. If you have more than one person at your company, this is not as big of a hurdle, but it can still be inconvenient. Also, go the extra mile and get your scale calibrated to ensure your scale is accurate at all times.

e. "Major equipment, transfer lines, containers and tanks are used for processing, filling or holding cosmetics. All are identified to indicate contents, batch designation, control status and other pertinent information."

> **Know your Steps:** Carry the same lot number and documentation all the way through every step of manufacturing. You should be able to clearly identify from a label on a batch of product at any phase of the production what it is, the lot number, what stage of manufacturing it is in, whether it has passed QC, and where it is going from there.

f. "Labels are examined for identity before labeling operations to avoid mix-up."

> **Avoid Mislabeling Tip:** Check your labeling, double check and check again. There is nothing worse than labeling lavender lotion as coffee shampoo!

g. "The equipment for processing, holding, transferring and filling of batch is labeled regarding identity, batch identification and control status."

> **Equipment Identifying Batch:** As your product moves through your processing, holding, transferring, and filling equipment, it should be clearly marked with the product name, batch number, and control status of that product at that moment.

h. "Packages of finished products bear permanent code marks."

> **Permanent Code Mark Tip:** You need to keep track of a product from start to finish. The finished product should have a permanent code mark that can help you identify the batch and logs associated with it.

i. "Returned cosmetics are examined for deterioration or contamination."

> **Returned Products Tip:** If a product is returned to you, do not throw it away. Even if the customer didn't like it, a returned product is an opportunity to evaluate how the product stands up under real life conditions.

6. "Laboratory Controls. Check whether:

a. Raw materials, in-process samples and finished products are tested or examined to verify their identity and determine their compliance with specifications for physical and chemical properties, microbial contamination, and hazardous or other unwanted chemical contaminants."

> **Compliance with Specifications of Physical and Chemical Properties Tips:** Does that statement terrify you? There are some easy steps you can add to aid in laboratory controls in your company. These are just examples that you can modify depending on your needs.

Tips for creating your own *incoming* Quality Control Log:
1. Name of Product
2. Supplier Name
3. Lot Number from Supplier
4. Lot Number assigned by your company (if not the same as from supplier)
5. Date Received
6. Invoice Number from supplier
7. Quantity receiving into inventory
8. QC checked by:
9. Date & Time of QC
10. Color of the product - indicate if there is any variance (which is common in natural products)
11. Micro-test Results - either micro-test in house or, if you received it from Essential Wholesale indicate "passed as per EW." Nothing leaves our building unless it has passed the micro-test, so you are guaranteed we have a record of every product passing micro-tests.
12. pH can be measured with pH strips or if your products come from Essential Wholesale you can indicate "EW" because we have records if it is ever needed.
13. Scent: Indicate if there is a variance and describe the aroma.
14. Viscosity: Describe it and indicate any variance.
15. Texture: Describe it and indicate any variance.
16. Approved or Rejected
17. Explanation and course of action if rejected

Tips for creating your own *finished* goods Quality Control Log:
1. Product name
2. Batch Size
3. Order number if production is to fill a specific order
4. End user to indicate if it is for stock, private label customer, specific store
5. Compounded by
6. Measurements Checked by
7. Compounding Date
8. Sample pulled & by whom
9. Micro test Results - either micro test in house or if you received it from Essential Wholesale indicate "passed as per EW". Nothing leaves our building unless it has passed micro testing so you are guaranteed we have a record of every product passing micro tests.
10. Viscosity, describe it and indicate any variance (unless you have a viscometer)
11. pH

12. QC'd by
13. Lot # Assigned
14. Filling Date
15. Filled by
16. Parent Product # if using a finished product to make other products. For example, if you make a product that you scent various ways to make other products.
17. Child Product Name
18. Child Product Lot # Assigned
19. Product Retest Date

b. "Reserve samples of approved lots or batches of raw materials and finished products are retained for the specified time period, are stored under conditions that protect them from contamination or deterioration, and are retested for continued compliance with established acceptance specifications."

Reserve Samples Tips: Make sure you hold onto all of your samples of every batch of product you make. The labeling on the lot sample should make it simple to find the paperwork attached to that lot number. Store your lot samples under similar conditions that your product will have in the stores. Don't hang onto them in the garage where they are sure to be destroyed.

c. "The water supply, particularly the water used as a cosmetic ingredient, is tested regularly for conformance with chemical, analytical and microbiological specifications."

Water Supply Tip: Your water source is critical. At Essential Wholesale we take our water source seriously because even if you take every step to ensure clean, raw materials, contaminated water can still destroy your product. You should use de-ionized water or distilled water to manufacture your products, not tap water.

d. "Fresh as well as retained samples of finished products are tested for adequacy of preservation against microbial contamination, which may occur user reasonably foreseeable condition of storage and consumer use."

Testing Tips: Even when you have your products tested at production, real life conditions can be the best indicator of a successful preservation system.

7. **"Records.** Check whether control records are maintained for:

a. Raw materials and primary packaging materials, documenting disposition of rejected materials.

b. Manufacturing of batches, documenting the:
    i. Kinds, lots and quantities of material used.
    ii. Processing, handling, transferring, holding, and filling.
    iii. Sampling, controlling, adjusting, and reworking.
    iv. Code marks of batches and finished products.

c. Finished products, documenting sampling, individual laboratory controls, test results and control status.

d. Distribution, documenting initial interstate shipment, code marks and consignees."

> **Records Tips:** Going through all the steps to be GMP compliant is essential, but you also must keep records of it all. That is why I've been repeating myself with log it, log it, and log it! You should always be able to find your documents, logs, product sample, and finished product. The trick is to follow all the other steps of GMP and keep accurate records on your compliance every day. You can't back log this kind of data; it must all be kept along the way.

8. **"Labeling.** Check whether the labels of the immediate and outer container bear:

a. On the principal display panel:
    i. In addition to the name of the product, the statements of identity and net contents,
    ii. The statement "Warning—The safety of this product has not been determined" if the safety of the respective product has not adequately been substantiated. Determine whether and what toxicological and/ or other testing the firm has conducted to substantiate the safety of its products. See 21 CFR 740.10.

b. On the information panel:
    i. The name and address of the firm manufacturing the product or introducing it into interstate commerce
    ii. The list of ingredients (only on outer container) if intended for sale or customarily sold to consumers for consumption at home
    iii. The warning statement(s) required at 21 CFR 740.11, 740.12 and 740.17.

iv. Any other warning statement necessary or appropriate to prevent a health hazard; determine the health hazard or their basis for a warning statement.

v. Any direction for safe use of product."

> **Labeling Tip:** The best investment you can make to ensure proper labeling and avoid misbranding is the book, *Soap & Cosmetic Labeling, How to Follow The Rules and Regs, Explained in Plain English* by Marie Gale. There are too many details to fit inside this book on labeling and Marie Gale literally wrote the book on Soap and Cosmetic labeling.

9. "Complaints. Check whether the firm maintains a consumer complaint file and determine:

a. The kind and severity of each reported injury and the body part involved.

b. The product associated with each injury, including the manufacturer and code number.

c. The medical treatment involved, if any, including the name of the attending physician.

d. The name(s) and location(s) of any poison control center, government agency, physician's group etc., to whom formula information and/or toxicity data are provided."

> **Complaints Tips:** We haven't had or known anyone who has had any complaints of bodily harm from cosmetics. But you should have protocol in place so you or your employees know exactly what to do if you ever receive such a complaint. It is easier to take the correct steps if you are prepared for the worst.
>
> **Create a log (that you pray always stays empty) that includes:** Customers name, date of injury, date of call, kind of injury, body part injured, product that caused injury, lot number of product, medical treatment needed, name of the attending physician, hospital, and whether you were contacted by poison control or a government agency. You never want to get this call but it is best to be prepared. You might want to designate who should take the call as well.

All of these GMP tips might have seemed a bit overwhelming for you, but don't disregard them altogether. Think big, dream big and aim high by working as many of the GMP compliance guidelines into your working business as possible.

:: Chapter 13 ::
Essential Oil Profiles

I am a National Association of Holistic Aromatherapy (NAHA) certified aromatherapist. Due to my long history with NAHA and my high respect for the organization, I used their standards for education and training for level one and two aromatherapy certification to determine what information and which profiles to include in this book. NAHA requires the profiles of clary sage (*Salvia sclarea*), eucalyptus, geranium, lavender, lemon, peppermint, roman chamomile, rose, rosemary, sweet orange, tea tree, and ylang ylang to be covered for level one aromatherapy training. I've included the ten essential oils chosen by NAHA along with eleven of my favorite essential oils including: bergamot, cedarwood (*Cedrus deodora*), frankincense, cistus, neroli, grapefruit, myrrh, laurel leaf, blue chamomile, patchouli, and ginger.

Bergamot (*Citrus bergamia*)

The aroma of bergamot is familiar to many Earl Grey tea drinkers, as it is added to all Earl Grey. A few sources of bergamot dark chocolate have been popping up recently as well. Bergamot is the easiest of all essential oils to blend with as it smells good with anything. This has made it one of the most popular essential oils used in perfuming.

Latin Name
Citrus bergamia

Common Name
Bergamot

CAS Number 8007-75-8
EINECS 296-429-8

Geographical Source
Ivory Coast, Italy, France

Family
Rutaceae

Plant Part
Fruit Peel

Method
Cold Expressed

Representative Constituents
Alcohols, Furanocoumarins, Ester, Terpene

Main Components
Limonene, Linalyl Acetate, Linalool, Gamma-Terpinene, Beta-Pinene

Minor Components of Note
Bergamot contains approximately 0.44% furocoumarins which accounts for its phototoxicity.

Properties
Antiseptic, anti-biotic, anti-spasmodic, anti-depressant, sedative, fever reducing, insect repellant, anti-inflammatory, analgesic, encourages skin cell growth, deodorant, expectorant, insecticide, tonic, and antiviral.

General Aromatherapy Uses
Depression, stress, tension, fear, hysteria, infection (all types including skin), anorexia, psoriasis, eczema, emotional crisis, convalescence, insomnia, wounds, acne, boils, varicose veins, ulcers, hemorrhoids, cold sores, shingles, chicken pox, tonic action on uterus, uplifts, balances, refreshes, decreases sympathetic nervous system action, and useful as a cat repellant. It is an excellent essential oil for oily and acneic skin types.

Perfume Note
Top

Category
Balancing, Refreshing

Scent
Citrus, "earl grey tea", fresh, sweet, refreshing, but with slightly spicy floral undertones

Appearance
Transparent light yellow to greenish hue

Blends Well
It blends well with all essential oils

Possible Substitutions
Mandarin, Sweet Orange, Lemon

Special Precautions and Warnings
Using more than 0.4% in a leave-on skin product in the presence of UV light is not recommended due to photosensitizing caused by furanocoumarin. Use furocoumarin free (FCF) to avoid phototoxicity.

IFRA Critical Effect
Phototoxicity

IFRA Fragrance Material Specifications
"For applications on areas of skin exposed to sunshine, excluding bath preparations, soaps and other products which are washed off the skin, bergamot oil expressed should not be used such that the level in the consumer products exceeds 0.4%."

IFRA Perfume Note: See remark on phototoxic ingredients in the introduction to the Standards (Appendix 8 to the IFRA Code of Practice) and the Standard on Citrus oil and other furocoumarins-containing essential oils.

It is further recommended that, for qualities of the expressed oil in which the less volatile components have been concentrated by partial or total removal of the terpene fraction, this limit should be reduced in proportion to the degree of concentration."

IFRA Recommended Usage Level
"The amount of bergamot used in a topical preparation should be limited to a maximum of 0.4%, except in bath preparations such as soap and other bath preparations which are washed off the skin."

RIFM Recommended Safety Limit
0.4% for expressed and 20% for rectified

European Union Allergen Declaration
Limonene, Linalool, Geraniol

Specs
Flash Point = 108 °F
Specific Gravity = 0.87600 to 0.88400 @ 25.00 °C.
Estimated Pounds per Gallon = 7.289 to 7.356 lbs.
Refractive Index = 1.46400 to 1.46600 @ 20.00 °C.
Optical Rotation = +8.00 to +24.00

Storage
Store in airtight dark glass bottles in a cool, dark area. This essential oil is prone to oxidation, so store in containers with minimum headspace.

Shelf Life
Two years or more if stored properly

Price Point
Medium

FCC
Yes

FDA
GRAS

Reactive in Soap
Yes, due to 30% linalyl acetate

Interesting Fact:
Two hundred pounds of bergamot yields one pound of essential oil.

Cedarwood (*Cedrus deodora*)

Cedarwood is an excellent example of why you should choose your essential oils by Latin name and not by common name. Cedarwood atlas (*Cedrus atlantica*) has a completely different scent profile than Himalayan cedarwood (*Cedrus deodora*). I don't like the scent of *Cedrus atlantica*; however, *Cedrus deodora* has one of my very favorite scent profiles. A very common "so called" cedar is Virginian cedar, which is actually a juniper (*Juniperus virginiana*) and a member of the cypress family. Other mistaken "cedars" are white cedar (*Thuja occidentalis*) and red cedar (*Thuja plicata*), which are both arborvitae from the cypress family and not cedar.

Latin Name
Cedrus deodora

Common Name
Cedarwood or Himalayan Cedarwood

CAS Number 8023-85-6
EINECS 91722-61-1

Geographical Source
India

Family
Pinaceae

Plant Part
Wood

Method
Steam Distilled

Representative Constituents
Alcohols, Sesquiterpenes

Main Components
Cis- and trans- atlantones, himalchenes, (+)-himachalol and
(+)-allohimachalol, alpha-cedrene, beta-cedrene, deodarone

Properties
Antiseptic, tonic, anti-fungal, helps control the products of sebum,
regenerative, astringent, sedative, diuretic, emollient, expectorant, and
insecticides

General Aromatherapy Uses
Chest infections, urinary infections, general tonic, cleansing, rheumatism,
asthma, anxiety, arthritis, regenerative and reduces sinus congestion.
Lymphatic tonic, aids in the removal of body fat. Indicated for retention of
fluid in the tissue and cellulite. Circulatory and lymphatic stimulant. Stress,
tension and nervous disorders. In skincare it is good for acne, general tonic,
cleansing, helps scalp disorders, cellulite, dries oily or blemished skin, natural
astringent, relieves eczema, psoriasis, skin inflammation, bug bites, hair loss,
dry or oily hair, softens skin.

Perfume Note
Base

Category
Relaxing

Scent
Soft, sweet, warm, woody and fruity with honey overtones

Appearance
Viscous clear to yellow

Blends Well
Bergamot, Cardamom, Cistus, Cypress, Frankincense, Grapefruit, Lavender,
Lemon, Mandarin, Myrrh, Orange, Patchouli, Tangerine, Vetiver, Ylang Ylang

Possible Substitutions
Sandalwood, Spruce

Specs
Flash Point = 197.00 °F
Specific Gravity = 0.97200 to 0.98300 @ 25.00 °C.
Estimated Pounds per Gallon = 8.088 to 8.180
Refractive Index = 1.51400 to 1.52900 @ 20.00 °C.
Boiling Point = 513 °F

Storage
Store in airtight dark glass bottles in a cool, dark area

Shelf Life
Two years or more if stored properly

Price Point
Medium

FDA
GRAS

Biblical References to Cedar Plant Material
"The priest shall order that two live clean birds and some cedar wood, scarlet yarn and hyssop be brought for the one to be cleansed." Leviticus 14:4. These cleansing instructions go on in Leviticus 14:6, 49, 51-52 and Numbers 19:6.

"Like valleys they spread out, like gardens beside a river, like aloes planted by the LORD, like cedars beside the waters." Numbers 24:6

"He described plant life, from the cedar of Lebanon to the hyssop that grows out of walls. He also taught about animals and birds, reptiles and fish."1 Kings 4:33

"So give orders that cedars of Lebanon be cut for me. My men will work with yours, and I will pay you for your men whatever wages you set. You know that we have no one so skilled in felling timber as the Sidonians." Kings 5:6

"I will put in the desert the cedar and the acacia, the myrtle and the olive. I will set pines in the wasteland, the fir and the cypress together," Isaiah 41:19

"his young shoots will grow. His splendor will be like an olive tree, his fragrance like a cedar of Lebanon." Hosea 14:6

There are an additional 75 references to cedar in the Bible

Important Note:
Lebanon cedar, *Cedrus libani*, from the Bible is a different species than *Cedrus deodora*.

Chamomile, Blue (*Maticaria chamomilla, Chamomilla recuita*)

Blue chamomile is worth every pretty penny that it costs. It has some of the best properties for skin care of all the essential oils out there. A great trick to using blue chamomile in small batch cosmetics and aromatherapy product is to mix it fifty-fifty with Roman chamomile. Be sure to list both out on your ingredient list. The two essential oils work synergically well together, allowing for measurement of precious blue chamomile into small batches.

Latin Name
Maticaria chamomilla, Chamomilla recuita

Common Name
Chamomile Blue or Chamomile

CAS Number 8002-66-2
EINECS 84082-60-0

Geographical Source
Bulgaria, Egypt, Nepal

Family
Compositae

Plant Part
Flower

Method
Steam Distilled

Representative Constituents
Esters, Sesquiterpenes, Alcohols, Oxides, Coumarins

Main Components
Farnesol, farnesene, chamazulene, alpha-bisabolol oxide b, alpha-bisabolol, alpha-bisabolol oxide a, delta-cadinene, alpha-muurolene, (e)-beta-ocimene, gamma-muurolene, cis-spiroethers, -en-yn-dicycloether, 7-methoxycoumarin

Properties
Anti-allergic, anti-fungal, anti-inflammatory, anti-spasmodic, promotes healing through the formation of scar tissue, decongestant, tonic, hormone-like

General Aromatherapy Uses
Headaches, rheumatism, ulcers, nausea, PMS, insomnia, nervous tension, migraine, menopause, arthritis, muscle aches, sprains. In skincare it is good for acne, wounds, eczema, skin problems, rosacea, and dermatitis

Perfume Note
Middle

Category
Relaxing

Scent
Herbaceous

Appearance
It has a dark blue appearance from chamazulene that is formed during steam distillation of the essential oil. The blue color can be destroyed from exposure to light and air and the oil can change to green and even yellow with age.

Blends Well
Lavender, Roman Chamomile, Tea Tree, Bergamot, Geranium, Ylang Ylang

Possible Substitutions
Roman Chamomile

IFRA
7-Methoxycoumarin $\geq$0.10%

RIFM Recommended Safety Limit
4%

European Union Allergen Declaration
Farnesol

Specs
Flash Point = 125.00 °F
Specific Gravity = 0.91300 to 0.95300 @ 25.00 °C.
Estimated Pounds per Gallon = 7.597 to 7.930
Refractive Index = 1.460-1.49 @ 20.00 °C
Density = 0.900-0.965

Storage
Store in airtight dark glass bottles in a cool, dark area

Shelf Life
2 years or more, if stored properly

Price Point
High

FDA
GRAS

Chamomile, Roman (*Anthemis nobilis, Chamaemelum nobile*)
The aroma of Roman chamomile is sometimes a bit too herbaceous for many. I have found that when you blend it with lavender essential oil, you can find a nice balance between the herbaceous chamomile and the flowery lavender that has a harmonious blend which not only smells great, but is highly effective.

Latin Name
Anthemis nobilis, Chamaemelum nobile

Common Name
Roman Chamomile

CAS Number 8015-92-7
EINECS 283-467-5

Geographical Source
United Kingdom, USA

Family
Compositae

Plant Part
Flower

Method
Steam Distilled

Representative Constituents
Alcohol, Ester, Sequiterpene

Main Components
Isoamyl angelate, isobutyl angelate, 2-methylbutyl 2-methylbutyrate, 3-methylpentyl angelate, 2-methylbutyl angelate, alpha-pinene, isobutyl tiglate, isoamyl tiglate, amyl angelate, amyl methacrylate, 2-methylbutyl 2-methylpropionate, butyl methacrylate, isobutyl isobutyrate, chamazulene

Properties
Analgesic, anti-spasmodic, antiseptic, anti-biotic, anti-inflammatory, anti-infectious, immunostimulant, sedative, reduces nerve pain, strengthens and tones the nerves and nervous system, anti-depressant, anti-allergenic, reduces swelling, relieves itching, relieves rheumatism, promotes healing through the formation of scar tissue, diuretic, emollient, promotes and regulates menstrual flow, fever reducing, aids digestion, increases perspiration, tonic.

General Aromatherapy Uses
Pain relief, fevers, menstrual problems, muscular spasms, sedative, rheumatism, depression, nervousness, migraines, headaches, insomnia and menopause. Good for skin care problems such as rashes, eczema, chilblains, cracked nipples, razor burn, boils, burns and wounds.

Perfume Note
Middle

Category
Relaxing

Scent
Sweet, herbaceous, fresh and fruity

Appearance
Yellow to pale blue as it ages

Blends Well
Bergamot, Calendula Absolute, Cardamom, Cedarwood (*Cedrus deodora*), Blue Chamomile, Cistus, Clary Sage (*Salvia sclarea*) Cypress, Geranium, Helichrysum, Hyssop, Jasmine, Juniper, Lavender, Lemon, Lime, Litsea, Orange, Tangerine, Ylang Ylang

Possible Substitutions
Blue Chamomile, Lavender

IFRA
dl-Citronellol < 0.7%, Geraniol < 0.7%

RIFM Recommended Safety Limit
4%

European Union Allergen Declaration
Citronellol, Geraniol

Specs
Flash Point = 138.00 °F.
Specific Gravity = 0.87900 to 0.90400 @ 25.00 °C.
Estimated Pounds per Gallon = 7.314 to 7.522 lbs.
Refractive Index = 1.43450 to 1.13990 @ 20.00 °C.
Vapor Pressure = 0.530000 mm/Hg @ 25.00 °C.

Storage
Store in airtight dark glass bottles in a cool, dark area

Shelf Life
2 years or more if stored properly

Price Point
Medium to Medium-High

FDA
GRAS

Reactive in Soap
Yes, due to 90 % Esters

Cistus (*Cistus ladanifer*)

Cistus essential oil is an example of essential oils that you simply need to smell to believe. It is among my top five favorite essential oils for aroma. However, it isn't one that I came across in my early aromatherapy education. I love to blend with Cistus because it contributes such uniqueness and mystery to an essential oil blend.

Latin Name
Cistus ladanifer

Common Name
Cistus or Rock Rose

CAS Number 8016-26-0
EINECS 89997-74-0

Geographical Source
Spain, Portugal and NW Africa

Family
Cistaceae

Plant Part
Branches, Leaf

Method
Steam Distilled

Representative Constituents
Alcohols, Esters and Terpenes

Main Components
Alpha-pinene, bornyl acetate, camphene, (3z)-hexen-1-ol 2,2,6-trimethylcyclohexanone, 2-methyl-3-methyleneheptan-6-one, borneol, 1,8-cineole, geraniol, linalyl acetate, beta-pinene, benzaldehyde, alpha-terpinene, beta-phellandrene, neral, carvotanacetone, acetophenone, alpha-phellandrene, thujone, limonene, delta-cadinene, fenchone, sabinene

Properties
Antiviral, antibacterial, anti-arthritic, supports and strengthens the immune and autoimmune systems, antimicrobial, antiseptic, alleviates or suppresses coughs, astringent, promotes and regulates menstrual flow, expectorant, tonic, great for skin with wrinkles, acneic skin and wound healing. Cistus is non-toxic, non-irritating and non-sensitizing.

General Aromatherapy Uses
Children's illnesses, whooping cough, inflammation of the arteries, bronchitis, cancer, aids with mucus production, skin ulcers, rhinitis, tumors, and ulcers. Used in perfumery as a fixative.

Perfume Note
Base

Category
Relaxing

Scent
Complex, rich, woody and dry

Appearance
Semi-viscous yellow to clear liquid

Blends Well
Frankincense, Myrrh, Bergamot, Lavender

Possible Substitutions
Myrrh

IFRA
Eugenol <2.80% and Geraniol <1.20%

European Union Allergen Declaration
Linalool, Geraniol, Limonene

Specs
Flash Point = 189.00 °F
Specific Gravity = 0.86800 to 0.89900 @ 25.00 °C.
Estimated Pounds per Gallon = 7.223 to 7.481 lbs.
Refractive Index = 1.49200 to 1.50700 @ 20.00 °C.
Optical Rotation = -15° / +15

Storage
Store in airtight dark glass bottles in a cool, dark area

Shelf Life
2 years or more if stored properly

Price Point
Medium High to High

FDA
GRAS

Biblical References
"I am a rose of Sharon, a lily of the valleys." Song of Solomon 2:1 (Rose of Sharon is thought to be Cistus)

"Then the LORD said to Moses, "Take fragrant spices--gum resin, onycha and galbanum--and pure frankincense, all in equal amounts," Exodus 30:34 (Onycha is also thought to be Cistus)

Clary sage (*Salvia sclarea*)

I depend heavily on clary sage (*Salvia sclarea*) in my essential oil blends for women; however, I can't stand the smell of it. It is the pillar of the essential oil blend that I created at Essential Wholesale known as Women's Balance Blend. That essential oil blend is one of the most beautiful and effective blends I ever created. Clary sage (*Salvia sclarea*) offered me challenges because I can't sell something I don't like, but I needed the powerful aromatherapy properties of it when I created a blend for women in all stages of their life. This is an excellent example of Synergy Blending, as earlier mentioned.

Latin Name
Salvia sclarea

Common Name
Clary sage

CAS Number 8016-63-5
EINECS 84775-83-7

Geographical Source
Russia, France, Indonesia, Bulgaria

Family
Labiatae

Plant Part
Flowering Plant

Method
Steam Distilled

Representative Constituents
Hydrocarbons, Alcohols, Aldehydes, Esters, Oxides, Ketones, Coumarins

Main Components
Linalyl acetate, linalool, alpha-terpineol, beta-caryophyllene, germacrene d, geranyl acetate, limonene, geraniol

Properties
Antiseptic, sedative, calming, tonic, promotes and regulates menstrual flow, anti-infectious, anti-spasmodic, increases perspiration, aphrodisiac, nerve tonic, strengthens and tones the nerves and nervous system, anti-convulsive, anti-depressant, reduces swelling, neurotonic, helpful during delivery in childbirth, sedative, aids digestion, tonic to the uterus, anti-fungal,

decongestant, detoxifying, guards from or prevents the spread or occurrence of disease or infection, regenerative

General Aromatherapy Uses
Muscular fatigue, menstrual problems, PMS, fertility, exhaustion, insomnia, menopausal problems, stress, depression, cramps, excessive perspiration, dermal fungus, pre-menopause, nervous fatigue, calming to the parasympathetic nervous system, varicose veins, hair growth, alopecia, anti-aging

Perfume Note
Top, Middle

Category
Euphoric

Scent
Herbaceous, nutty, heady, warm and mildly intoxicating

Appearance
Colorless to pale yellow

Blends Well
Jasmine, Litsea, Ylang Ylang

Possible Substitutions
Roman Chamomile

Special Precautions & Warnings
Clary sage (*Salvia sclarea*) is mildly intoxicating. Clary sage has historically carried the contraindication of "Avoid during pregnancy and estrogen dependent conditions such as endometriosis, cancers, and cysts." However, Robert Tisserand has debunked that myth. In reality, Tisserand points out that clary sage oil contains only 4 % of a constituent called sclareol, and that this does not promote estrogen, in fact it blocks estrogen receptors in the body and has been shown to inhibit the growth of breast and uterine cancers.

IFRA
Geraniol <2.20% and (E)-2-hexen-1-al trace to <0.10%, Coumarine <0.1%

RIFM Recommended Safety Limit
8%

European Union Allergen Declaration
Geraniol, Limonene, Linalool

Specs
Flash Point = 142.00 °F
Specific Gravity = 0.88900 to 0.92300 @ 25.00 °C.
Estimated Pounds per Gallon = 7.397 to 7.680 lbs.
Refractive Index = 1.45800 to 1.47300 @ 20.00 °C.
Boiling Point = 440 °F

Storage
Store in airtight dark glass bottles in a cool, dark area

Shelf Life
Two years or more if stored properly

Price Point
Medium

FCC
Yes

FDA
GRAS

Reactive in Soap
Yes, due to 60% Linalyl Acetate

Eucalyptus (*Eucalyptus globules*)
Eucalyptus is probably one of the top five familiar aromas in aromatherapy. The memory that came to mind the first time I smelled it was of my mother rubbing Vicks® VapoRub® on my chest during one of my many childhood respiratory infections. As a matter of fact, eucalyptus is listed among the active ingredients in the drug facts of Vicks® VapoRub®. Currently, one of my favorite uses of eucalyptus is to take the itch out of insect bites.

Latin Name
Eucalyptus globulus

Common Name
Eucalyptus

CAS Number 8016-26-0
EINECS 84625-32-1

Geographical Source
China, Spain, France, Madagascar, Australia, Portugal

Family
Myrtaceae

Plant Part
Leaf

Method
Steam Distilled

Representative Constituents
Oxides, Hydrocarbons, Alcohols, Ketones, Aldehydes, Esters

Main Components
1,8-cineole, alpha-pinene, myrcene, citronellal, menthone, limonene

Properties
Antiseptic, expectorant, anti-fungal, fever reducing, reduces nerve pain, relieves chest or respiratory tract disorders, antibacterial, analgesic, relieves rheumatism, reduces swelling, anti-spasmodic, antiviral, encourages skin cell growth, decongestant, deodorant, purifies the blood and fluids of the body, diuretic, stimulant, breaks down mucus

General Aromatherapy Uses
Athlete's foot, cold sores, dandruff, insect bites, wound healing, aids with mucus production, bronchitis, colds, flu, fever, sinusitis, muscular aches and pains, headaches, sluggishness, mental exhaustion, rheumatism, asthma, insect bites, rashes, skin ulcers, sore throat, coughs, sinusitis, respiratory tract infections, migraine, asthma, combats fever, insect repellant

Perfume Note
Top

Category
Stimulating

Scent
Pungent, sharp, strong and camphor-like with woody sub-notes

Appearance
Colorless

Blends Well
All citrus and mint essential oils

Possible Substitutions
Eucalyptus radiata, Rosemary

Special Precautions & Warnings
It is contraindicated for use on babies or small children.

RIFM Recommended Safety Limit
10%

European Union Allergen Declaration
Limonene

Specs
Flash Point = 120.00 °F
Specific Gravity = 0.90500 to 0.92500 @ 25.00 °C.
Estimated Pounds per Gallon = 7.531 to 7.697 lbs.
Refractive Index = 1.45800 to 1.46500 @ 20.00 °C.
Optical Rotation = +1.00 to +4.00

Storage
Store in airtight dark glass bottles in a cool, dark area

Shelf Life
Two years or more if stored properly

Price Point
Medium

FCC
Yes

FDA
GRAS

Frankincense (*Boswellia carteri*)

Most people's first thought of frankincense includes myrrh and the Bible. Frankincense is referenced in the Bible twenty four times. It is cited twenty-two times in the Old Testament, but it is most famous for being brought to the baby Jesus by the Magi. "Then they opened their treasures and presented him with gifts of gold, frankincense and myrrh." Matthew 2:11

Latin Name
Boswellia carteri

Common Name
Frankincense

CAS Number 8016-36-2
EINECS 8050-07-5

Geographical Source
Somalia

Family
Burseraceae

Plant Part
Resin

Method
Steam Distilled

Representative Constituents
Hydrocarbons, Alcohols, Ketones, Esters

Main Components
a-pinene, a-phellandrene, limonene, b-pinene and myrcene

Properties
Analgesic, tonic, stimulant, expectorant, anti-depressant, antiseptic, revitalizer, astringent, anti-tumor, diuretic, sedative, antioxidant, anti-infectious, anti-inflammatory, energizing

General Aromatherapy Uses
Deepens breathing, aids asthmatic coughs, used for colds and bronchitis, skin diseases or disorders, circulation problems, burns including sunburns, anti-aging, wounds. Used as aid for rheumatism, tonic to the uterus, urinary tract infections, breast inflammations, cramps, and sports injuries. Helpful to combat anxiety, nervous exhaustion, stress, nightmares, and has a calming sedative effect. Boosts immune system, sedative, and has a diuretic effect. Used for dry, mature, aging skin, acne, pimples, scars, smoothes out wrinkles, balances out oily skin, tonic to all skin types.

Perfume Note
Base

Category
Balancing, Relaxing

Scent
Warm, mild, soothing, complex, balsamic

Appearance
Viscous liquid

Blends Well
Sandalwood, Myrrh, Lavender, Lemon, Bergamot, Sweet Orange, Cedarwood (*Cedrus deodora*), Cistus, Grapefruit, Mandarin And Ylang Ylang

Possible Substitutions
Cistus

RIFM Recommended Safety Limit
8% essential oil and 3% absolute

European Union Allergen Declaration
Linalool, Limonene

Specs
Flash Point = 96.00 °F
Specific Gravity = 0.86000 to 0.89000 @ 25.00 °C.
Estimated Pounds per Gallon = 7.156 to 7.406 lbs.
Refractive Index = 1.46600 to 1.47700 @ 20.00 °C.
Optical Rotation = -0.05 to 0.00
Boiling Point = 137.00 to 141.00 °C. @ 760.00 mm Hg

Storage
Store in airtight dark glass bottles in a cool, dark area

Shelf Life
Two years or more if stored properly

Price Point
High

FDA
GRAS

Biblical References

"Then the LORD said to Moses, "Take fragrant spices—gum resin, onycha and galbanum—and pure frankincense, all in equal amounts, and make a fragrant blend of incense, the work of a perfumer. It is to be salted and pure and sacred. Grind some of it to powder and place it in front of the Testimony in the Tent of Meeting, where I will meet with you. It shall be most holy to you. Do not make any incense with this formula for yourselves; consider it holy to the LORD." Exodus 30: 34-37

"...cargoes of cinnamon and spice, of incense, myrrh and frankincense, of wine and olive oil, of fine flour and wheat; cattle and sheep; horses and carriages; and bodies and souls of men." Revelation 18:13

"On coming to the house, they saw the child with his mother Mary, and they bowed down and worshiped him. Then they opened their treasures and presented him with gifts of gold, frankincense and myrrh. And having been warned in a dream not to go back to Herod, they returned to their country by another route. When they had gone, an angel of the Lord appeared to Joseph in a dream. "Get up," he said, "take the child and his mother and escape to Egypt. Stay there until I tell you, for Herod is going to search for the child to kill him. So he got up, took the child and his mother during the night and left for Egypt, where he stayed until the death of Herod. And so was fulfilled what the Lord had said through the prophet: 'Out of Egypt I called my son.'" Matthew 2:11-15

Frankincense is also implied in all references to holy incense or anointing oil in the Bible, due to the instructions given in Exodus 30: 34-37. For example, "The smoke of the incense, together with the prayers of the saints, went up before God from the angel's hand." Revelation 8:4

Geranium (*Pelargonium x asperum*)

Geranium essential oil is not one of my first loves as a single note, but it is essential in blending for both properties and perfuming. The scent is overwhelming alone in my opinion, but when blended with other essential oils it is a fundamental piece of the scent and property puzzle. I almost always am drawn to it when I blend essential oils for women's issues.

Latin Name
Pelargonium x asperum

Common Name
Geranium, Rose Geranium

CAS Number 8000-46-2
EINECS 90082-51-2

Geographical Source
Egypt, France, Morocco, India

Family
Geraniaceae

Plant Part
Leaf

Method
Steam Distilled

Representative Constituents
Hydrocarbons, Alcohols, Esters, Aldehydes, Ketones, Oxides

Main Components
Citronellol, geraniol, linalool, citronellyl formate, isomenthone, 10-epi-gamma-eudesmol, geranyl formate, citronellyl propionate, geranyl butyrate, geranyl propionate, geranyl tiglate, cis-rose oxide, citral

Properties
Astringent, diuretic, anti-depressant, regenerative, tonic, anti-spasmodic, anti-infectious, anti-fungal, analgesic, promotes healing through the formation of scar tissue, encourages skin cell growth, diuretic, deodorant, insecticidal, relaxant

General Aromatherapy Uses
Female reproductive disorders, promotes fertility, circulatory disorders, anti-depressant, menopause, bruising, ulceration, hemorrhoids, nervous fatigue, emotional balance, rheumatism, athletes foot, candida, acne, wounds, arthritis, painful menstruation, varicose veins, burns, cuts, stretch marks, breast congestion, lymph congestion, anxiety, nervous fatigue

Perfume Note
Middle

Category
Balancing

Scent
The scent is extremely powerful. Has prominent rosy perfume notes, green floral along with earthy undertones, sweet, dry citrus undertone

Appearance
Varies from yellow to greenish

Blends Well
Lavender, Ylang Ylang, Clary Sage (*Salvia sclarea*), All Citrus

Possible Substitutions
Clary Sage (*Salvia sclarea*), Rose, Palmarosa

IFRA Critical Effect
Sensitization

IFRA
Citral <1.50%, Citronellol <30.00%, Geraniol <20.00%

European Union Allergen Declaration
Citral, Geraniol, Citronellol and Linalool

Specs
Flash Point =   165.00 °F
Specific Gravity = 0.88700 to 0.89200 @ 25.00 °C
Pounds per Gallon = 7.381 to 7.422 lbs.
Refractive Index = 1.46600 to 1.47000 @ 20.00 °C.
Boiling Point = 387 °F

Storage
Store in airtight dark glass bottles in a cool, dark area

Shelf Life
Two years or more if stored properly

Price Point
Medium

FCC
Yes

FDA
GRAS

Ginger (*Zingiber officinale*)

Not all ginger essential oils have the same aroma. Many have an earthy, almost musky aroma, but there are a handful of Gingers in which the spicy scent of fresh ginger survives the distillation process. As a huge fan of the scent of fresh-cut ginger I searched the world for a ginger essential oil with that wonderful strong aroma and found it for Essential Wholesale. Don't give up on ginger until you have found one that is pleasing to your nose.

Latin Name
Zingiber officinale

Common Name
Ginger

CAS Number 8007-08-7
EINECS 84696-15-1

Geographical Source
Sri Lanka, Madagascar, Indonesia, Nigeria, India

Family
Zingiberaceae

Plant Part
Rhizome

Method
Steam Distilled

Representative Constituents
Hydrocarbons, Alcohols, Aldehydes, Oxides

Main Components
Beta-bisabolene, camphene, ar-curcumene, alpha-phellandrene, beta-phellandrene, limonene, alpha-pinene, p-cymene, borneol, 1,8-cineole, myrcene, beta-farnesene, beta-eudesmol, limonene, linalool, citral

Properties
Analgesic, aids with mucus production, expectorant, general tonic, sexual tonic

General Aromatherapy Uses
Rheumatism, chronic bronchitis, nausea, impotence, colic, motion sickness

Category
Stimulating

Scent
Peppery, sharp, fresh, pungent, earthy aromatic and warm

Appearance
Clear to pale yellow

Blends Well
All Citrus, Lavender, Ylang Ylang, Litsea, Jasmine

Possible Substitutions
Cardamom

Perfume Note
Middle, Base

IFRA
Limonene, Linalool, Citral

European Union Allergen Declaration
Limonene, Linalool, Citral

Specs
Flash Point = > 200.00 °F
Specific Gravity = 0.870 to 0.882 @ 25deg. C
Refractive Index = 1.488 to 1.494 @ 20 deg. C
Saponification Value = 8.51

Storage
Store in airtight dark glass bottles in a cool, dark area

Shelf Life
Two years or more if stored properly

Price Point
Medium

FDA
GRAS

Grapefruit (*Citrus paradisi*)

According to a study by Dr. Alan Hirsch of the Smell and Taste Institute the aroma of grapefruit makes men perceive women as almost five years younger. That is reason enough to love grapefruit! Over years of watching the reaction people have when they smell essential oils, I have found that grapefruit brings a smile to the faces of 99 % of the people who smell it.

Latin Name
Citrus paradisi

Common Name
Grapefruit

CAS Number 8016-20-4
EINECS 289-904-6

Geographical Source
USA, Israel, South Africa

Family
Rutaceae

Plant Part
Fruit Peel

Method
Cold Expressed

Representative Constituents
Terpenes

Main Components
Limonene, Myrcene

Properties
Anti-fungal, astringent, euphoric

General Aromatherapy Uses
Athlete's foot, acne, oily skin, tones congested skin, tightens skin, increases circulation, stimulates lymphatic detoxification, cellulite, depression, headache, PMS, stress

Perfume Note
Top

Category
Stimulating, euphoric

Scent
Clean, warm, sweet and fresh citrus with slight floral undertone

Appearance
Yellow to pale orange

Blends Well
All Citrus essential oils, Frankincense, Myrrh, Cistus, Cedarwood (*Cedrus Deodora*), Lavender, Rosemary

Possible Substitutions
Lemon

IFRA Critical Effect
Phototoxicity

IFRA Other Specification
< 20 moles / L of peroxides

IFRA
Citral <0.10%

IFRA Fragrance Material Specifications
May be used in cosmetic products, provided that the total concentration of furocoumarin-like substances in the finished cosmetic product do not exceed 1ppm. For qualities of the expressed oil in which the less volatile components have been concentrated by partial or total removal of the terpene fraction, this limit should be reduced in proportion to the degree of concentration.

European Union Allergen Declaration
Citral

Specs
Specific Gravity = 0.85200 to 0.86000 @ 25.00 °C.
Refractive Index = 1.47400 to 1.47900 @ 20.00 °C.
Flash Point = 111.00 °F

Storage
Store in airtight dark glass bottles in a cool, dark area. This essential oil is prone to oxidation, so store in containers with minimum headspace.

Shelf Life
One year or more if stored properly

Price Point
Medium Low

FCC
Yes

FDA
GRAS

Laurel Leaf (*Laurus nobilis*)

Laurel leaf is my go-to essential oil during cold and flu season. After a lifetime of chronic respiratory issues that have sent me searching for cures, I can honestly give laurel leaf credit as my number one favorite respiratory, fatigue and immunity essential oil. According to Dr. Kurt Schnaubelt, "Its positive effects on the lymphatic system are undeniable. Rubbing a few drops of Bay Laurel on swollen lymph nodes will produce an immediately noticeable relieving effect." I always carry it with me when I travel. One time, when I arrived in Alabama to speak at a conference, I was surprised to find that the small airport I landed at diffused laurel leaf essential oil throughout the building, only to find that my very own laurel leaf had leaked in my suitcase and I was the source of the aroma.

Latin Name
Laurus nobilis

Common Name
Laurel Leaf, Bay Laurel

CAS Number 8006-78-8
EINECS 84603-73-6

Geographical Source
Turkey, Yugoslavia, Morocco, Italy

Family
Lauraceae

Plant Part
Leaf

Method
Steam Distilled

Representative Constituents
Oxides, Esters, Alcohols, Phenols

Main Components
1,8-cineole, alpha-terpinyl acetate, sabinene, alpha-pinene, methyl eugenol, beta-pinene, linalool, alpha-terpineol, eugenol, terpinen-4-ol, gamma-terpinene, geraniol

Properties
Antibacterial, anti-rheumatic, antiseptic, antiviral, promotes perspiration, digestive, diuretic, expectorant, fungicidal, lowers blood pressure, sedative, warming, narcotic-like

General Aromatherapy Uses
asthma, bronchitis, bruises, colds, colic, digestion, earache, fever, flu, gout, hair loss after infection, hysteria, indigestion, lice, menstrual promotion, migraine headaches, palpitations, rheumatic aches and pains, scanty periods, sprains, tonsillitis, viral infections, sinus infections, muscular pain

Perfume Note
Top

Category
Stimulating, euphoric

Scent
Medicinal, fresh, herbaceous

Appearance
Pale yellow to clear liquid

Blends With
All Citrus essential oils, Rosemary, Peppermint, Lavender, Eucalyptus, Ginger

Special Precautions & Warnings
Avoid overuse because it has a narcotic-like effect.

IFRA
Eugenol <3.00%, Geraniol <0.30%, (E)-2- hexen-1-al trace to <0.10%, Methyl eugenol <4.00%

RIFM Recommended Safety Limit
2%

European Union Allergen Declaration
Eugenol, Geraniol, Eugenol

Specs
Flash Point = 128.00 °F
Specific Gravity = 0.90500 to 0.92900 @ 25.00 °C.
Estimated Pounds per Gallon = 7.531 to 7.730
Refractive Index = 1.46500 to 1.47000 @ 20.00 °C.

Storage
Store in airtight dark glass bottles in a cool, dark area

Shelf Life
Two years or more if stored properly

Price Point
Medium High

FDA
GRAS

Biblical References
"I have seen a wicked, ruthless man, spreading himself like a green laurel tree"
Psalm 37:35

"He cuts down cedars for his use, or he takes a cypress or an oak. He lets it grow strong among the trees of the forest. He plants a laurel, and the rain makes it grow." Isaiah 44:14

Lavender (*Lavandula angustifolia*)

What would the world be like without lavender? I'd hate to find out. If you haven't incorporated lavender essential oil into your aromatherapy collection, you have barely begun to see the miraculous properties of essential oils. I remember being moved to tears as I read *The Chemistry of Essential Oils* by David G. Williams while studying for my aromatherapy registration exam as. The overwhelming complexity and planning in God's creation of the lavender plant made me think of all the thought, love, and care that He had in mind for us with the creation of lavender on the third day. "Then God said, 'Let the land produce vegetation: seed-bearing plants and trees on the land that bear fruit with seed in it, according to their various kinds.' And it was so. The land produced vegetation: plants bearing seed according to their kinds and trees bearing fruit with seed in it according to their kinds. And God saw that it was good. And there was evening, and there was morning—the third day." Genesis 1:11-13

Latin Name
Lavandula angustifolia

Common Name
Lavender

CAS Number 8000-28-0
EINECS 90063-37-9

Geographical Source
Eastern Europe, France, Tasmania, England, USA

Family
Labiatae

Plant Part
Flower

Method
Steam Distilled

Representative Constituents
Hydrocarbons, Alcohols, Esters, Oxides, Ketones, Aldehydes

Main Components
Linalool, linalyl acetate, terpinen-4-ol, 1,8-cineole, camphor, beta-caryophyllene, limonene, borneol, alpha-terpineol, (z)-beta-ocimene, para-cymene, alpha-pinene, coumarin, geraniol, 7- methoxycoumarin, 1- octen-3-yl acetate

Properties
Antiseptic, analgesic, encourages skin cell growth, anti-spasmodic, tonic, promotes the formation of a cicatrix to aid healing of sore or wound, anti-inflammatory, promotes and regulates menstrual flow, anti-venomous, anti-toxic, anti-parasitic, relieves or suppresses coughs, diuretic, restorative, decongestant, anti-depressant, a sedative, sedative, anti-biotic, anti-infectious, muscular relaxant

General Aromatherapy Uses
Cuts, grazes, burns, rheumatism, chilblains, dermatitis, eczema, sunburn, insect bites, headaches, migraine, insomnia, infections, arthritis, anxiety, tension, panic, hysteria, fatigue, inflammatory conditions, rashes, nervous conditions, aids with menstruation that is painful and difficult, spasms, muscle aches, candida, athlete's foot, acne, sinusitis, infectious skin conditions. Can be used safely on children and it is non-toxic, non-irritating.

Perfume Note
Top, Middle

Category
Relaxing, balancing

Scent
Floral, light, powdery, sweet, camphoraceous freshness, herbaceous, with slight spicy warmth and sweetness

Appearance
Colorless to pale yellow

Blends Well
All Citrus, Cedarwood (*Cedrus deodora*), Clary Sage (*Salvia sclarea*), Frankincense, Geranium, Neroli, Rose, Rosemary

Possible Substitutions
Lavandin

IFRA Other Specification
< 20 moles / L of peroxides

IFRA
Coumarin <0.10%, Geraniol <1.00%, 7- Methoxycoumarin <0.02%, 1- Octen-3-yl Acetate <1.00%

European Union Allergen Declaration
Coumarin, Geraniol, Linalool

Specs
Flash Point = 160.00 °F
Specific Gravity = 0.87500 to 0.88800 @ 25.00 °C.
Estimated Pounds per Gallon = 7.281 to 7.389 lbs.
Refractive Index = 1.45900 to 1.46900 @ 20.00 °C.
Optical Rotation = -3.00 to -10.00
Boiling Point = 399 °F

Storage
Store in airtight glass dark bottles in a cool dark area

Shelf Life
Two years or more if stored properly

Price Point
Medium

FCC
Yes

FDA
GRAS

Reactive in Soap
Yes, due to 40% Esters

Lemon (*Citrus limon*)

Lemon is a universally loved aroma. There are very few people who will turn up their nose to the scent of lemon essential oil. When I think of lemon essential oil, my first thought is to use it a room freshener, not only for its fresh scent, but also because it is the best essential oil for disinfecting the air.

Latin Name
Citrus limon

Common Name
Lemon

CAS Number 84929-31-7
EINECS 84929-31-7

Geographical Source
Argentina, Israel, Italy, USA

Family
Rutaceae

Plant Part
Fruit Peel

Method
Cold Expressed

Representative Constituents
Hydrocarbons, Alcohols, Aldehydes, Esters

Main Components
Limonene, beta-Pinene, gamma-Terpinene, Myrcene, alpha-Pinene, Citral, Geraniol, Limonene, Linalool

Properties
Anti-biotic, sedative, diuretic, arrests bleeding, astringent, digestive, immunostimulant, anti-depressant, stimulant, antiseptic, fever reducing, anti-spasmodic, prevents hardening of tissue, promotes the formation of a cicatrix to aid healing of sore or wound, astringent, insect bites, tonic, insecticide, lowers blood pressure, emollient, relieves itching, relieves rheumatism, reduces nerve pain

General Aromatherapy Uses
General tonic, infections, detoxification, general fatigue, obesity, acne, physical exhaustion, depression, rheumatism, colds and flu, skin care, athlete's foot, stress, hypertension, varicose veins, boils, anti-aging, warts, insomnia, edema, asthma, endocrine stimulant, aids concentration

Perfume Note
Top

Category
Stimulating

Scent
Citrus, fresh, sharp

Appearance
Clear with a yellow hue

Blends Well
Blends well with all essential oils

Possible Substitutions
Lime, Grapefruit, Litsea

Special Precautions and Warning
Phototoxic

IFRA

Citral <3.00%, geraniol <0.20%

IFRA Critical Effect

Phototoxicity

IFRA fragrance material specification

May be used in cosmetic products, provided that the total concentration of furocoumarin-like substances in the finished cosmetic product do not exceed 1ppm. For qualities of the expressed oil in which the less volatile components have been concentrated by partial or total removal of the terpene fraction, this limit should be reduced in proportion to the degree of concentration.

European Union Allergen Declaration

Citral, Geraniol, Limonene, Linalool

Specs

Flash Point = 115.00 °F

Specific Gravity = 0.84900 to 0.85500 @ 25.00 °C.

Estimated Pounds per Gallon = 7.065 to 7.114 lbs.

Refractive Index = 1.47200 to 1.47400 @ 20.00 °C.

Optical Rotation = +57.00 to +65.50

Boiling Point = 349 °F

Storage

Store in airtight dark glass bottles in a cool, dark area. This essential oil is prone to oxidation, so store in containers with minimum headspace.

Shelf Life

1 year or more if stored properly

Price Point

Low

FDA

GRAS

Myrrh (*Commiphora myrrha*)

Everyone's first thought when they have a cough is to turn to eucalyptus for relief, but don't discount myrrh. It is my go-to inhalation therapy essential oil for persistent coughs. Myrrh is most famous for multiple references in both the Old and the New Testament of the Bible. Perhaps the most interesting of all the Biblical references to the plant material myrrh are Psalm 69:21 and Mark 15:

22-23. In Psalm 69:21 it is foretold that the Messiah would be given, "poison for food; they offered me sour wine for my thirst." In Mark 15: 22-23 it says, "They brought Jesus to the place of Golgotha (which means The Place of the Skull). Then they offered him wine mixed with myrrh, but he did not take it." Myrrh is toxic in high concentrations and poisonous if taken internally.

Latin Name
Commiphora myrrha

Common Name
Myrrh

CAS Number 8016-37-3
EINECS 9000-45-7

Family
Burceraceae

Plant Part
Resin

Method
Steam Distilled

Geographical Source
Somalia

Representative Constituents
Hydrocarbons, Ketones, Aldehydes, Phenols, Alcohols, Acids

Main Components
Curzerene, heerabolene, sesquiterpenoid, beta-elemene, gamma-elemene

Properties
Relieves chest or respiratory tract disorders, antiseptic, promotes the formation of a cicatrix to aid healing of sore or wound, balsamic, anti-fungal, astringent, prevents tissue degeneration and arrests bleeding in wounds, antiviral, aphrodisiac, anti-inflammatory, antimicrobial, reduces swelling, diuretic, stimulant, aid digestion, increases perspiration, tonic.

General Aromatherapy Uses
Coughs, aids with mucus production, bronchitis, ulcerations, colds, wounds, feeling cold, eczema, ringworm, sores, skin care, inflamed skin, asthma

Perfume Note
Base

Category
Euphoric

Scent
Very light, warm, smoky, slightly musty and earthy

Appearance
Yellow amber to brown clear viscous liquid

Blends Well
Cistus, Frankincense, Lavender, Lemon, Bergamot

Possible Substitutions
Frankincense

RIFM Recommended Safety Limit
8% essential oil and 3% absolute

Specs
Flash Point = > 200.00 °F
Specific Gravity = 0.98800 to 1.01700 @ 25.00 °C.
Estimated Pounds per Gallon = 8.221 to 8.462 lbs.
Refractive Index = 1.51700 to 1.52800 @ 20.00 °C.
Boiling Point = 428 °F

Storage
Store in airtight glass dark bottles in a cool dark area

Shelf Life
2 years or more if stored properly

Price Point
High

FDA
GRAS

Bible References
"As they sat down to eat their meal, they looked up and saw a caravan of Ishmaelites coming from Gilead. Their camels were loaded with spices, balm

and myrrh, and they were on their way to take them down to Egypt." Genesis 37:25

"Then their father Israel said to them, "If it must be, then do this: Put some of the best products of the land in your bags and take them down to the man as a gift—a little balm and a little honey, some spices and myrrh, some pistachio nuts and almonds." Genesis 43:11

"All your robes are fragrant with myrrh and aloes and cassia; from palaces adorned with ivory the music of the strings makes you glad. Psalm 45:8

"I have perfumed my bed with myrrh, aloes and cinnamon." Proverbs 7:17

"Before a young woman's turn came to go in to King Xerxes, she had to complete twelve months of beauty treatments prescribed for the women, six months with oil of myrrh and six with perfumes and cosmetics." Esther 2:12

Also: Exodus 30: 23-25 and 34, 1 Kings 10:25, Song of Solomon 1:13, 3:6, 4:6, 4:14, 5:1, 5:5,
Matthew 2:11, 27: 33-34, 27:59, Mark 14:8, 15: 22-24, Psalms 69:21, Acts 9:37, John 11:44, 12:3-7, 19:39-40, 20:7, 2 Chronicles 9:24, 16:14, Revelation 18:13

Neroli (*Citrus aurantium var. amara*)

When I first started in aromatherapy, I wasn't a fan of neroli; it smelled synthetic to me. Well, it turned out my nose was so good, that before I really knew anything about adulterated essential oils, I could pick one out blindly. I had been buying neroli from a well-known aromatherapy supplier long before we started Essential Wholesale and it was a blend of synthetics and natural aromas. Needless to say, I learned these important lessons early: to trust my nose, to check our sources of supplies thoroughly, and to not be afraid to have my essential oils tested.

Latin Name
Citrus aurantium var. amara

Common Name
Neroli or Orange Blossom

CAS Number 8016-38-4
EINECS 72968-50-4

Geographical Source
Spain, Italy, Morocco, Tunisia

Family
Rutaceae

Plant Part
Flower

Method
Steam Distilled

Representative Constituents
Hydrocarbons, Alcohols, Esters, Aldehydes, Ketone, Oxides

Main Components
Linalool, limonene, beta-pinene, (e)-beta-ocimene, geraniol, linalyl acetate, sabinene, nerolidol, alpha-terpineol, geranyl acetate, myrcene, alpha-pinene, gamma-terpinene, farnesol, citral, farnesol

Properties
Antibacterial, anti-depressive, anti-parasitic, neurotonic, guards from or prevents the spread or occurrence of disease or infection, immuno-stimulant

General Aromatherapy Uses
Nervous depression, mildly tranquillizing, hypertension, fatigue, aids sleep, varicose veins, scars, stretch marks, acne, mature skin, improves elasticity, good for circulation, aphrodisiac, PMS, menopause, aids labor, shock, stress, anxiety, mild hypnotic, tranquilizes sympathetic nervous system

Perfume Note
Middle

Category
Relaxing

Scent
Floral, rich, fruity, spicy, sweet with highly radiant fragrance

Appearance
Pale yellow

Blends Well
All Citrus, Clary Sage (*Salvia sclarea*), Geranium, Jasmine, Lavender, Rose, Ylang Ylang

Possible Substitutions
Petitgrain

IFRA
Citral <0.60%, farnesol <4.00%, geraniol <3.50%

European Union Allergen Declaration
Citral, Farnesol, Geraniol, Linalool, Limonene

RIFM Recommended Safety Limit
4% essential oil and 3% absolute

Specs
Flash Point = 154.00 °F
Specific Gravity = 0.86000 to 0.87900 @ 25.00 °C.
Estimated Pounds per Gallon = 7.156 to 7.314
Optical Rotation = +2.50 to +11.50

Storage
Store in airtight glass dark bottles in a cool dark area

Shelf Life
2 years or more if stored properly

Price Point
High

FDA
GRAS

Orange, Sweet (*Citrus sinensis*)

I clean all of my hard surfaces of my house with sweet orange essential oil so my scent-association with the aroma is clean. It is the 'wonder' essential oil of the cleaning world due to the high content of limonene. Since sweet orange is so inexpensive, it also makes a great essential oil to blend with because it is good for your bottom line, smells great, and blends even better.

Latin Name
Citrus sinensis

Common Name
Orange Sweet

CAS Number 8028-48-6
EINECS 8028-48-6

Geographical Source
Brazil, USA

Family
Rutaceae

Plant Part
Fruit Peel

Method
Cold Expressed

Representative Constituents
Terpenes

Main Components
Limonene, Myrcene, Linalool

Properties
A sedative, diuretic, tonic, anti-spasmodic, antiseptic, anti-biotic, anti-depressant, fever reducing

General Aromatherapy Uses
Diuretic, constipation, helps eliminate toxins, overindulgence, nervous anxiety, general body tonic

Perfume Note
Top

Category
Relaxing

Scent
Citrus, sweet, fresh, fruity, tangy and sweet. A perky and lively scent

Appearance
Yellow to orange clear liquid

Blends Well
Blends well with all essential oils

Possible Substitutions
Tangerine, Mandarin

Special Precautions and Warning
Phototoxic

IFRA
Citral < 0.1%

RIFM Recommended Safety Limit
10%

European Union Allergen Declaration
Limonene, Linalool

Specs
Boiling Point = 347 °F
Specific Gravity = 0.84000 to 0.86000 @ 20.00 °C
Estimated Pounds per Gallon = 6.998 to 7.164 lbs.
Refractive Index = 1.45500 to 1.47500 @ 20.00 °C.
Optical Rotation = +70.00 to +90.00

Storage
Store in airtight dark glass bottles in a cool, dark area. This essential oil is prone to oxidation, so store in containers with minimum headspace.

Shelf Life
1 year or more if stored properly

Price Point
Low

FDA
GRAS

Patchouli *(Pogostemon cablin)*

When I first started in the aromatherapy world I thought patchouli smelled like dirt and mold, but now I love it. I discovered, in one of my informal non-scientific research studies, that how people feel about patchouli essential oil is directly related to their scent-memory of it. When we had an aroma-party plan I used to pass around patchouli essential oil when I talked about scent-memories. I found that those who responded positively to the aroma had a good to great scent-memory associated with it. And those that responded very negatively to it had bad scent-memories associated with patchouli. I and many others, who had almost no scent memory of it, were indifferent to the aroma of it. There is nothing formal about my research, but I have continued to ask questions in my 13 years in the aromatherapy world, and I get the same result today as I did then.

Latin Name
Pogostemon cablin

Common Name
Patchouli

CAS Number CAS8014-09-03
EINECS 84238-39-1

Geographical Source
Indonesia, India, Brazil, Malaysia

Family
Labiatae

Plant Part
Leaf, Flower

Method
Steam Distilled

Representative Constituents
Hydrocarbons, Alcohols, Ketones, Oxides

Main Components
Patchouli alcohol, alpha-bulnesene, beta-caryophyllene, alpha-guaiene, bulnesene oxide, caryophyllene oxide, elemene, pogostol, guaioxide, norpatchoulenol

Properties
Tonic, anti-infectious, antiseptic, decongestant, anti-fungal, anti-depressant, aphrodisiac, astringent, a sedative, strengthens or tones the nerves and nervous system, reduces swelling, promotes healing through the formation of scar tissue, deodorant, diuretic, insecticide

General Aromatherapy Uses
Fungal infections, bacterial infections, tonic to the uterus, dandruff, insect repellent, insect bites, stress-related emotional disorders, substance addictions, dermatitis, athlete's foot, ringworm, helps eliminate toxins, acne, allergies, inflamed skin, seborrheic eczema, scar tissue, varicose veins

237

Perfume Note
Base

Perfuming Note of Caution
Patchouli is highly odoriferous and can easily take over a blend, use sparingly.

Category
Euphoric

Scent
Earthy, heavy, musty musk, penetrating, herbaceous, and smoky

Appearance
Dark amber viscous liquid

Blends Well
All Citrus, Vetiver, Cedarwood (*Cedrus deodora*), Clary Sage (*Salvia sclarea*), Lavender, Geranium, Rose, Neroli

Possible Substitutions
Vetiver

RIFM Recommended Safety Limit
10%

Specs
Flash Point = 190.00 °F
Specific Gravity = 0.95000 to 0.97500 @ 25.00 °C.
Estimated Pounds per Gallon = 7.905 to 8.113 lbs.
Refractive Index = 1.49900 to 1.51500 @ 20.00 °C.
Optical Rotation = 48.00 to -65.00
Boiling Point = 549 °F

Storage
Store in airtight dark glass bottles in a cool, dark area.

Shelf Life
Patchouli gets better with age

Price Point
Medium

FDA
GRAS

Peppermint (*Mentha x piperita*)

I love peppermint essential oil. Have you ever really wondered about the difference between peppermint 3rd and peppermint natural essential oils? One of the most interesting aromatherapy classes I've taken over the years was *Chemistry of Essential Oils* taught by Dr. Rob Pappas. In that class he taught that isovaleraldehyde is the component of peppermint that is distilled off in the manufacturing of peppermint 3rd essential oil. The fascinating part is that isovaleraldehyde is a scent component of vomit and blue cheese as well. Now that you know this, take the time to smell the difference between peppermint 3rd and peppermint natural and see if you can pick up the faint scent component difference.

Latin Name
Mentha x piperita

Common Name
Peppermint

CAS Number 8006-90-4
EINECS 98306-02-6

Geographical Source
USA, France, England

Family
Labiatae

Plant Part
Flowering Herb

Method
Steam Distilled

Representative Constituents
Hydrocarbons, Alcohols, Ketones, Oxides, Esters, Coumarins

Main Components
Menthol, menthone, 1,8-cineole, methyl acetate, methofuran, isomenthone, limonene, alpha-pinene, beta–pinene, germancrene-d, trans-sabine hydrate

Properties
Antiseptic, anti-biotic, anti-infectious, aids digestion, anti-spasmodic, purifies the blood and fluids of the body, stimulant, tonic, promotes and regulates menstrual flow, anti-parasitic, expectorant, analgesic, digestive, decongestant,

hormone-like, antibacterial, anti-fungal, anti-inflammatory, blocks lactation, reduces fevers, anti-spasmodic, expectorant, neurotonic, reproductive stimulant, tones uterine muscle

General Aromatherapy Uses
Headaches, nausea, fatigue, apathy, coughs, digestive problems, bowel disorders, flatulence, muscular pain, sinus congestion, shock, faintness, travel sickness, mouth or gum infections, mental tiredness, poor circulation, ringworm, bronchitis, sinusitis, prevents milk from forming, migraine, fever, colic, herpes, bronchial asthma, bronchitis, ovarian stimulant, insect repellent, impotence, facilitates delivery

Perfume Note
Top

Category
Stimulating

Scent
Minty fresh, slightly camphor-like, candy-like

Appearance
Colorless to pale yellow clear liquid

Blends Well
All Citrus, Rosemary, Spearmint, Eucalyptus, Lavender

Possible Substitutions
Spearmint, Rosemary

IFRA
(E)-2- hexen-1-al trace to <0.10%

RIFM Recommended Safety Limit
8%

European Union Allergen Declaration
Limonene

Specs
Flash Point = 160.00 °F
Specific Gravity = 0.89600 to 0.90800 @ 25.00 °C.
Estimated Pounds per Gallon =7.456 to 7.555 lbs.
Refractive Index = 1.45900 to 1.46500 @ 20.00 °C.

Optical Rotation = -18.00 to -32.00
Boiling Point = 408 °F

Storage
Store in airtight dark glass bottles in a cool dark area

Shelf Life
2 years or more if stored properly

Price Point
Medium

FCC
Yes

FDA
GRAS

Biblical Reference of Plant Material
"Woe to you Pharisees, because you give God a tenth of your mint, rue and all other kinds of garden herbs, but you neglect justice and the love of God. You should have practiced the latter without leaving the former undone." Luke 11:42

"Woe to you, teachers of the law and Pharisees, you hypocrites! You give a tenth of your spices—mint, dill and cummin. But you have neglected the more important matters of the law—justice, mercy and faithfulness. You should have practiced the latter, without neglecting the former." Matthew 23: 23

Rose Absolute (*Rosa damascene*)
Rose Absolute is one of my favorites when blending for mature skin. It is extremely expensive but also very potent, so a little bit goes a long way.

Latin Name
Rosa damascene

Common Name
Rose Absolute

CAS Number 8007-01-0
EINECS 90106-38-0

Geographical Source
Bulgaria, Morocco, Turkey, Egypt

Family
Rosaceae

Plant Part
Flower

Method
Solvent Extracted

Representative Constituents
Hydrocarbons, Alcohols, Aldehydes, Esters, Oxides

Main Components
Citronellol, geraniol, phenyl ethanol, nerol, stearopten, ethanol, linalool, neral, geranyl acetate, methyl eugenol, benzyl benzoate, citral, farnesol

Properties
Anti-infectious, tonic, astringent, aphrodisiac, promotes the formation of a cicatrix to aid healing of sore or wound, relieves chest or respiratory tract disorders, anti-depressant, sedating, emollient, reduces swelling, anti-spasmodic, diuretic, promotes and regulates menstrual flow, anti-inflammatory, neurotonic, sexual tonic

General Aromatherapy Uses
Female reproductive problems, aids, infertility, scarring, poor circulation, childbirth, nervous tension, calming, emotional crisis, general tonic, blotchy skin, wounds, frigidity

Perfume Note
Middle, Base

Category
Euphoric, balancing

Scent
Intense, sweet and floral

Appearance
Dark amber to orange-ish

Blends Well
Citrus and Florals, Cedarwood (*Cedrus deodora*), Patchouli

Possible Substitutions
Palmarosa, Geranium

IFRA Critical Effect
Potential carcinogenic activity

IFRA
Benzyl benzoate <0.30%, citral <1.00%, citronellol <42.00%, eugenol <1.50%, farnesol <2.50%, geraniol <22.00%, methyl eugenol <3.50%

RIFM Recommended Safety Limit
2%

European Union Label Declaration
Citronellol, geraniol, linalool, eugenol

Specs
Flash Point = 139.00 °F
Specific Gravity = 0.84800 to 0.86800 @ 25.00 °C.
Estimated Pounds per Gallon = 7.056 to 7.223 lbs.
Refractive Index = 1.45900 to 1.47200 @ 20.00 °C.
Optical Rotation = -4.00 to +2.00
Melting Point = 85.00 °C. @ 760.00 mm Hg

Storage
Store in airtight glass dark bottles in a cool dark area

Shelf Life
1 year or more if stored properly

Price Point
High

FDA
GRAS

Biblical References to Plant Material
"The wilderness and the solitary places shall be glad, and the desert shall rejoice, and blossom as the rose." Isaiah 35:1

Rosemary (*Rosmarinus officinale cineole*)

In small settings when I have taught non-aromatherapists about the amazing properties of rosemary essential oil it never fails that someone will pipe up and say, "Well, I guess I'm going to eat more rosemary." The reality is that eating rosemary is good for you, but it would require that you eat over 31 pounds of rosemary in order to get the equivalent to 1 ounce of rosemary essential oil.

Latin Name
Rosmarinus officinale cineole

Common Name
Rosemary (Cineole type)

Other Chemotypes
Cineole type, bornyl acetate type, verbenone type

CAS Number 8000-25-7
EINECS 84604-14-8

Geographical Source
Spain, France, Tunisia

Family
Labiatae

Plant Part
Flowering Herb

Method
Steam Distilled

Representative Constituents
Hydrocarbons, Alcohols, Esters, Oxides, Ketones, Aldehydes

Main Components
Alpha-pinene, 1,8-cineole, camphene, bornyl acetate, camphor, borneol, limonene, beta-pinene, verbenone, linalool, myrcene, para-cymene, sabinene, linalyl acetate, beta-caryophyllene

Properties
Antiseptic, anti-spasmodic, stimulant, analgesic, anti-depressant, anti-toxic, relieves chest or respiratory tract disorders, promotes and regulates menstrual flow, diuretic, decongestant, relieves rheumatism, astringent, stimulates and clearers the mind, diuretic, dissolves boils and swelling, stimulant, aid digestion, increases perspiration, tonic, neurotonic

244

General Aromatherapy Uses
Muscular pain, rheumatism, arthritis, muscular weakness, coughs, colds, bronchitis, helps eliminate toxins, memory enhancement, overwork, general debility, infections, overindulgence, hangovers, acne, exhaustion, poor circulation, cellulite, migraine, headaches, sinus problems, general tonic, chills, burns, wounds, bruises

Perfume Note
Middle

Category
Stimulating

Scent
Woody, fresh, herbaceous, powerful, sharp, piney-resinous, camphoraceous, spicy

Appearance
Colorless to pale yellow clear liquid

Blends Well
All Citrus, Basil, Lavender, Peppermint, Eucalyptus

Possible Substitutions
Peppermint, Eucalyptus, Camphor

RIFM Recommended Safety Limit
10%

European Union Label Declaration
Linalool

Specs
Flash Point = 104.00 °F
Specific Gravity = 0.90000 to 0.91500 @ 25.00 °C.
Estimated Pounds per Gallon = 7.489 to 7.614 lbs.
Refractive Index = 1.45700 to 1.47500 @ 20.00 °C.
Optical Rotation = -5.00 to +10.00
Boiling Point = 549 °F

Storage
Store in airtight dark glass bottles in a cool, dark area

Shelf Life
2 years or more if stored properly

Price Point
Medium

FDA
GRAS

Tea Tree (*Melaleuca alternifolia*)
Tea tree will always be near and dear to my heart since it was the essential oil that launched my aromatherapy career and business. It has a medicinal aroma that some people can't quite get over, but once you've experienced the near-miraculous healing property of tea tree essential oil, the aroma will become a non-issue.

Latin Name
Melaleuca alternifolia

Common Name
Tea Tree

CAS Number 68647-73-4
EINECS 85085-48-9

Geographical Source
Australia

Family
Myrtaceae

Plant Part
Leaf

Method
Steam Distilled

Representative Constituents
Hydrocarbons, Alcohols, Oxides

Main Components
See chart below

Properties
Anti-infectious, anti-biotic, balsamic, anti-fungal, antiviral, anti-parasitic, anti-inflammatory, expectorant, immunostimulant, decongestant, analgesic, protective against sores from radiation

General Aromatherapy Uses
Tea tree has historic uses for rashes, insect bites, nail fungus, dermatitis, ringworm, head lice, sore throats, boils, and fatigue, useful for a wide spectrum of infections, bronchial congestion, scabies, ulcers, wounds, arthritis, cold sores, acne, candida, abscesses and varicose veins. For treating acne it acts as an oil-controlling agent and has high germicidal value. It also has the property to penetrate pus by mixing with it, which liquefies the pus causing it to slough off, leaving a healthy surface.

Perfume Note
Middle

Category
Stimulating

Scent
Medicinal, strong, warm, spicy, slightly earthy, peppery-smell, sharp

Appearance
Pale yellow to clear liquid

Blends Well
Peppermint, Eucalyptus, Rosemary, Lemon

Possible Substitutions
Niaouli, Manuka

RIFM Recommended Safety Limit
1%

European Union Label Declaration
Limonene, Linalool

Specs
Flash Point = 122.00 °F
Specific Gravity = 0.88800 to 0.90900 @ 25.00 °C.
Estimated Pounds per Gallon: 7.389 to 7.564 lbs.
Refractive Index = 1.47500 to 1.48200 @ 20.00 °C.
Optical Rotation = +5.00 to +15.00
Boiling Point = 329 °F

Storage

Store in airtight dark glass bottles in a cool, dark area

Shelf Life

2 years or more if stored properly

Price Point

Medium

Standards

Tea tree oil has set international stands and identical Australian standards.

Tea Tree ISO4730 and AS 2782-1997 Standards

The chemical composition of tea tree oil is defined by international standard ISO 4730 (2004) and the identical Australian standard AS 2782-2009 ("Oil of Melaleuca, Terpinen-4-ol type"), which specifies levels of 15 of the more than 100 components in pure Australian tea tree oil. Any batch of oil sold by an Australian Tea Tree International Association (ATTIA) member must be accompanied by an independently tested certificate of analysis demonstrating conformance to these standards. ATTIA also recommends that the country of origin is clearly declared when purchasing tea tree oil from any supplier.

AS 2782 – 2009 Oil of Melaleuca, terpen-4-ol type (Tea Tree Oil)

Essential oil obtained by steam distillation of the foliage and terminal branchlets of *Melaleuca alternifolia (Maiden et Betche) Cheel, Melaleuca linariifolia Smith*, and *Melaleuca dissitiflora F. Mueller*, as well as other species of Melaleuca provided that the oil obtained conforms to the requirements given in this International Standard.

Appearance	Clear, mobile liquid	
Colour	Colorless to pale yellow	
Odour	Characteristic	
Relative density (20° C)	Min: 0.885	Max: 0.906
Refractive index (20° C)	Min: 1.475	Max: 1.482
Optical rotation (20° C)	Between + 5° and + 15°	
Miscibility in ethanol (20° C)	Not necessary to use more than 2 volumes of ethanol, 85% (volume fraction) to obtain a clear solution with 1 volume of essential oil.	
Flashpoint (closed cup)	mean value	mean value
Min volume of test sample	50 ml	

Chromatographic Profile		
Component	Min %	Max %
α-Piniene	1	6
Sabinene	Trace	3.5
α-Terpinene	5	13
Limonene	0.5	1.5
p-Cymene	0.5	8
1,8-Cineole	Trace	15
γ-Terpinene	10	28
Terpinolene	1.5	5
Terpinen-4-ol	30	48
α-Terpineol	1.5	8
Aromadendrene	Trace	3
Ledene (syn. viridiflorene)	Trace	3
δ-Cadinene	Trace	3
Globulol	Trace	1
Viridiflorol	Trace	1

From the Australian Tea Tree Oil, ISO4730 and AS 2782-1997 Standards

---

Ylang Ylang (*Cananga odorata var. genuina*)

Ylang ylang is considered one of the most important essential oils in perfume blending, and I have to agree. I am not fond of ylang ylang alone, because it is so syrupy sweet to me, but it has the ability to create delicious blends.

Latin Name
Cananga odorata var. genuina

Common Name
Ylang Ylang

Pronounced
"ilang-ilang"

CAS Number 8006-81-3
EINECS 838636-30-3

Geographical Source
China, Madagascar, Philippines, Comoros Islands

Family
Annonaceae

Plant Part
Flower

Method
Steam Distilled

Grades

"Extra" or "Bourbon" is top grade within a few hours (1.5 hours) of distilling
"1" (2-2.5 hours)
"2" (3-5 hours)
"3" (6 hours) are from further distilling
"Complete" is a blend of "1" and "2".
The chemical composition varies in different grades of Ylang Ylang.

Representative Constituents

Hydrocarbons, Alcohols, Phenols, Esters, Phenyl methyl ethers

Main Components (Ylang Ylang Extra)

Farnesene, benzyl acetate, linalool, delta-cadinene, p-cresyl methyl ether, beta-caryophyllene, benzyl benzoate, geranyl acetate, methyl benzoate, alpha-humulene, gamma-cadinene, benzyl salicylate

Main Components (Ylang Ylang III)

Farnesene, beta-caryophyllene, alpha-humulene, delta-cadinene, gamma-cadinene, benzyl benzoate, linalool, geranyl acetate, (E)-nerolidol.

Properties

Sedative, antiseptic, aphrodisiac, anti-depressant, helps control the products of sebum, anti-spasmodic, balancing, calming, tonic, and reproductive stimulant.

General Aromatherapy Uses

Commonly used for physical exhaustion, stress, nervous tension, irritability, anxiety, PMS, regulate circulation, tonic to the uterus, hair growth promoting and is relaxing. Has a narcotic scent. It is one of the most relaxing fragrances to mind and body. Used for cramps, colic, insomnia, hypertension and frigidity.

Perfume Note

Middle, Base

Category

Euphoric, Relaxing

Scent

Floral, jasmine-like, flowery, syrupy sweet, fruity

Appearance

Pale yellow

Blends Well
Bergamot, Black Pepper, Orange, Cedarwood (*Cedrus deodora*), Clary Sage (*Salvia sclarea*), Grapefruit, Ginger, Jasmine, Lavender, Lemon, Lime, Litsea, Mandarin, Neroli, Rose, Tangerine.

Possible Substitutions
Jasmine absolute and one ylang ylang grade for another

Special Precautions and Warning
Excessive exposure may lead to headache and nausea, possible skin sensitization

IFRA Critical Effect
Sensitization

IFRA
Benzyl alcohol <0.50 %, benzyl benzoate <9.20 %, benzyl salicylate <4.00 %, eugenol <0.50 %, iso eugenol <0.50 %, farnesol <3.00 %, geraniol <2.60 %
.

IFRA Perfume Notes
(1) IFRA would recommend that any material used to impart perfume or flavour in products intended for human ingestion should consist of ingredients that are in compliance with appropriate regulations for foods and food flavourings in the countries of planned distribution and, where these are lacking, with the recommendations laid down in the Code of Practice of IOFI (International Organisation of the Flavor Industry). Further information about IOFI can be found on its website (www.iofi.org).

(2) Category 11 includes all non-skin contact or incidental skin contact products. Due to the negligible skin contact from these types of products there is no justification for a restriction of the concentration of this fragrance ingredient in the finished product.

European Union Allergen Declaration
Linalool, Benzyl benzoate, Benzyl salicylate, Eugenol, Isoeugenal

General Specs
Specific Gravity = 0.904 - 0.920
Refractive Index = 1.495 - 1.505
Optical Rotation = -15.0 to -30.0°
Boiling Point = 507 °F

Storage
Store in airtight dark glass bottles in a cool, dark area

Shelf Life
2 years or more if stored properly

Price Point
Medium to High

FDA
GRAS status

Reactive in Soap
Yes, due to 30% Esters

Essential Oil Crop Calendar

CROP CALENDAR														
Product	Country	Jan	Feb	Mar	Apr	May	Jun	Jul	Aug	Sep	Oct	Nov	Dec
Almond	USA	▒	▒	▒	▒	▒	▒	▒	▒	▒			▒
Amyris	Haiti	▒	▒	▒	▒	▒	▒	▒	▒	▒	▒	▒	▒
Aniseed	Spain	▒	▒	▒	▒	▒	▒	▒	▒	▒			▒
Aniseed	Turkey	▒	▒	▒	▒	▒	▒	▒	▒	▒			▒
Anise, Star	China	▒	▒	▒	▒	▒			▒	▒	▒	▒	▒
Balsam, Copaiba	Brazil	▒	▒	▒	▒	▒	▒	▒	▒	▒	▒	▒	▒
Balsam Peru	El Salvador	▒	▒	▒	▒	▒	▒	▒			▒	▒	▒
Basil	Egypt	▒	▒	▒	▒	▒	▒	▒			▒	▒	▒
Basil	India	▒	▒	▒	▒	▒	▒	▒	▒	▒	▒	▒	▒
Bay	W. Indies	▒	▒	▒	▒								
Bergamot	Brazil		▒	▒	▒	▒							▒
Bergamot	Italy	▒	▒	▒		▒	▒	▒	▒				▒
Cabreuva	Brazil	▒	▒	▒	▒	▒	▒	▒					
Camphor	China	▒	▒	▒	▒	▒	▒	▒	▒	▒	▒	▒	▒
Camphor	Taiwan		▒	▒	▒	▒	▒	▒	▒	▒	▒	▒	▒
Cananga	Indonesia	▒	▒	▒	▒	▒	▒	▒	▒	▒	▒	▒	▒
Caraway Oil	Holland							▒	▒	▒			
Cardamom	Guatemala		▒	▒									
Cardamom	India								▒	▒	▒	▒	▒
Cassia	China	▒	▒	▒	▒	▒	▒	▒	▒	▒	▒	▒	▒
Cedarleaf	Canada		▒	▒	▒	▒	▒	▒	▒	▒	▒		▒
Cedarwood	China	▒	▒	▒	▒	▒	▒	▒	▒	▒	▒	▒	▒
Cedarwood	USA (Texas)	▒	▒	▒	▒	▒	▒	▒	▒	▒	▒	▒	▒
Celery	China	▒	▒	▒	▒	▒	▒	▒	▒	▒	▒	▒	▒
Celery	India	▒	▒	▒	▒	▒	▒	▒	▒	▒	▒	▒	▒
Cinnamon	Madagascar	▒	▒	▒	▒	▒	▒	▒	▒	▒	▒	▒	▒
Cinnamon	Sri Lanka	▒	▒	▒	▒	▒	▒	▒	▒	▒	▒	▒	▒
Citronella	Argentina	▒	▒	▒	▒	▒			▒	▒			
Citronella	China				▒	▒	▒	▒	▒	▒	▒		
Citronella	Indonesia	▒	▒	▒	▒	▒	▒	▒	▒	▒	▒	▒	▒
Citronella	Sri Lanka	▒	▒	▒	▒	▒	▒	▒	▒	▒	▒	▒	▒
Clove	Brazil								▒	▒	▒		
Clove	Indonesia						▒	▒	▒	▒			
Clove	Madagascar			▒	▒					▒	▒	▒	
Clove	Zanzibar						▒	▒	▒	▒			
Coriander	Europe						▒	▒	▒	▒			
Coriander	Morocco				▒	▒	▒						
Cumin	India	▒	▒	▒	▒								▒
Dill Weed	Europe						▒	▒	▒	▒			
Dill Weed	USA						▒	▒	▒				
D'Limonene	Brazil	▒	▒	▒	▒	▒	▒	▒	▒	▒	▒	▒	▒
D'Limonene	USA (Florida)	▒	▒	▒	▒	▒	▒		▒	▒	▒	▒	▒
Eucalyptus	Australia	▒	▒	▒	▒	▒	▒	▒	▒	▒	▒	▒	▒
Eucalyptus	Chile	▒	▒	▒	▒	▒	▒	▒	▒	▒	▒	▒	▒
Eucalyptus	China			▒	▒	▒	▒	▒	▒	▒	▒		
Eucalyptus	Portugal			▒	▒	▒	▒	▒	▒	▒	▒	▒	
Eucalyptus	Spain			▒	▒	▒	▒	▒	▒	▒	▒		
Eucalyptus Citr.	China							▒	▒	▒			
Fennel	China			▒	▒	▒	▒			▒	▒		
Fennel	Egypt				▒	▒	▒						
Fennel	India			▒	▒	▒	▒						
Fir Needle	Austria			▒	▒	▒	▒	▒	▒	▒	▒	▒	
Fir Needle	Canada			▒	▒	▒	▒	▒	▒	▒	▒		
Geranium	China						▒	▒	▒				
Geranium	Egypt			▒	▒				▒	▒			
Geranium	Morocco			▒	▒				▒	▒	▒		
Geranium	Reunion			▒	▒				▒	▒	▒		▒

CROP CALENDAR

Product	Country	Jan	Feb	Mar	Apr	May	Jun	Jul	Aug	Sep	Oct	Nov	Dec
Ginger	China	■											■
Ginger	India	■	■	■	■	■							
Gingergrass	India	■											■
Grapefruit	Australia	■						■	■	■	■	■	■
Grapefruit	Belize	■	■	■									
Grapefruit	Brazil	■						■	■				
Grapefruit	Israel	■	■	■	■	■					■	■	■
Grapefruit	South Africa	■		■	■	■	■	■	■	■			
Grapefruit	USA (Florida)	■	■	■	■	■	■	■	■				
Guaiacwood	Paraguay	■	■	■	■	■	■	■	■	■	■	■	■
Ho Leaf	Taiwan	■	■	■	■	■	■	■	■	■	■	■	■
Ho Wood	China	■	■	■	■	■	■	■	■	■	■	■	■
Ho Wood	Taiwan	■	■	■	■	■	■	■	■	■	■	■	■
Juniperberry	Europe	■	■	■	■	■	■	■	■	■	■		■
Lavender	France							■	■	■	■	■	■
Lemon	Argentina							■	■	■	■	■	■
Lemon	Australia	■						■	■	■	■	■	■
Lemon	Brazil			■	■	■	■	■	■	■			
Lemon	Israel	■	■	■	■	■					■	■	■
Lemon	Italy	■	■	■	■	■	■	■					
Lemon	South Africa		■	■	■								
Lemon	USA (California)	■	■	■	■	■	■	■					
Lemon	Argentina					■	■	■	■				
Lemon	USA (Arizona)									■			
Lemongrass	China							■	■	■	■		
Lemongrass	Guatemala	■	■	■	■	■	■	■	■	■	■	■	■
Lemongrass	India							■	■	■	■	■	■
Lime	Brazil	■	■	■	■								
Lime	Peru	■									■	■	■
Lime	USA (Florida)	■	■	■	■								
Lime	Haiti						■	■	■	■	■	■	■
Lime	Mexico					■	■	■	■	■	■	■	■
Lime	Ivory Coast						■	■	■	■	■	■	■
Listea Cubeba	China							■	■				
Marjoram	France							■	■				
Mandarin	Brazil		■	■	■	■							
Mandarin	Italy	■	■	■							■	■	■
Murcot	Brazil							■	■	■			
Nutmeg	Indonesia	■	■	■	■	■	■	■	■	■	■	■	■
Ocotea Cymbarium	Brazil	■											
Orange	Belize	■	■	■	■								■
Orange	South Africa					■	■	■	■				
Orange	USA (California)	■	■	■	■	■	■						
Orange, Bitter	Brazil	■	■	■	■	■	■	■					
Orange, Midseason	USA (Florida)	■	■	■									■
Orange, Navel	Australia	■						■	■	■	■	■	■
Orange, Navel	Israel	■	■									■	■
Orange, Pera	Brazil	■	■								■	■	■
Orange, Shamouti	Israel	■	■	■								■	■
Orange, Valencia	Australia							■	■	■	■	■	■
Orange, Valencia	Brazil							■	■	■	■	■	■
Orange, Valencia	Israel				■	■	■	■					
Orange, Valencia	USA (Florida)		■	■	■	■	■						
Oregano Oil	Turkey							■	■	■	■		
Oregano Oil	Spain							■	■	■			
Palmrosa	Brazil	■	■	■	■						■	■	■
Parsley	USA	■	■	■	■	■	■	■	■		■	■	■
Patchouli	China	■	■	■	■	■	■	■	■	■	■	■	■
Patchouli	Indonesia	■	■	■	■	■	■	■	■	■	■	■	■
Pennyroyal	Spain	■	■	■	■	■	■						
Pepper, Black	Brazil	■	■	■									
Pepper, Black	India	■	■	■									
Peppermint, Crude	China							■	■	■	■		
Peppermint, Crude	India					■	■	■	■				

CROP CALENDAR		Jan	Feb	Mar	Apr	May	Jun	Jul	Aug	Sep	Oct	Nov	Dec
Product	Country												
Peppermint, Crude	Paraguay	X											X
Peppermint, F. West	USA								X				
Peppermint, M. West	USA							X					
Petitgrain	Paraguay	X	X	X	X	X	X	X	X	X	X	X	X
Pimento Leaf	Jamaca					X				X			
Pine Needle	Europe				X	X	X	X	X				
Rose	Bulgaria					X	X						
Rose	Turkey					X	X						
Rosemary	Spain				X	X							
Rosemary	Tunisia	X	X	X	X	X							
Rosewood	Brazil				X	X	X	X	X	X			
Sage	Albania						X	X	X	X	X		
Sage	Dalmatian						X	X					
Sage	Spain					X	X	X					
Sage, Clary	France							X	X				
Sage, Clary	USA						X	X					
Sage, Clary	Russia							X					
Sandalwood	India	X	X	X	X	X	X	X	X	X	X	X	X
Sassafrass	China	X	X	X	X	X	X	X	X	X	X	X	X
Spearmint	China							X	X				
Spearmint, F. West	USA							X	X				
Tangerine	Brazil				X	X	X						
Tangerine	USA (Florida)	X	X									X	X
Tarragon	Argentina												
Teatree	Australia	X	X	X	X	X	X	X	X	X	X	X	X
Thyme	Spain				X	X	X	X	X	X	X		
Vetivert	China	X	X	X	X	X	X	X	X	X	X	X	X
Vetivert	Haiti	X	X	X	X						X	X	X
Vetivert	Indonesia				X						X		
Vetivert	Reunion							X	X	X	X	X	X
Ylang	Madagascar	X	X	X	X	X	X	X	X	X	X	X	X

"Essential oil production has been divided into cultivated and wild-gathered woodyperennial sources (trees, bushes) accounting for approx 65% of the world output, cultivated herbal sources accounting for the remaining 30.6% and wild-gathered herbal sources accounting for just 1.4%, with other sources accounting for the remaining 3.0% (Verlet 1993). To put this in context, it has to be born in mind that the world production of orange oil at 26,000 t/y is some four to six times the annual production volume of any other essential oil, and that the production of many minor essential oils is under 100 Kg/y, with some even at under 10 Kg/y." Tony Burfield

Crop Watch by Tony Burfield of Crop Watch reports the following in *Updated List of Threatened Aromatic Plants Used in Aroma and Cosmetic Industries:*

Critically Endangered: agarwood (*Aquilaria crassna*), arnica syn. mountain tobacco (*Arnica Montana L.*), civet (animal sourced *Civetticus civetta, Viverra civettina, Viverra zibetha* and *Viverricula indica*), and in Jammu and Kasmir *Saussurea lappa.*

Endangered: in Kenya East African sandalwood (*Osyris lanceolata*), in victoria and Queensland *Santalum lanceolatum*, spikenard (*Nardostachys grandiflora*), in Iran asafoetida (*Ferula assa-foetida L.*), in Pakistan calamus oil (*Acorus*

calamus L.), cedarwood Kenya (*Juniperus procera*), in India *Coleus forskohlii*, *Commiphora wrightii*, in India *Saussurea lappa*, ginger lily (*Hedychium coronaium*), gurjun (*Dipterpcarpus spp*), in Jordan *Juniperus Phoenicia L.*, melanje cedarwood (*Widdringtonia whytei*), *Michelia champaca L.*, and rosewood a.k.a. Bois de Rose (*Aniba spp.*).

Threatened Species: *Aglaia odorata*, ambergris (animal source sperm whale *Physeter catadon L.*), *Aquilaria cumingiana*, *Aquilaria khasiana* (agarwood), *Aquilaria microcarpa*, *Aquilaria rostrata*, in Tanzania East Africa sandalwood (*Osyris lanceolata*), sandalwood East Indian (*Santalum album*), *Santalum austrocaledonicum*, *Santalum fernandezianum F. Philippi*, *Santalum haleakalae*, *Santalum macgregaorii*, siam wood (*syn Pe Mou*), Norway spruce (*Picea mariana*), styrax (*Liquidambar styraciflua L. var. macrophylla*), *Thymus moroderis*, *Thymus zygis*, in Pakistan *Valeriana jatamansi*, white sage oil (*Salvia apiana*), boldo (*Peumus boldus Molina*), *Canarium zeylanicu*, cedarwood atlas (*Cedrus atlantica*), cedarwood Himalayan (*Cedrus deodara*) production is down, *Hydnocarpus nana*, in Nepal *Cinnamomum cedidoaphne*, *Commiphora guidottii*, *Commiphora parvifolia*, *Commiphora pseudopaoli*, in Pakistan *Saussurea lappa*, balsam fir (*Abies balsamea L. mill.*), nordman fir (*Abies nordmanniana* and *Abies nordmanniana subsp. Nordmanniana*), silver fir (*Albies alba L. Mill.*), *Gentiana spp.*, hinoki wood (*Chamaecyparis obtuse*), incense juniper (*Juniperus trurifera L.*), *Juniperus oxycedrus L.*, larch (*Larix decidua Miller.*), Brazilian sassafras (*Ocotea pretosia*), alleppo pine (*Pinus halepensis Miller*), arolla pine (*Pinus cembra L.*), merkus pine (*Pinus merkusii*), Monterey pine (*pinus radiata*), Oregon pine (*Pseudotsuga menziessii*), Siberian dwarf pine (*Pinus pumila*), Scotch pine (*Pinus silvestris L.*), Siberian pine (*Pinus sibirica*), slash pine (*pinus elliottii*), Eastern white pine (*pinus strobus L.*), poplar (*Propulus nigra*), *Prostanthera spp.*, *Pterocarpus santalinus L. f.*, and rosewood (*Ocotea caudate*).

Potentially Threatened: holy wood (*Bursera glabrifolian*), and in China musk (animal product *Moschus spp.*)

Nearly Threatened: *Cinnamomum tamala*

Volnerable Crop: amyris "sandalwood" (*Amyris balsamifera L.*), aniseed myrtle (*Anetholia anisata*), *Santalum insulare var. hendersonensis*, *Santalum insulare var. marchionense*, Asian styrax (*Liquidambar orientalis var orientalis* and *Liquidamber orentalis var integriloba*), in Nepal *Valeriana Jatamansi*, in Morocco argan (*Argania spinosa*), in some Eastern European areas common mugwort (*Artemisia vulgaris L*), buchu oils (*Agathosma betulina*), cypress cedar (*Cedrus bevifolia*), chaulmoogra (*Hydnocarpus pentadra* and *Hydnocarpus macrocarpa*), certain Chinese essential oils bearing *Cinnamomum spp*, in Oman *Commiphora spp.*, dragons blood (diterpene acids from *Daemonorops genus*), elemi (*Canarium luzonicu*), *Gonystylus bancanus*, *Gonystylus macrophyllus*, in Jammu and Kashir, India inula racemosa (*Poshkar moola*), spiked ginger-lily (*Kaempferia rotunda L.*), spiked ginger lily (*Kedychium spicatum*), frankincense (*Boswellia aff. Ameero, Boswellia bullata, Boswellia dioscoride, Boswelia elongat, Boswellia nana, Boswellia ogadensis, Boswellia papyrifer, Boswellia pirottae*, and *Boswellia socotrana*), *Origanum spp.*, in Brazil, Columbia, and in Surinam threated species rosewood a.k.a. Bois de Rose (*Aniba spp.*).

Depleted Crop: sandalwood New Caledonia (*Santalum austrocaledonicum Vieill. Var. austrocaledonicum*) and *Santalum yasi*.

Depleted (in Wild): wintergreen oil (*Gaultheria fragrantissam*), emu (animal sourced *Dromaius novaehollandiae*) and *Jurinea dolmiaea*.

Diminishing Accessibility: aniroba (*Carapa guianesis* Aublet) and *Copaiba spp.*

Much Reduced (in wild): Australian sandalwood (*Santalum spicatum*)

In Decline: Spanish lemon thyme (*Thymus baeticus*)

Protected: Western Australia sandalwood (*Santalum acuminatum*) and *Santalum murrayanum* protected by the Australian government.

Scarce: *Cedrela odorata*

Becoming Rare: in India calamus oil (*Acorus calams L.*), candeia plant (*Eremanthus erythropappus*) and *Kaempferia rotunda L.*

Rare: Greater wormwood (*Artemisia gracilis*) and orchids *Orchidaceae*.

Destructive Harvesting: *Ravensara aromatica* not to be confused with ravensara leaf essential oil *Cinnamomum camphora spp.*

Locally Extinct: in Iran galbanum (*Ferula gummosa Boiss.*)

Facing Extinction: *Kaempferia galangal*

Not Threatened: frankincense (*Boswellia bhau-dajiana, Boswellia. frereana, Boswellia microphylla, Boswellia multifoliolata, Boswellia neglecta* and *Boswellia rivae.*)

:: Appendix 2 ::
Weights and Measurement Guides

When you are measuring your ingredient either chose to measure by weight or by volume. As much as possible, do not switch back and forth. Eventually, you will have to make larger batches and will need to convert your formulas. It is best if you start all of your formulas measuring by weight. When you are ready to make larger batches you will not want to have to measure out your ingredients by the cup. Every ingredient has a different specific gravity, meaning 1 cup of feathers does not weigh the same as 1 cup of water. In the long run it is easier and more accurate to use weight for all of your measurements.

BY WEIGHT EQUIVALENTS			
1 ounce	.0625 lb	28.3495231 gram	.0283495 kilograms
1 lbs	16 ounces	453.59237 gram	.453592 kilograms
1 kilogram	2.2046 lbs	35.2739619 ounce	1000 grams
1 gram	.035274 ounces	.564384 lbs	0.001 kilogram
1 gallon (H$_2$O)	8.3453 lbs (H$_2$O)	133.5248 ounces*	

*Specific Gravity Varies

BY VOLUME EQUIVALENTS						
.17 fl ounce	1 teaspoon	60 drops	5 milliliters			
.5 fl ounce	1 tablespoon	180 drops	15 milliliters			
1 fl ounce	480 drops	6 teaspoons	2 tablespoons	29.57 milliliters		
8 fl ounce	3840 drops	48 teaspoons	16 tablespoons	1 cup	236.56 milliliters	
16 fl ounces	7680 drops	96 teaspoons	32 tablespoons	2 cups	1 pint	473.12 milliliters
64 fl ounce	½ gallon	30,720 drops	1892.48 milliliters			
128 fl ounce	1 gallon	64,440 drops	3784.96 milliliters			

COMMON PERCENTAGES BY WEIGHT AND VOLUME

This is a tool to determine how much of an ingredient to add based on percentages. We have left all measurements for you to decide if you would like to round up or round down. We are aware of the fact that you cannot put in 2.4 drops, but we left it up to you to decide if you want to round down to two or round up to three drops. Also, the specific gravity of every ingredient is different. We have given you the specific gravity of water. If you need to determine a different percentage than we have given you simply multiply the percentage you want to use by the amount of product you are adding it to. For instance, to add .8 % essential oil to 1 lb of product by weight the equation would be: 1 lb x .8 % = .008 lbs. If you needed to determine how many ounces .008 lbs equaled, you would multiply .008 lbs by 16 ounces: .008 x 16 = .128 ounces.

BY WEIGHT				
.5% of 1 ounce	.005 ounce	2.4 drops		
.5% of 1 lbs	.08 ounces	.005 lbs	38.4 drops	
.5% of 1 kilogram	.005 kilograms	.011 lbs	.175 ounce	5 grams
.5% of 1 gram	.000177 ounce	.0002822 lbs	.000005 kilograms	
.5% of 1 gallon (H$_2$O)	.041727 lbs (H$_2$O)	.667624 ounces*		
1% of 1 ounce	ounce	4.8 drops		
1% of 1 lbs	ounces	.01 lbs	76.8 drops	
1% of 1 kilogram	kilograms	.022 lbs	.35 ounce	10 grams
1% of 1 gram	ounce	.005644 lbs	.00001 kilograms	
1% of 1 gallon (H$_2$O)	lbs (H$_2$O)	1.335248 ounces*		
1.5% of 1 ounce	ounce	7.2 drops		
1.5% of 1 lbs	ounces	.015 lbs	115.2 drops	
1.5% of 1 kilogram	kilograms	.033 lbs	.525 ounce	15 grams
1.5% of 1 gram	ounce	.0059262 lbs	.000015 kilograms	
1.5% of 1 gallon (H$_2$O)	lbs (H$_2$O)	2.002872 ounces*		
2% of 1 ounce	ounce	9.6 drops		
2% of 1 lbs	ounces	.02 lbs	153.6 drops	
2% of 1 kilogram	kilograms	.044 lbs	.7 ounce	20 grams
2% of 1 gram	ounce	.011288 lbs	.00002 kilograms	
2% of 1 gallon (H$_2$O)	lbs (H$_2$O)	2.670496 ounces*		
2.5% of 1 ounce	ounce	12 drops		
2.5% of 1 lbs	ounces	.025 lbs	192 drops	
2.5% of 1 kilogram	kilograms	.055 lbs	.875 ounce	25 grams
2.5% of 1 gram	ounce	.01411 lbs	.000025 kilograms	
2.5% of 1 gallon (H$_2$O)	lbs (H$_2$O)	3.33812 ounces*		
3% of 1 ounce	ounce	14.4 drops		
3% of 1 lbs	ounces	.03 lbs	153.6 drops	
3% of 1 kilogram	kilograms	.066 lbs	1.05 ounce	30 grams
3% of 1 gram	ounce	.016932 lbs	.00003 kilograms	
3% of 1 gallon (H$_2$O)	lbs (H$_2$O)	4.005744 ounces*		

*Specific Gravity Varies

BY VOLUME			
.5% of 1 teaspoon	.00085 fl ounces	.3 drops	.025 milliliters
.5% of 1 tablespoon	.0025 fl ounces	.9 drops	.075 milliliters
.5% of 1 fl. ounce	2.4 drops	.14785 milliliters	
.5% of 8 fl. ounces	.04 fl ounces	19.2 drops	1.1828 milliliters
.5% of 16 fl. ounces	.08 fl ounces	38.4 drops	2.3656 milliliters
.5% of 64 fl. ounces or ½ gallon	.32 fl ounces	153.6 drops	9.4624 milliliters
.5% of 128 fl. ounces or 1 gallon	.64 fl ounces	322.2 drops	18.9248 milliliters
1% of 1 teaspoon	.0017 fl ounces	.6 drops	.05 milliliters
1% of 1 tablespoon	.005 fl ounces	1.8 drops	.15 milliliters
1% of 1 fl. ounce	4.8 drops	.2957 milliliters	
1% of 8 fl. ounces	.08 fl ounces	38.40 drops	2.3656 milliliters
1% of 16 fl. ounces	.16 fl ounces	76.8 drops	4.7312 milliliters
1% of 64 fl. ounces or ½ gallon	.64 fl ounces	307.2 drops	18.9248 milliliters
1% of 128 fl. ounces or 1 gallon	1.28 fl ounces	644.4 drops	37.8496 milliliters
1.5% of 1 teaspoon	.00255 fl ounces	.9 drops	.075 milliliters
1.5% of 1 tablespoon	.0075 fl ounces	1.35 drops	.225 milliliters
1.5% of 1 fl. ounce	7.2 drops	.44355 milliliters	
1.5% of 8 fl. ounces	.12 fl ounces	57.6 drops	3.5484 milliliters
1.5% of 16 fl. ounces	.24 fl ounces	115.2 drops	7.0968 milliliters
1.5% of 64 fl. ounces or ½ gallon	.96 fl ounces	4608 drops	28.3872 milliliters
1.5% of 128 fl. ounces or 1 gallon	1.92 fl ounces	966.6 drops	56.7744 milliliters

BY VOLUME			
2% of 1 teaspoon	.0034 fl ounces	1.2 drops	.1 milliliters
2% of 1 tablespoon	.01 fl ounces	3.6 drops	.3 milliliters
2% of 1 fl. ounce	9.6 drops	.5914 milliliters	
2% of 8 fl. ounces	.16 fl ounces	76.8 drops	4.7312 milliliters
2% of 16 fl. ounces	.32 fl ounces	153.6 drops	9.4624 milliliters
2% of 64 fl. ounces or ½ gallon	1.28 fl ounces	614.4 drops	37.8496 milliliters
2% of 128 fl. ounces or 1 gallon	2.56 fl ounces	1288.8 drops	75.6992 milliliters
2.5% of 1 teaspoon	.00425 fl ounces	1.5 drops	.125 milliliters
2.5% of 1 tablespoon	.00125 fl ounces	4.5 drops	.375 milliliters
2.5% of 1 fl. ounce	12 drops	.73925 milliliters	
2.5% of 8 fl. ounces	.2 fl ounces	96 drops	5.914 milliliters
2.5% of 16 fl. ounces	.4 fl ounces	192 drops	11.828 milliliters
2.5% of 64 fl. ounces or ½ gallon	1.6 fl ounces	768 drops	47.312 milliliters
2.5% of 128 fl. ounces or 1 gallon	3.2 fl ounces	1661 drops	94.624 milliliters
3% of 1 teaspoon	.0051 fl ounces	1.8 drops	.15 milliliters
3% of 1 tablespoon	.015 fl ounces	5.4 drops	.45 milliliters
3% of 1 fl. ounce	14.4 drops	.8871 milliliters	
3% of 8 fl. ounces	.24 fl ounces	115.2 drops	7.0968 milliliters
3% of 16 fl. ounces	.48 fl ounces	230.4 drops	14.19636 milliliters
3% of 64 fl. ounces or ½ gallon	1.92 fl ounces	921.6 drops	56.7744 milliliters
3% of 128 fl. ounces or 1 gallon	3.84 fl ounces	1933.2 drops	113.5488 milliliters

:: *Appendix 3* ::
Aromatherapy Schools

Since I am a Registered and Certified Aromatherapist I am often asked to recommend a good certification program. I am a member of the National Association of Holistic Aromatherapists (NAHA) and have been for many years. I referred to their list of NAHA approved schools when I chose the program that worked best for me at the time. Another great source for a solid aromatherapy education is the Alliance of International Aromatherapists (AIA) schools.

The advice I normally give is that any one of the NAHA or AIA approved schools is going to give you a great Level I and II foundation in aromatherapy. You have to find the one that will work best for you. There are many factors to consider. I am including a list of the NAHA and AIA approved schools, and their description of the program along with a few notes from me on what I know about the schools. These are in no order of preference – just simply alphabetized.

NAHA and/or AIA Approved Aromatherapy Certification Programs

American College of Healthcare Sciences
www.achs.edu
NAHA - Accredited Certificate and Diploma in Aromatherapy. American College of Health Sciences is the only nationally accredited, NAHA-approved Level I and II professional clinical Aromatherapy training available online. ACHS also offers a specialized Certificate in Aromatherapy Chemistry course along with a wide variety of online, professional holistic health programs meeting all of your accredited holistic health education needs. CEU´s (Continuing Education Units) are available for many professionals including Registered Aromatherapists (RA). Contact: Admissions to apply for the next intake of one of ACHS accredited online holistic health programs.

AIA - ACHS is the only nationally accredited, AIA Level II and III professional clinical aromatherapy training available in the United States. ACHS offers specialized training in aromatherapy chemistry, along with a wide variety of online, professional holistic health certificate and diploma programs. ACHS also offers the only accredited AAS with an aromatherapy major and MS in CAM degree with a graduate level course in aromatherapy in the United States. CEUs are available for many health professionals including Registered Aromatherapists (RA), RNs and LMTs.

Kayla's Notes: I have worked with the President and founder of ACHS, Dorene Petersen, on a committee that reviewed questions to be added to the test to become a Registered Aromatherapist. She is extremely knowledgeable and passionate about aromatherapy. Dorene serves as Chair of Aromatherapy Registration Council. There is no doubt in my mind that the education from ACHS would be wonderful. This program is approved by AIA and NAHA.

Aroma Apothecary Healing Arts Academy
www.learnaroma.com
Offering professional clinical aromatherapy courses in distant learning or in-classroom format. Approved for Clinical Aromatherapy Level I and Level II. Level I is a 50-hour comprehensive foundation of clinical aromatherapy and therapeutic blending, Level II is a 240-hour (an in-depth continuation of the Materia Aromatica (55 essential oil profiles), advanced study of anatomy and physiology, five elements and acupressure meridians, integrative medicine and a holistic approach to health and disease, in-depth clinical study of stress related and auto immune conditions, client consultation and assessment, 30 case studies, professional ethics, business development, and advanced blending and formulating twenty organic products).

Other courses being offered include: Chi Nei Tsang: Internal Organ Rejuvenation, Five Element Reflexology, Women's Essence, and Aromatherapy First Aid. Instructor has 30 years of holistic clinical training and experience. Aroma Apothecary is an approved provider by the National Certification Board for Therapeutic Massage and Bodywork (NCBTMB) and the Texas Department of Health Services for continuing massage education.

Kayla's Notes: I don't formally know Shanti Dechen, Director of Aroma-apothecary Healing Arts Academy. The program is approved for Continuing Education credits by NAHA and the National Certification Board for Therapeutic Massage and Bodywork. This could be a definite plus if your interest in aromatherapy is related to your Massage Therapy business.

Aromahead Institute School of Essential Oil Studies
www.aromahead.com
Aromahead Institute offers a 200-hour and 400-hour Aromatherapy Certification Program designed to meet both the National Association for Holistic Aromatherapy (NAHA) and the Alliance of International Aromatherapists (AIA) requirements, respectively. Additionally the Institute offers a 5-day Teacher Training Program, a 3-day Business Class, and several Advanced Workshops in Essential Oil Chemistry and Medicinal Blending. Aromahead Institute also offers the 200-hour certification as an online, home study program.

All classes provide an in-depth exploration into the art and science of essential oil therapies. Andrea Butje is approved by the National Certification Board for Therapeutic Massage and Bodywork (NCBTMB) as a Continuing Education Provider. In additional, all programs are approved in Florida for CEU's in Massage Therapy.

Kayla's Notes: I have heard several aromatherapists mention Aromahead Institute. If you are on the East Coast their location could be a definite plus. The continuing education classes and certification classes that are taught at the Institute look great. This program is approved by NAHA and AIA.

Aroma Studio, LLC
www.aromastudio.com
Aroma Studio, LLC™ is a full service aromatherapy school for professionals. Aroma Studio, LLC™ specializes in Home Study Certification, Live Training, Therapeutic Essential Oils and Hydrosols, and Special Events. The program includes Foundation, Advanced, Master, and Teacher Level Training for aromatherapists totaling 300 hours. Aroma Studio was founded in 1999 by Katherine Graf who has over 20 years experience in the aromatherapy field. Katherine is the author of The Business of Aromatherapy: The Insider's Guide To Success. Kathy is a Provence-trained aromatherapist who teaches European, Ayurvedic, Five Element, and other creative blending techniques.

Aroma Studio, LLC tm specializes in mentoring professionals with a passion for aromatherapy to help them to achieve their aromatherapy goals and dreams. Aroma Studio, LLC tm is "your aromatherapy mentor tm."

Kayla's Notes: I received my certification in aromatherapy through The Aroma Studio in the late 90's. I chose this program because the price was affordable, all of the important elements were thoroughly covered and there was a focus on the business of aromatherapy. I found Katherine Graf very easy to learn from and work with. We have referred several people to the Aroma Studio and sent some of our own employees through this program.

Ashi Aromatics Inc.-Flower Power for Pets(sm)
Instructor: Kelly Holland Azzaro, RA, CCAP, CBFP, LMT
www.ashitherapy.com
Do want to learn more about aromatherapy for animals? Ashi Aromatics Inc. Flower Power for Pets(sm) offers educational studies in Animal Aromatherapy and Bach Flowers for Pets for all levels. NCBTMB Approved Continuing Education is available for Licensed Massage Therapists. ARC RA renewal hours are available for Aromatherapists. Learn about safe use of essential oils, botanicals and flowers essences for use for you and your animal friends. Additional course topics and online classes are also available.

Kayla's notes: I left aromatherapy for pets completely out of this book because I believe it is another animal in and of itself (pun intended.) Kelly Holland Azzaro offers the most authoritative source for aromatherapy training for pets.

Astralessence School of Aromatherapy

www.astralessence.com
Quality education for beginners and Professional Level certification with Shellie Enteen, RA, BA, LMT. Classes cover the spectrum from physical to subtle aspects of this spiritual science. Online classes coming soon!

Atlantic Institute of Aromatherapy

www.AtlanticInstitute.com
The Aromatherapy Practitioner Course is a very detailed 200 hour course for self-study with over 500 pages of text and complete back-up documentation. The Practitioner Module (optional 100 hours) includes case studies and a publishable research paper. Geared toward professional medical health care providers, the course is also easily assimilated by business owners, student beginners or the lay-person who simply desires a better quality of life. This course is considered the most well-referenced, wide-ranging, comprehensive and detailed course available, and stands alone in the marketplace. NAHA (Level I and II).

Practitioner Module: (Optional 100 hours) Contents: Setting up a practice and clinic. Consultation and treatment program design. The basics of business development Legal business and ethical issues Requirements: 1. Student must complete a 20-25 page research paper of REAL research, (a clinical trial), that is publishable in medical journals. 2. Student must complete a minimum of 10 case histories

Kayla's Notes: I took a Continuing Education course from Sylla Sheppard Hanger from the Atlantic Institute of Aromatherapy, when she came to Portland for a weekend course. I enjoyed her teaching style and passion for aromatherapy. Her book The Aromatherapy Practitioner Reference Manual is one of my favorite go-to books to check facts.

Certification Academy for Holistic Aromatherapy (CAHA)

www.aromaacademy.com
CAHA offers certification programs. (USA and Korea) NAHA approved Level One and Level Two professional clinical Aromatherapy training course. The completion of these classes qualifies students to take the ARC test to become Registered Aromatherapist title in the USA. CAHA offers very exciting aromatherapy D.I.Y. certification courses. (USA and Korea) Natural Soap making course (I and II), Natural cosmetic DIY, Spa DIY, Pets DIY, Aromatherapy Gift making.

East-West School for Herbal and Aromatic Studies

www.theida.com

NAHA-approved Level 1 and Level 2 professional clinical Aromatherapy training available live and distance learning. The EWSHAS offers classes throughout the United States for Aroma101 and Aroma 201 as well as other specialized modules. Specialized topics include: Chemistry by and for the Aromatherapists, Aromatic applications for the skin, Aromatherapy and Hospice Care, Aromatherapy and Energetic Healing, and a variety of workshops for the general public and practitioner. CEU hours are available for massage therapists (NCBTMB approved provider) and for Registered Aromatherapists (RA).

Kayla's Notes: I have heard Jade Shutes name for as long as I have been in aromatherapy. Jade has played an important role in setting the standards for aromatherapy education in America. While I have never taken one of her courses her history as an educator speaks volumes.

Essential Education International, Inc.

www.essentialeducationinternational.com

Become a professionally qualified Aromatherapist in their 235 hour Certification Program in the art and science of Aromatherapy. This NAHA Approved School (Level I and II in one program) offers a creative hands-on approach to learning in a comfortable setting in Gainesville, Florida. Becoming certified provides you with new career opportunities – whether you are interested in offering consultations, complementing your existing practice, or creating an all natural organic product line. Classes are approved for Massage Therapy Continuing Education Credit by the Florida Board of Massage and NCBTMB. Also offers 1 and 2 day introductory workshops for health professionals and the general public.

Essential Elements School of Aromatic Studies

www.essentialelementssite.com

The ACP (Aromatherapy Certification Program) is designed to prepare students to become qualified professionals in the therapeutic uses of Essential Oils. Their 235-hour course of study includes three 5-day classroom sessions, over three months. Students learn through a fun, intensive program taught in a relaxed nurturing environment with lots of hands-on activities. In our NAHA approved program (level one and two combined) students learn the therapeutic uses of 60 oils and how to safely use them at home or in a professional setting. Also offers Introduction to Essential Oils class with Continuing Education Credit for Massage Therapy and Acupuncture in Florida.

Floracopeia

www.floracopeia.com

Floracopeia offers Level I Approved Curriculum.

Institute of Integrative Aromatherapy

www.floramedica.com

The Certificate Program in Integrative Aromatherapy is a comprehensive correspondence course for health professionals and non-professionals. You will be personally mentored by author and Holistic Nurse Aromatherapist, Valerie Cooksley. The certification is fully endorsed by the American Holistic Nurses Association, The National Certification Board for Therapeutic Massage and Bodywork and NAHA (Level I and II). 325 CEU's for nurses and massage therapists.

Kayla's Notes: Valerie Cooksley was one of the Board members of the Aromatherapy Registration Council and on the Advisory Board for NAHA. She has written several books on aromatherapy. I have read many of the books and articles that Valerie has written. Her course is designed for health professionals and non-professionals. Valerie is a Holistic Nurse Aromatherapist which would provide a very unique perspective as a teacher.

Institute for Integrative Healthcare Studies

www.integrative-healthcare.org

The Institute for Integrative Healthcare Studies provides post-graduate, distance training for certified massage therapists and other healthcare professionals. The more than 35 CE distance learning courses offered are convenient, cost-effective, self-paced and easy to follow. Student Advisory services are also available from the Institute's knowledgeable staff at no additional charge. The Institute is approved by the NCBTMB as a CE Approved Provider and by the Florida and Louisiana Boards of Massage Therapy. The CE Hours are also accepted by the Texas Board of Massage, AMTA, ABMP and most other state boards. The Institute has been providing this valuable service since 1996 and to date, the Institute has had over 100,000 course enrollments.

Institute of Spiritual Healing and Aromatherapy, Inc.

www.ishaaromatherapy.com

The Institute of Spiritual Healing and Aromatherapy, Inc offers two programs: The Healing Touch Spiritual Ministry program in energy healing and the Certification in Clinical Aromatherapy program which is a NAHA and AIA approved school of aromatherapy. Offering both Level 1 and 2 in aromatherapy, the ISHA courses present both the British and French models of aromatherapy. The 240 hour coursework includes three classes, required reading, homework packets, a research project and written exams. Contacts hours are awarded to nurses, massage therapists and chaplains. Courses include hands-on energy treatments, anatomy and physiology, organic chemistry, introduction to botany, toxicity and safety, vibrational frequencies, professional issues, description of 55 oils for physical, emotional and spiritual clearing. This program is a holistic approach to the study of essential oil therapy and prepares students to take the ARC exam. Their faculty is all certified aromatherapists, and certified energy practitioners and instructors.

Kayla's Notes: This course blends both British and French approaches to aromatherapy. I have not personally studied the spiritual healing side of aromatherapy. I don't have enough personal history to give any accurate recommendations on this school. This program is also approved by AIA.

JennScents® Institute of Aromatherapy
www.jennscents.com
Level I (24 hours) and Level II (218 hours) approved. Holistic Aromatherapy Correspondence Courses include workbook/DVD. Level I includes history, safety, quality, limbic and immune systems, essential oil production, application methods, 10 carrier oils, blending introduction, aroma-chemistry introduction, 25 essential oils. Level II aromatherapy courses - Advanced, Specialized, Body Systems, Herbal Integration, Emotional Healing, Business Building and Skin Care. Courses address fundamentals of aromatherapy, modern development, safety, quality, limbic system, practical applications, basic botany, extraction methods, aroma-chemistry, anatomy/physiology, herbal integration, emotional healing, skin care formulations, 25 carrier oils, 35 essential oils, business development, ethics and legal issues.

Kayla's Notes: What stands out to me is that the courses here are taught on DVD. Everyone learns differently and for some DVD's could be a great method of learning. The course is taught by Holistic Aromatherapist, Jennifer Hochell Pressimone.

Natural Options Aromatherapy
www.naturaloptions.us
NAHA Approved School Level I. Natural Options Aromatherapy provides a 30 hour clinical aromatherapy certification program. This is very much a "how to seminar" with the focus on how to achieve desired outcomes. It is also accredited by NCBTMB for 30 CE hours, ideal for LMT's, Reflexologists, Nurses, practitioners of any type, as well as anyone with a desire to learn how to use aromatherapy safely and effectively. Six "labs" are included. In each lab you will make two blends for two distinct issues. Case studies are required to complete the course.

Ohana Healing Institute

www.ohanahealinginst.com

Ohana Healing Institute offers two programs. AROMA –Aromatherapy school for professional and the general public. They provide 200 hours NAHA-approved Level 1 and Level 2 Professional clinical Aromatherapy training and a variety of bodywork workshop for the general public and massage therapists.

Online Continuing Ed, LLC

www.onlineCE.com

Online Continuing Ed, a division of OnlineContinuingEd, LLC is a leading provider of distance based continuing education programs. You start your Aromatherapy studies with their Aromatherapy Level 1: Fundamentals of Aromatherapy, a 40 hour course offered entirely online. You can then continue your studies with Aromatherapy Level 2: Professional Aromatherapy Certification, a 160 hour course which is completed by distanced based learning using an online format, but you also communicate by email/fax with a personal tutor. OnlineContinuingEd, LLC is an approved NCBTMB provider for Massage Therapy, the Board of Certification for Athletic Trainers, and their HandCredits division is an approved provider of AOTA (American Occupational Therapy Association).

Kayla's Notes: Online Continuing Education Courses teaches continuing education for Aromatherapy, athletic trainers, Chiropractic Physicians, Hand Therapists, Motorcycle Safety, Massage Therapists, Naturopathic Physicians, Occupational therapists/Assistants, and Legal Secretary/Word Processor.

Reiki Center of Venice

www.reikicenterofvenice.com

The Reiki Center of Venice offers both on-site and long distance learning opportunities for students wishing to learn more about Aromatherapy and the use of essential oils. The Center offers a 200 hour NAHA approved Certification Program in two levels of training: Level One-Basic Aromatherapy (30 hours) and Level Two-Holistic Aromatherapy (170 hours).

Level One is a 30-hour comprehensive basic foundation of aromatherapy and therapeutic blending procedures. Course includes client consultation and assessment, blending and formulating techniques. Level Two is a 170-hour detailed course covering professional ethics, a holistic approach to health and disease, essential oils used in the systems of the body, case studies, and the basics of business development. Students must complete a minimum of 10 case histories and a book report.

Portions of these classes are approved by NCBTMB and FL Board of Massage Therapy for Ce's (Continuing Education). Additional classes for Ce's

(Continuing Education) include "Aromatherapy Massage" and "Aroma Lava Shell Massage." Instructing alternative therapy courses since 1998, the Center is open to the public and offers essential oils, bottles, salts, dried herbs, flower essences, and more at its Venice location.

RJ Buckle and Associates, LLC

Dr. Jane Buckle—Clinical Aromatherapy for licensed health professionals—not open to the lay public. Taught course (250 CEUs) - 4 classroom weekends plus student-work comprising 33 case-studies plus small mentored research project. Successful completion leads to CCAP (Certified Clinical Aromatherapy Practitioner). Program endorsed by AHNA. CEUs through AACN and NCBTMB. $375. Home-study available for aromatherapists interested in exploring Clinical Aromatherapy. Can lead to Certificate in Clinical Aromatherapy. Two CDs plus mentoring $550. The 'M' Technique®. method of touch suitable for the critically ill, very fragile or novice massage giver. Video/DVD (4.5 CEUs) $45. Certification course (14 CEUs) Two days plus case-studies. $375. Available in the USA.

Kayla's Notes: This course if for health professionals only. Dr. Jane Buckle has a long list of publications and is highly regarded in the industry.

International Schools

NAHA and AIA both have an extensive list of Internationals schools for aromatherapy. I have added all of them to the Aromatherapy and Business Resources in Appendix 4.

How to Become a Registered Aromatherapist

Everything you ever needed to know about becoming a Registered Aromatherapist can be found on the Aromatherapy Registration Council (ARC) website. ARC started in 1999. It is a non-profit that is independent from any membership body, organization, or educational facility.
The Aromatherapy Registration Examination is held twice per year. In order to be eligible to sit for the exam you must fit the following requirements:

- The ARC Registration Examination in Aromatherapy is open to anyone who has completed a minimum of a one year Level 2 program in aromatherapy from a college or school that is in compliance with the current NAHA Educational Guidelines or anyone who could provide evidence of equivalent training (transcripts must be enclosed with Application).
- Agreement to adhere to the Disciplinary Policy.
- Completion and filing of Application for ARC Registration Examination in Aromatherapy.
- Payment of required fees.

No matter where you are in your aromatherapy education becoming a Registered Aromatherapist is a great goal. The Frequently Asked Questions page at ARC is worth a careful read through to understand the requirements, continuing education and how started ARC and why.

:: Appendix 4 ::
Aromatherapy and Business Resources

A

A Consumer's Dictionary of Cosmetic Ingredients: Complete Information About the Harmful and Desirable Ingredients Found in Cosmetics and Cosmeceuticals by Ruth Winter, M.S.

All Business Resource
www.allbusiness.com
All Business, A DandB Company
650 Townsend Street, Suite 450
San Francisco, CA 94103
Telephone: 415-694-5000
Fax: 415-694-50001

Alliance of International Aromatherapists
www.alliance-aromatherapists.org
Alliance of International
Aromatherapists
Suite 323
9965 W. Remington Place – Unit A10
Littleton, Colorado 80128
E-Mail: info@alliance-aromatherapists.org
Telephone: 303-531-6377
Toll Free: 1-877-531-6377
Fax: 303-979-7135

American Cancer Society
www.cancer.org
Telephone: 1-800-227-2345 (or 1-866-228-4327 for TTY)

American Botanical Council (ABC)
abc.herbalgram.org
American Botanical Council
6200 Manor Rd.
Austin, TX 78723
E-Mail: abc@herbalgram.org
Telephone: 512-926-4900
Fax: 512-926-2345

American College of Healthcare Sciences
www.achs.edu
5940 SW Hood Ave
Portland, Oregon, 97239
E-Mail: achs@achs.edu
Telephone: 800-487-8839

American Council on Truth and Science
www.acsh.org
American Council on Science and Health
1995 Broadway, Second Floor
New York, NY 10023-5860
E-Mail: acsh@acsh.org
Telephone: 212-362-7044
Toll Free: 866-905-2694
Fax: 212-362-4919

American Herbal Products Association
www.ahpa.org
American Herbal Products
Association
8630 Fenton Street, Suite 918
Silver Spring, MD 20910
E-Mail: ahpa@ahpa.org
Telephone: 301-588-1171
Fax: 301-588-1174

American Massage Therapy Association
www.amtamassage.org

American Medical Association
www.ama-assn.org

Aroma Apothecary Healing Arts Academy
www.learnaroma.com
PO BOX 690
Crestone, CO 81131
E-Mail: info@learnaroma.com
Telephone: 1-888-AROMAS-8
(1-888-276-6278)

Aroma Art International Pte Ltd
www.aromaart.com.sg
Singapore

Aroma Harvest International College of Aromatherapy
Taipei, Taiwan
www.aromaharvest.com.tw

Aromahead Institute, School of Essential Oil Studies
www.aromahead.com
Sarasota, Florida
E-Mail: andrea@aromahead.com
Telephone: 941-323-3483

Aromatic Plant Project
www.aromaticplantproject.com
219 Carl Street
San Francisco, CA 94117
Telephone: 415-564-6785
Fax: 415-564-6799

Aromatherapists Society
www.thearomatherapistssociety.net

Aromatherapy & Allied Practitioners' Association
www.aapa.org.uk
14 Orleans Road
Upper Norwood
London SE19 3TA

Aromatherapy Alliance
www.aromatherapyalliance.org

Aromatherapy Council
www.aromatherapycouncil.co.uk

Aromatherapy Global Online Research Archives
www.nature-helps.com/agora/agora.html

Aromatherapy Registration Council
www.aromatherapycouncil.org
Aromatherapy Registration Council
C/- 5940 SW Hood Ave.
Portland, OR 97039
E-Mail: info@aromatherapycouncil.org
Telephone: 503-244-0726
Fax: 503-244-0727

Aromatherapy Environment Association of Japan
www.aromakankyo.or.jp/english/index.html

Aromatherapy Supplies
www.essentialwholesale.com
Essential Wholesale
8850 SE Herbert Court
Clackamas, Oregon 97015
E-Mail: info@essentialwholesale.com
Telephone: 503-722-7557
Fax: 503-296-5631

Aroma Harvest International College of Aromatherapy
www.aromaharvest.com.tw
Taipei, Taiwan

Aroma Heals Aromatherapy Institute
www.aromahealsinstitute.com
B.C. Canada

Aroma Studio, LLC
www.aromastudio.com
P.O. Box 37 Warwick, NY 10990
E-Mail: aromastudio@yahoo.com
Telephone: 845-651-1225
Toll-Free: 888-432-0292

Artiscent Aromatherapy Ltd.
www.artiscent.com
Burnaby, B.C.

Ashi Aromatics Inc.-Flower Power for Pets(sm)
www.ashitherapy.com
Instructor: Kelly Holland Azzaro, RA, CCAP, CBFP, LMT
PO BOX 1858, Banner Elk, NC 28604
E-Mail: ashitherapy@skybest.com
Phone: 828-898-5555

Asia-Pacific Aromatherapy
Hong Kong
E-Mail: aroma@netvigator.com

Astralessence School of Aromatherapy
www.astralessence.com

Associated Bodywork and Massage Professionals
www.abmp.com/home

Atlantic Institute of Aromatherapy
www.atlanticinstitute.com

B

Basali Dermal Institute
www.basali.com

Bastyr Center for Natural Health
3670 Stone Way N.
Seattle, WA 98103
Telephone: 206-834-4100
Fax: 206-834-4107
Bastyr Center for Natural Health Dispensary
Telephone: 206-834-4114
Bastyr Center for Natural Health Chinese Herbal Medicine Dispensary
Telephone: 206-834-4169

Bastyr University Natural Medicine Education
Kenmore, WA 98028-4966
Telephone: 425-823-1300
Fax: 425-823-6222

BDIH
Natural Cosmetics Certifier
www.kontrollierte-naturkosmetik.de/e/index_e.htm

Better Business Bureau
www.bbb.org/online

The Council of Better Business Bureaus
4200 Wilson Blvd., Suite 800
Arlington, VA 22203-1838

British Columbia Alliance of Aromatherapy
www.bcaoa.org
20729 93A Ave
Langley, BC V1M 2W7
Telephone: 604-515-2226
Toll Free: 1-866-339-2226

British Columbia Association of Practicing Aromatherapists
www.bcapa.org
49719 Prairie Central Rd,
Chilliwack, BC, V2P 6H3
Telephone: 604-794-7299

C

California Safe Cosmetics Program
www.cdph.ca.gov/programs/cosmetics/Pages/default.aspx
Telephone: 916-558-1784

Canadian Council of Better Business Bureaus
2 St. Clair Ave. East
Toronto, ON M4T 2T5
Telephone: 703-276-0100
Fax: 703-525-8277

Canadian Cosmetic, Toiletry and Fragrance Association (CCTFA)
www.cctfa.ca/site/cctfa
420 Britannia Road East, Suite 102
Mississauga, Ontario, L4Z 3L5
E-Mail: cctfa@cctfa.ca
Telephone: 905-890-5161
Fax: 905-890-2607

Canadian Federation of Aromatherapists
www.cfacanada.com
110 Thorndale Place,
Waterloo, ON N2L 5Y8
E-Mail: cfamanager@cfacanada.com
Telephone: 519 746-1594
Fax: 519 746-9493

Canadian Institute of Aromatherapy
www.canadaroma.com
Canada

Canadian Institute of Aromatherapy (CIA)
www.aromatherapyinstitute.com
Canada

Caveman Chemistry
www.cavemanchemistry.com

Colipa
European Cosmetics Association
www.colipa.eu

Contract Manufacturing/Packaging

Essential Labs
www.essentiallabs.com
8850 SE Herbert Court
Clackamas, Oregon 97015
E-Mail: info@essentiallabs.com
Telephone: 503-905-3273

Cosmetic Ingredient Review Panel
www.cir-safety.org
1101 17th St. N.W., Suite 412
Washington D.C. 20036-4702
E-Mail: cirinfo@cir-safety.org
Telephone: 202-331-0651
Fax: 202-331-0088

Cosmetic Bench Reference
dir.cosmeticsandtoiletries.com
Allured Business Media
336 Gundersen Drive, Suite A
Carol Stream, IL 60188-2403
E-Mail: cbr@allured.com
Telephone: 630-653-2155
Fax: 630-653-2192

Cosmetics Info
www.cosmeticsinfo.org

Cosmetics Toiletry and Perfume Association
dir.cosmeticsandtoiletries.com
Allured Business Media
336 Gundersen Drive, Suite A
Carol Stream, IL 60188-2403
E-Mail: cbr@allured.com
Telephone: 630-653-2155
Fax: 630-653-2192

D

Disaster Information Management Research Center (DIMRC)
One Democracy Plaza, Suite 1030
6701 Democracy Blvd., MSC 4876
Bethesda, MD 20892

Dr. Dukes's Phytochemical and Ethnobotanical Databases
www.ars-grin.gov/duke/chem-activities.html

E

East-West School for Herbal and Aromatic Studies
www.theida.com
335 Amber Lane
Willow Springs, NC 27592
E-Mail: info@theida.com
Telephone: 919-894-7230

Ecocert
www.ecocert.com

Environmental Health and Toxicity
sis.nlm.nih.gov/enviro.html
Specialized Information Services (SIS)
Two Democracy Plaza, Suite 510
6707 Democracy Blvd., MSC 5467
Bethesda, MD 20892-5467

E-mail: tehip@teh.nlm.nih.gov
Telephone: 301-496-1131 (local and international)
Toll Free: 1-888-FINDNLM
Fax: 301-480-3537

Essential Education International, Inc.
www.essentialeducationinternational.com
PO Box 141363
Gainesville, Florida 32614
E-Mail: christinapolnyj@mac.com
Telephone: 352-222-1747

Essential Elements School of Aromatic Studies
www.essentialelementssite.com
3001 First Avenue South
St. Petersburg, FL 33712
E-Mail: essential.elements@mac.com
Phone: 727-327-1309
Fax: 727-327-1409

Essential Oils
Essential Wholesale
www.essentialwholesale.com
8850 SE Herbert Court
Clackamas, Oregon 97015
E-Mail: info@essentialwholesale.com
Telephone: 503-722-7557
Fax: 503-296-5631

Essential U Blog
www.essentialublog.com

Etsy
www.etsy.com
Set up your store under "Bath and Beauty"

European Commission CosIng
*ec.europa.eu/consumers/cosmetics/
cosing*
European Commission
Health and Consumers Directorate-
General
B – 1049 Brussels
Belgium

**Europa, Summaries of EU
Legislation**
*europa.eu/legislation_summaries/
consumers/product_labelling_and_
packaging/l21191_en.htm*

eWomen Network
www.ewomennetwork.com
14900 Landmark Blvd.
Suite 540
Dallas, TX 75254
E-Mail: info@ewomennetwork.com
Telephone: 972-620-9995
Fax: 972-720-9995

F

Fairtrade International
www.fairtrade.net
Fairtrade International (FLO)
Bonner Talweg 177
53129 Bonn, Germany
E-Mail: info@fairtrade.net
Telephone: +49 228 949230
Fax: +49 228 2421713

**Federal Communications
Commission**
www.fcc.gov
45 12ths Street, SW
Washington, DC 20554

Fioravanti, Kayla
www.kaylafioravanti.com

Flower Essence Society
www.flowersociety.org

**Food and Drug Administration
(FDA)**
www.fda.gov/Cosmetics/default.htm
10903 New Hampshire Ave.
Silver Spring, MD 20993-0002
Telephone: 888-463-6332, 301-
796-8240 (Emergency Operations),
or 866-300-4374 (Emergency
Operations)

Fragrance Foundation
www.fragrance.org

**Fragrance Materials Association of
the United States**
www.fmafragrance.org

Free Conference Calling
www.freeconferencecalling.com

Free Small Business Help
www.buzgate.org
Buzgate.org
c/o P.O. Box 219
E. Kingston, NH 03827

G

Give more Media, Inc.
www.givemore.com
2500 Gaskins Rd.
Richmond, VA 23238
E-Mail: sparker@givemore.com
Telephone: 804-762-4500 ext. 303

Global Trade Item Number
www.gtin.info
Bar Code Graphics
Inc. 875 N Michigan Ave
Ste 2650
Chicago, IL 60611
Toll Free: 800-662-0701 x240

H

Handcrafted Soapmakers Guild
www.soapguild.org

H.A.S.A.P. Aromatherapy Center
www.hasap.kr
Seoul, Korea

Health Canada
www.hc-sc.gc.ca/cps-spc/index-eng.php
Health Canada
Address Locator 0900C2
Ottawa, Ontario
KIA OK9
E-Mail: Info@hc-sc.gc.ca
Telephone: 613-957-2991
Toll Free: 1-866-225-0709
Fax: 613-941-5366
Teletypewriter: 1-800-267-1245
(Health Canada)

Herb Research Foundation
www.herbs.org/herbnews
1007 Pearl St. Suite 200
Boulder, CO 80302b
Phone: 303-449-2265
Fax: 303-449-7849
E-Mail: info@herbs.org

Household Products Data Base
hpd.nlm.nih.gov/index.htm
U.S. National Library of Medicine
8600 Rockville Pike
Bethesda, MD 20894
E-Mail: tehip@teh.nlm.nih.gov

How to Follow the Rules and Regs Explained in Plain English by Marie Gale
www.mariegale.com/purchase-soap-cosmetic-labeling-book/

I

IARA International Aromatherapy
www.eduaroma.com
Research Association
Mapogu Seoul, Korea

INCI Dictionary
www.essentiallabs.com/PDF/INCI_NAMES_3col.pdf

Independent Cosmetic Manufacturers and Distributors (ICMAD)
www.icmad.org
1220 W. Northwest Hwy
Palatine, IL 60067
E-Mail: info@icmad.org
Toll Free: 800-334-2623
Fax: 847-991-8161

Indie Beauty Network
www.indiebeauty.com
E-Mail: indiebusiness@gmail.com
Telephone: 704-291-7280
Send an email to request the mailing address

Institute of Integrative Aromatherapy
www.floramedica.com
PO Box 130166
The Woodlands, TX 77393
E-Mail: Valerie@floramedica.com
Telephone: 877-363-3422

Institute for Integrative Healthcare Studies
www.integrative-healthcare.org
2311 State Route 17K
Montgomery, NY 12549
E-Mail: info@natural-wellness.com
Telephone: 800-364-5722
Fax: 845-361-1118

Institute of Spiritual Healing and Aromatherapy, Inc.
www.ishaaromatherapy.com
PO Box 741239
Arvada, CO 80006
E-Mail: Staff@ISHAhealing.com
Telephone: 303-467-7829
Fax: 303-467-2328

International Aromatherapy & Aromatic Medicine Association
www.iaama.org.au
PO Box 215
Burwood, NSW
Australia 1805
Telephone: +61 2 9715 6622

International Aromatherapy Society (I.A.S.)
www.aromaday.co.kr
Mapogu Seoul, Korea

International Cosmetology Training Institute
www.icti.com.hk
Hong Kong, China

International Federation of Aromatherapist (IFPA)
www.ifaroma.org
International Federation of Aromatherapist, UK Head Office
7B Walpole Court
Ealing Green
Ealing, London
W5 5ED
Telephone: 020 8567 2243 or 020 8567 1923
Fax: 020 8840 9288

International Fragrance Association
www.ifraorg.org
IFRA Operations
Avenue des Arts, 6 1210

Brussels Belgium
IFRA Head Office
Chemin de la Parfumerie 5CH-1214
Vernier, Geneva Switzerland
IFRA Operations
Telephone: +32-2214 20 60
Fax: +32-2 214 2069
IFRA Head Office
Telephone: +41-22 431 82 50
Fax: +41-22 431 88 06

International Fragrance Association North America
1620 Street NW, Suite 925
Washington D.C. 20006
E-Mail: info@ifrana.org
Telephone: 202-293-5800
Fax: 202-463-8998

International Journal of Clinical Aromatherapy
www.ijca.net

International Institute of Chinese Medicinal Aromatherapy
www.yangsen.com.tw
Taipei, Taiwan

International Spa and Beauty College
www.isbc.com.hk
Hong Kong China

IRS Small Business and Self-Employed Tax Center
www.irs.gov/businesses/small/index.html

J

Jamu Spa School
Traditional Indonesian Therapies
www.jamuspaschool.com

Jalan By Pass Ngurah Rai 99x Tuban
Bali - Indonesia
E-Mail: info@jamuspaschool.com
Telphone: +62 361 704581
Fax: +62 361 704582

JennScents® Institute of Aromatherapy
www.jennscents.com
702 West Montrose Street
Clermont, Florida 34711
E-Mail: jh@jennscents.com
Tepehone: 352-243-9627

Joyessence Aromatherapy Centre Inc.
www.joyessence.on.ca
Canada

Joyessence Aromatherapy Centre Inc.
www.royalbeautyedu.com
Taipei, Taiwan

Just Sell Resources
www.justsell.com

K

Kitchen Chemistry TV
Do-It-Yourself Instructional Videos
www.youtube.com/user/ essentialwholesale

L

Ladies Who Launch
www.ladieswholaunch.com
46 Shopping Plaza #190
Chagrin Falls, OH 44022
E-Mail: info@ladieswholaunch.com
Telephone: 440-247-2239

LiLing International College of Aromatherapy
www.liling.com.tw
Taipei County, Taiwan

M

Mexican Association for the Investigation and Practice of Aromatherapy
www.amipaa.org.mx

N

National Association for the Self-Employed
www.nase.org
P.O. Box 241
Annapolis Junction, MD 20701-0241
Toll Free: 1-800-649-6273
(Continental US) or 1-800-232-6273
(Alaska and Hawaii)

Natural Association of Holistic Aromatherapy
www.naha.org
P.O. Box 1868
Banner Elk, NC 28604
E-Mail: info@naha.org
Telephone: 828-898-6161
Fax: 828-898-1965

National Association of Women Business Owners
www.nawbo.org
601 Pennsylvania Ave. NW
South Building, Suite 900
Washington, DC 20004
E-Mail: national@nawbo.org
Toll Free: 800-556-2926
Fax: 202-403-3788

National Certification Board for Therapeutic Massage and Bodywork NCBTMB
www.ncbtmb.org
1901 South Meyers Road, Suite 240
Oakbrook Terrace, IL 60181
630-627-8000

Natrue
www.natrue.org

Natural Options Aromatherapy
www.naturaloptions.us
1540 Honeycreek Road
Bellville, OH 44813
E-Mail: natoptaroma@aol.com
Phone: 419-886-3736

Natural Products Association
www.npainfo.org

National Federation of Independent Business
www.nfib.com
53 Century Blvd. – Suite 250
Nashville, TN 37214
Telephone: 615-872-5800
Toll Free: 800-634-2669

Natural Planter Company, Ltd.
www.natural-planter.com.tw
Taichung City, Taiwan

O

U.S. Department of Labor Occupational Safety and Health Administration
www.osha.gov
200 Constitution Avenue
Washington, D.C. 20210
Toll Free: 1-800-321-6742

Ohana Healing Institute
www.ohanahealinginst.com
1225 W. 190th Street #455-C
Gardena, CA 90248
E-Mail: ohanahealing_usa@yahoo.co.jp
Phone: 323-345-7188
Fax: 310-295-2468

Online Continuing Ed, LLC
www.onlineCE.com
Po Box 15 1940 Silas Deane Hwy.
Rocky Hill, CT 06067
E-Mail: info@onlinece.com
Telephone: 860-463-9003

Organic Consumers Association
www.organicconsumers.org
6771 South Silver Hill Drive
Finland, MN 55603
Telephone: 218-226-4164
Fax: 218-353-7652

Organic Monitor
www.organicmonitor.com

Oregon Tilth
www.tilth.org

P

Personal Care Products Council
www.ctfa.org
1101 17th Street NW, Suite 300
Washington D.C. 20036-4702
Telephone: 202-331-1770
Fax: 202-331-1969

Personal Care Truth
www.personalcaretruth.com

Phytotherapy Institute
www.jimmharrison.com/Aromatherapy.html
Jim Harrison

Press Release Info
toolkit.prnewswire.com/score/index.shtml#

Private Label Cosmetics
Essential Labs
www.essentiallabs.com
8850 SE Herbert Court
Clackamas, Oregon 97015
Telephone: 503-905-3273

Product Insurance
Indie Beauty Network
http://www.indiebeauty.com
E-Mail: indiebusiness@gmail.com
Telephone: 704-291-7280

Pub Med
www.ncbi.nlm.nih.gov/sites/entrez
National Center of Biotechnology
Information
National Library of Medicine
8600 Rockville Pike, Building 38A
Bethesda, MD 20894
E-Mail: info@ncbi.nlm.nih.gov
Telephone: 301-496-2475

R

Ran Herbs College of Phytotherapy
www.ranherbs.com
Israel

Ready to Publish
readytopublish.blogspot.com
Publish your book or pamphlet,
hire a proof-reader, retain an ebook
publishing coach. Their editors
reviewed this book!
Portland, Oregon
E-Mail: beth@fit2b.us
Telephone: 503-255-2845

Reiki Center of Venice
www.reikicenterofvenice.com
5073 Seagrass Drive
Venice, FL 34293
E-Mail: francinemilford@verizon.net
Telephone: 941-497-7795

R J Buckle Associates LLC
www.rjbuckle.com
1310 Brandt Avenue
New Cumberland, PA 17070
E-Mail: rjbinfo@aol.com
Phone: 717-645-1900

Research Institute for Fragrance
Materials (RIFM)
www.rifm.org

S

Sense of Smell Institute
www.senseofsmell.org
545 5th Avenue Suite 900
New York, NY 10017
E-Mail: info@senseofsmell.org
Scientific Affairs Director
Craig Warren
E-Mail: cwarren@senseofsmell.org
Telephone: 212-725-2755 x107
Fax: 212-779-9058

Safe Cosmetics Alliance
www.safecosmeticsalliance.org

Scientific Committee on Cosmetic
Products and Non-Food Products
Intended for Consumers
ec.europa.eu/health/ph_risk/
*committees/sccp/documents/out131_*
en.pdf

SCORE
www.score.org
Toll Free: 800-634-0245

Sense About Science
www.senseaboutscience.org.uk
25 Shaftesbury Avenue
London W1D 7ET
E-Mail: enquiries@senseaboutscience.org
Telephone: +44 (0) 20 7478 4380

Siyanli Professional Beauty Academy
www.siyanlischool.cn
Shang Hai, China

Small Business Loan Sources
www.ibank.com

Spa Association
www.thespaassociation.com

Spark Academy and Consultants
www.learninspark.com
Taipei, Taiwan

Soapmaking Supplies
Essential Wholesale
www.essentialwholesale.com
8850 SE Herbert Court
Clackamas, Oregon 97015
E-Mail: info@essentialwholesale.com
Telephone: 503-722-7557
Fax: 503-296-5631

Social Security Online
www.socialsecurity.gov/employer
Social Security Administration
Office of Public Inquires
Windsor Park Building
6401 Security Blvd.
Baltimore, MD 21235
Toll Free: 800-772-1213 or
1-800-325-0778 (TTY)

Society of Cosmetic Chemists
www.scconline.org
Society of Cosmetic Chemists
120 Wall Street, Suite 2400
New York, NY 10005-4088
E-Mail: scc@scconline.org
Telephone: 212-668-1500
Fax: 212-668-1504

Society of Cosmetic Scientists
www.scs.org.uk
SCS / IFSCC
Suite 6
Langham House East
Mill Street
LUTON
Bedfordshire LU1 2NA, UK
E-Mail: lorna.weston@ifscc.org
(Lorna Weston, Secretary General,
IFSCC), gem.bektas@btconnect.com
(Gem Bektas, Secretary General,
SCS), or mel.cheekoory@btconnect.
com (Mel Cheekoory, Admin.
Assistant)
Telephone: 01582 726661
Fax: 01582 405217

Start a Business Today
www.bizfilings.com
BizFilings
8040 Excelsior Dr., Suite 200
Madison, WI 53717
Telephone: 608-827-5300
Toll Free: 800-981-7183

Statistical Assessment Service
www.stats.org
2100 L. Street, Suite 300
Washington D.C. 20037
Telephone: 202-223-2942
Fax: 202-872-4014

T

Tisserand, Robert
www.roberttisserand.com
Expert in Aromatherapy and
Essential Oil Research
407 Park Road
Ojai, CA 93023
E-Mail: robert@roberttisserand.com
Telephone: 805-640-9012
Fax: 805-640-9012

ToxNet
toxnet.nlm.nih.gov
Specialized Information Services (SIS)
Two Democracy Plaza, Suite 510
6707 Democracy Blvd., MSC 5467
Bethesda, MD 20892-5467
E-Mail: tehip@teh.nlm.nih.gov
Telephone: 301-496-1131
(local and international)
Toll Free: 1-888-FINDNLM
Fax (SIS): 1-301-480-3537
Fax (DIMRC): 1-301-480-968

U

United Aromatherapy Effort
www.unitedaromatherapy.org
Helping Our Heroes

US Association for Small Business and Entrepreneurship
www.usasbe.org
Belmont University
1900 Belmont Blvd.
Nashville, TN 37212
E-Mail: usasbe@belmont.edu
Telephone: 615-460-2615
Fax: 615-460-2614

US Chamber of Commerce
www.uschamber.com
U.S. Chamber of Commerce
1615 H Street, NW
Washington DC, 20062-2000
Telephone: 202-659-6000
Toll Free: 800-638-6582

US Consumer Product Safety Commission
www.cpsc.gov
4330 East West Highway
Bethesda, MD 20814
Telephone: 301-504-7923
Toll Free: 800-638-2772
Fax: 301-504-0124 and 301-504-0025

US Department of Agriculture
www.usda.gov/wps/portal/usda/usdahome
1400 Independence Ave., S.W.
Washington, DC 20250
Telephone: 202-720-2791

US Department of Commerce
www.commerce.gov
U.S. Department of Commerce
1401 Constitution Avenue, NW
Washington, DC 20230
E-Mail: TheSec@doc.gov
Telephone: 202-482-2000

US Small Business Administration
www.sba.gov
409 3rd Street, SW
Washington, DC 20416
E-Mail: answerdesk@sba.gov
Telephone: 704-344-6640 (TTY)
Toll Free: 800-827-5722

W

West Coast Institute of Aromatherapy Inc.
www.westcoastaromatherapy.com
Canada

Supplies and Equipment

Contract Manufacturing

Essential Labs
www.essentiallabs.com
E-Mail: info@essentiallabs.com
Telephone: 503-905-3273

Diffusers

Amazon
www.amazon.com

Essential Wholesale
www.essentialwholesale.com
Reed Diffuser DIY Supplies
8850 SE Herbert Court
Clackamas, Oregon 97015
E-Mail: info@essentialwholesale.com
Telephone: 503-722-7557

Essential Oils

Essential Wholesale
www.essentialwholesale.com
Essential Oils DIY Supplies
8850 SE Herbert Court
Clackamas, Oregon 97015
E-Mail: info@essentialwholesale.com
Telephone: 503-722-7557

Insurance

Indie Beauty Network
www.indiebeauty.com
E-Mail: indiebusiness@gmail.com
Telephone: 704-291-7280

Manufacturing Equipment

Indco Mixers
www.indco.com

Jiffy Mixer Co, Inc
www.jiffymixer.com

Packaging

You can find a complete list of Packaging Suppliers here:
www.essentialwholesale.com/ Packaging-Resources

Private Label Manufacturing

Essential Labs
www.essentiallabs.com
E-Mail: info@essentiallabs.com
Telephone: 503-905-3273

Soapmaking Supplies

Certified Lye
www.certified-lye.com

Essential Wholesale
www.essentialwholesale.com
8850 SE Herbert Court
Clackamas, Oregon 97015
E-Mail: info@essentialwholesale.com
Telephone: 503-722-7557

Soap Equipment
www.soapequipment.com

Soap Molds.com
www.soapmolds.com
2138 Humboldt St
Bellingham, WA 98226
Telephone: 360-671-0201

Tradeshows and Conferences

Aliance of International Aromatherapists Conference
www.alliance-aromatherapists.org

Beauty Expo
www.beautyexpousa.com

Cosmoprof
www.cosmoprofnorthamerica.com

HBA Global Expo
www.hbaexpo.com

Global Spa Summit
www.globalspasummit.org

Handcrafted Soapmakers Guild Annual Conference
www.soapguild.org

Health and Nutrition Show
www.healthyharvestshow.com

In-Cosmetics
www.in-cosmetics.com

Indie Cruise
www.indiebusinessblog.com/category/cruise/

Integrative Healthcare Symposium
www.ihsymposium.com/12/public/enter.aspx

International Beauty Show
www.ibsnewyork.com

International Congress of Esthetics and Spa
www.lneonline.com/tradeshows

International Esthetics, Cosmetics & Spa Conferences
www.iecsc.com

ISPA Conference & Expo
www.experienceispa.com/events

Natural Products Expo
www.expowest.com/ew12/public/enter.aspx

Natural Beauty Summit
www.naturalbeautysummit.com

Natural & Organic Products Europe
www.naturalproducts.co.uk

New York International Gift Fair EX·TRACTS
www.nyigf.com

Sustainable Cosmetics Summit
www.sustainablecosmeticssummit.com

The World of Aromatherapy
www.naha.org/conference.htm

Glossary

A

Abhyanga is an oil massage in Ayurveda that is recommended for increasing flexibility of muscle and joints, rejuvenating skin, and keeping impurities from accumulating in the body by using massage and herb infused oil to stimulate various tissues.

Absorption is the route by which substances can enter the body via skin.

Adenosine triphosphate (ATP) is an important carrier of energy in cells in the body and a compound that is important in the synthesis of RNA. The body produces ATP from food and then ATP produces energy as needed by the body.

Alpha hydroxy acids (AHA) are any of various carboxylic acids with a hydroxyl group attached at the alpha position. Examples include: malic, lactic, glycolic, citric and tartaric acid. AHA are used in cosmetics for its exfoliating effect on the surface layer of skin. The FDA requires that you include this warning on any product made with AHAs: **Sunburn Alert:** This product contains an alpha hydroxy acid (AHA) that may increase your skin's sensitivity to the sun and particularly the possibility of sunburn. Use a sunscreen and limit sun exposure while using this product and for a week afterwards.

Amygdala is the one of the four basal ganglia in each cerebral hemisphere that is part of the limbic system and consists of an almond-shaped mass of gray matter in the anterior extremity of the temporal lobe.

Analgesic is a substance that reduce pain without resulting in a loss of consciousness.

Anosmia is a temporary or permanent lack of functioning olfaction, the inability to perceive odors.

Anti-allergy is a substance that exerts energy in the opposite direction of an allergy reaction.

Anti-fungal: destroying fungi or inhibiting their growth.

Anti-inflammatory: counteracting inflammation.

Anti-microbial: destroying or inhibiting the growth of microorganisms and especially pathogenic microorganisms.

Antiviral: destroying or inhibiting virus'.

Aphrodisiac: an agent or substance that arouses or is held to arouse sexual desire.

Aroma Chemicals are used to create a complex blend for compounded flavors and fragrances. Many times a flavor or fragrance will include aromachemicals, essential oils, natural extac ts, diluents and carriers. An aroma chemical can be synthetic or from natural sources.

Aromatic: having a strong smell.

Ayurveda: a form of holistic alternative medicine that is the traditional system of medicine of India.

B

Bactericidal: destroying bacteria

Benzene ring is a structural arrangement of atoms in benzene and other aromatic compounds that consists of a planar symmetrical hexagon of six carbon atoms which derives added stability from the delocalization of certain bonding electrons over the entire ring.

Bio-Terge 804 has the INCI name: Sodium C14-16 Olefin Sulfonate, Sodium Laureth Sulfate, and Lauramide DEA. Below is a closer look at the ingredients that make up Bio-Terge 804.

Blood-brain barrier: a naturally occurring barrier created by the modification of brain capillaries that prevents many substances from leaving the blood and crossing the capillary walls into the brain tissues.

Bone-char is a granular material produced by charring animal bones. Bone-char is used to refine crude oil into petroleum jelly.

C

Calcium Sulfate is a white salt $CaSO_4$ that occurs especially as anhydrite, gypsum, and plaster of Paris and that in hydrated form is used as a building material and in anhydrous form is used as a drying agent.

California Safe Cosmetics Program Chemical List is a list of chemicals that require mandatory reporting under the California Safe Cosmetics Act of 2005.

Camphoraceous: being or having the properties of camphor; "camphoraceous odor"

Carbomer is a water soluble thickener, suspending agent and stabilizer often used in cosmetics. Carbomer is a synthetic high molecular weight crosslinked polymers of acrylic acid. It has excellent thickening efficiency at high viscosity and sparkling clear transparency in aqueous solutions. Carbomer is a high molecular weight polymer. It is not absorbed by body tissues and is totally safe for human oral consumption. Test for toxicological tolerance have shown that it does not have pronounced physiological action and is non -toxic. Carbomer is used in conjunction with TEA to adjust the pH and thicken the product to a stable viscosity.

Carboxylic acid is an organic acid containing one or more carboxyl groups.

Carrier oil is another term for base oil or vegetable oil commonly used to dilute essential oils into.

CAS Number is a registry number given to more than 63 million organic and inorganic substances. Each registry number is a unique numeric identifier that designates only one substance.

Certificate of Analysis (C of A) is an authenticated document that is issued by an appropriate authority that certifies the quality and purity of pharmaceuticals as well as plant and animal products being exported.

Citric Acid is commonly used in hair and skincare products. It has astringent and antioxidant properties and can also be used as a stabilizer and preservative, and to neutralize odor. It is derived from citrus fruits by fermentation of crude sugars. It is used to adjust acid-alkali balance. When citric acid is used to adjust the pH of a cosmetic product the FDA does not require that it be included on the ingredient list.

Cocoamidopropyl Betaine is a fairly mild and gentle surfactant used in melt and pour soaps, shampoos, conditioners, and body washes. It has been valued for its foaming qualities and, ability to serve as a thickening agent. Cocoamidopropyl betaine leaves hair and skin soft and smooth. It is compatible with other cationic, anionic, and nonionic surfactants making it a favorite of cosmetic formulators. Cocoamidopropyl betaine has an exceptional safety profile and performs markedly well.

Cocamidopropyl betaine is a long chain surfactant derived from coconut oil. Skeptics are alarmed by the fact that during the synthesis of this ingredient, some of the reagents involved in the reaction may be potentially harmful. A solid comprehension of the chemistry involved in reagents will help clarify this debate. A reagent is a substance that is used in a chemical reaction to produce other substances. It is not in the final product. An example of this could be the Sodium Hydroxide when it is used to cause a reaction called saponification to create soap. Sodium Hydroxide is an ingredient with multiple hazard warnings, but when combined with other constituents it creates an effective, safe, and diverse cleaning agent. There is no un-reacted sodium hydroxide in the finished soap because a new product has been formed.

The Cosmetic Ingredient Review (CIR) Expert Panel reviewed Cocamidopropyl betaine and found it to be safe for use as used in rinse of products and limited it to 3% for leave-on products. According to the general provisions of the Cosmetics Directive of the European Union, Cocamidopropyl betaine may be used in cosmetics and personal care products marketed in Europe. In tests Cocoamidopropyl betaine was found to be readily biodegradable, slightly orally toxic, moderately irritating to the eyes, mildly irritating to the skin, and no delayed contact hypersensitivity or evidence of sensitization was observed. It is not a mutagenic, nor is it a carcinogen

Contact Dermatitis is an inflammation of the skin caused by direct contact with an irritating or allergy-causing substance.

Contraindication is a condition which makes a particular treatment or procedure inadvisable.

Cosmeceuticals is a term meant to imply that a product has the properties of both a cosmetic and a pharmaceutical. The FDA does not recognize the term, however if you use it you must then comply with all OTC drug regulations.

Crème of Tartar is the common name for potassium hydrogen tartrate, which is an acid salt commonly used in cooking. In bubble bars and foaming bath bombs it is used to stabilize the foaming action during use of the product.

D

Decongestant is an agent that relieves congestion.

Dermis is the second of the three major layers of skin. It varies in thickness depending on the location of the skin. The dermis is composed of three types of tissue that are present throughout it including: collagen, elastic tissue, and reticular fibers.

Dipropylene glycol is produced as a byproduct of the manufacture of propylene glycol. It works well as a solvent of essential and fragrance oils. Dipropylene glycol is not acutely toxic by oral, dermal, or inhalation exposure. Dipropylene glycol is not toxic to genetic material based on in vitro and in vivo study findings. Dipropylene glycols low toxicity and solvent properties make it an ideal additive for perfumes, reed diffusers and skin and hair care products. It is also a common ingredient in commercial fog fluid, used in entertainment industry smoke and haze machines.

Dilute: to diminish the strength.

E

Eczema is a chronic skin disorder that involves scaly and itchy rashes.

EINECS stands for European Inventory of Existing Commercial Chemical Substances. It is a comprehensive list of all the existing substances.

Emmenagogic: promoting menstruation.

Endometriosis: the presence and growth of functioning endometrial tissue in places other than the uterus.

Epidermis is outer layer of the two main layers of cells that make up the skin.

Essential Wholesale Basic Concentrate Crème is a simple concentrate crème that can be used for multiple purposes. It can be added to another lotion or crème base to thicken a product. It can also be mixed with herbal tinctures, essential oils, de-ionized or distilled water, fragrance oils or aloe juice to create a variety of different lotions or crèmes. It accepts additives up to one part Basic Crème Concentrate to one part added liquids total weight.

Essential Wholesale Body Linen Spray Base is an unscented stably preserved base that can be used for body, air or linen sprays.

Esterification is the reaction between alcohols and carboxylic acids to make esters.

European Union Allergen Declaration is from the 7th Amendment to the Cosmetic Directive of the European Union (EU) which requires that has added 26 fragrance ingredients be declared on the label when used at 0.001% in leave-on prod– ucts and 0.01% in rinse-off products.

Expectorant is a substance that helps bring up mucus and other material from the lungs, bronchi and trachea.

F

Fair Packaging and Labeling Act is a law in the United States that requires labels on consumer products identify the product; the name and place of business of the manufacturer, packer, or distributor; and the net quantity of contents in metric and U.S. customary units.

Fixative in perfumery is a substance that is used to reduce the evaporation rate and improve stability when added to volatile components.

Flash Point is the lowest temperature at which a volatile material can vaporize to form an ignitable mixture in air.

Food, Drug and Cosmetic Act is a set of laws passed in 1938 that gave authority of the U.S. Food and Drug Administration (FDA) to oversee the safety of food, drugs and cosmetics. It has since been updated, expanded and changed over the years. The online version contains all of the updates: *www.fda.gov/regulatoryinformation/legislation/federalfooddrugandcosmeticactfdcact/default.htm*

G

Gangrene: death of tissue in part of the body. Gas gangrene is the form that Gattefosse had after his burn. It is a potentially deadly form of gangrene.

Glycerin, Kosher Vegetable also referred to as Glycerol, is a sugar alcohol that is obtained by adding alkalies to fats and fixed oils. Glycerin is a soothing humectant that draws moisture from the air to the skin. It is an emollient, which makes the skin feel softer and smoother. Glycerin has a high hydrophilic (water) factor and a low lipophilic (fat) factor. It is completely miscible with water. The FDA includes Glycerin on its list of direct food additives considered Generally Recognized As Safe (GRAS), and on its list of approved indirect food additives. According to the general provisions of the Cosmetics Directive of the European Union, Glycerin may be used in cosmetics and personal care products marketed in Europe. Glycerin derived from raw materials of animal origin must comply with European Union animal by-products regulations. The Joint FAO/WHO Expert Committee on Food Additives has not specified an acceptable daily intake for Glycerin. Glycerol is considered to be readily biodegradable in the aquatic environment.

Glycolic Acid is a constituent of sugar cane juice. Glycolic acid is form of an alpha hydroxy acid that is extremely strong and must be handled with extreme care. Please be cautious in your formulations that contain glycolic acid. It is not necessary to use large percentages of glycolic acid in order to have a positive effect on the skin.

While the FDA does allow the use of 10% in "at home" products, I advise that you experiment with percentage ranges of 1-5% in your formulations. We have found that smaller percentages used more often can be more effective and less traumatic to the skin than high doses used irregularly. Recovery time should be a matter of hours and not days or weeks as with some glycolic acid products on the market.

According to the FDA, "the panel concluded that AHA's are 'safe for use in cosmetic products at concentrations less than or equal to 10 percent, at final formulation pH's greater than or equal to 3.5, when formulated to avoid increasing the skin's sensitivity to the sun, or when directions for use include the daily use of sun protection.' For salon use products, the panel said that the products are 'safe for use at concentrations less than or equal to 30 percent, at final formulation pH's greater than or equal to 3.0, in products designed for brief, discontinuous use followed by thorough rinsing from the skin, when applied by trained professionals, and when application is accompanied by directions for the daily use of sun protection.'"

H

Head lice are tiny insects that live on the scalp. They spread from close contact with people who have head lice.

Hepatotoxicity is a general term for liver damage. Hepatoxicants are substances that cause liver damage.

Hin is a liquid measure used by the ancients Hebrews that equaled about five liters.

Hippocampus is an area buried deep in the forebrain that helps regulate emotion and memory. Functionally, the hippocampus is part of the olfactory cortex, that part of the cerebral cortex essential to the sense of smell. Hyaluronic Acid was discovered by Karl Meyer in 1934 and has been successfully used in personal care and wound healing. Until the 1990's the only method of producing hyaluronic acid was extracting it from rooster combs. Currently there are two forms of hyaluronic acid on the market; one derived from rooster comb and the other derived by the fermentation of yeast. I only recommend the 100% vegan approved material.

Hyaluronic acid is naturally found in the extracellular matrix of human tissue. Topically applied hyaluronic acid forms an air permeable layer and penetrates into the dermis, thus boosting the elasticity and hydration of the skin. The protective breathable barrier on the skin locks in moisture which gives the skin a youthful appearance. The cuticular layer of the skin normally contains 10-20% water, however as we age it can drop to below 10%. Hyaluronic acid comes to the rescue with its unique ability to hold more than 1000 ml of water per gram of hyaluronic acid, which is a key factor in allowing the skin to retain more water. Amazingly, hyaluronic acid adjusts its moisture absorption based on the relative humidity in the air. It is the ideal ingredient in skin care products as it adjusts to the skin's need for a moisturizing effect depending on the relative humidity of seasons and climate of an area. Hyaluronic acid also protects the epidermis by scavenging reactive oxygen species generated by ultra violet light which would normally cause sunspots.

Hydrosol, also known as distillates are commonly sold under the terms distillate waters, hydrosols, hydrolates, hydrolats, plant waters and floral waters. They are the aromatic by-product created during the steam distillation of plant material in the manufacturing of essential oils. The hydrosols are the condensed water collected in the process of steam distillation. While hydrosols are aromatic in nature their aroma is very subtle.

Hypoallergenic means "least likely to cause a reaction." When it comes to cosmetics the FDA has not set standards or definitions of the terms. There is no requirement to submit substantiation of any hypoallergenic claim on cosmetics which leaves the meaning of the label up to the definition of the manufacturer.

I

Incense is derived from the Latin, incedere which means to burn. It is composed of fragrance materials that release a fragrant smoke while it burns.

Inorganic chemistry is the study of the properties and reactivity of all chemical elements.

Internal Use when referring to aromatherapy is the practice of using internal (oral, vaginal or rectal) application of essential oils. This author never recommends the use of essential oils under any circumstances.

Irritant is a substance or agent that induces a state of irritation.

K

Keystone pricing is a method of setting retail prices based on doubling the wholesale price.

L

Lauramide DEA (from Bio-Terge surfactant blend) is a fatty acid derivative of diethanolamine (DEA*). It is a nonionic surfactant used in the formulation of shampoos, hair dyes, bath products and lotions as a viscosity booster and, to increase and stabilize the foaming capacity of a formula. Lauramide DEA also thickens the aqueous portion of a formula. Lauramide DEA is produced from naturally occurring lauric acid.

The CIR Expert Panel concluded that Lauramide DEA was safe as a cosmetic ingredient. The CIR Expert Panel reviewed data on Lauramide DEA showing that: it is slightly toxic to non-toxic via acute oral administration; it is not a dermal toxin in acute and sub-chronic studies; it is a mild skin irritant but not a sensitizer or photosensitizer; it is a mild to moderate eye irritant; it does not demonstrate mutagenic activity.

Lauramide DEA is listed under Fatty Acid Dialkylamides and Dialkanolamides in the Cosmetics Directive of the European Union (see Annex III, Part I) and may be used with a maximum secondary amine concentration of 0.5%. It may not be used with nitrosating systems. In the Cosmetics Directive of the European Union, Lauramide DEA was lumped into the Fatty Acid Dialkylamides and Dialkanolamides along with Cocamide DEA, Linoleamide DEA and Oleamide DEA. The CIR Expert Panel determined that only Cocamide DEA should not be used with nitrosating systems.

*Since Lauramide DEA is a fatty acid derivative of diethanolamine (DEA) I wanted to take a moment to address the safety data regarding DEA. DEA has been assessed by the CIR Expert Panel and concluded they that DEA is safe for use in cosmetics and personal care products designed for discontinuous, brief use followed by thorough rinsing from the surface of the skin. In products intended for prolonged contact with the skin, the concentration of DEA should not exceed 5%.

Limbic system is a complex set of structures that lies in the brain on both sides of the thalamus, just under the cerebrum. The limbic system is often referred to as the "emotional center" of the brain.

M

Malic acid is an alpha hydroxy fruit acid, can be used in skin care products to rejuvenate and improve skin conditions. Malic acid is a natural constituent of many fruits and vegetables that are preserved by fermentation. This acid may be broken down during fermentation by certain bacteria into lactic acid and carbon dioxide.

Melting Point is the temperature at which a solid melts to become a liquid.

MSM, Methylsulfonylmethane, is a naturally occurring nutrient found in plants, meats, dairy products, fruits, and vegetables. MSM is therefore found in the normal human diet. It is an odorless, tasteless, white water soluble, crystalline solid in its purified form. MSM supplies sulfur to the body which allows it to heal itself. It produces muscle relaxation and reportedly a whole host of beneficial qualities. It has been used with great success in eliminating chronic back pain, muscle pain, repairing cut, scraped, burned and damage skin. We've seen reports of MSM eliminating wrinkles, brown spots, skin tumors, and spider veins. MSM is being used for burn victims and repairing scar tissue. Many people report relief from allergies after using MSM. Other reports indicate that MSM will remove parasites from the body, and help the body to detoxify itself.

MSM is anti-inflamatory and anti-microbial. MSM feeds the formation of collagen and elastin while preventing and reducing cross-linking between cells, which is the primary cause of wrinkles and scar tissue. MSM is a natural sulfur compound that contributes to healthy skin, hair and nails. MSM has been used orally and topically to aid skin disorders. When used topically, in the form of a cream or lotion, sulfur is helpful in treating skin disorders including acne, psoriasis, eczema, dermatitis, dandruff, scabies, diaper rash and certain fungal infections.

Multiple Fruit Blend Tincture is a hydro-alcohol mixture prepared from organic plant materials (lemon, orange, cane sugar, maple, bilberry, cranberry), organic alcohol and de-ionized water. The Multiple Fruit Acids Tincture contains naturally occurring alpha hydroxy acids (AHA's). The AHA's are water soluble components of the Multiple Fruits which maximized the stimulation of cell renewal while minimizing irritation associated with the use of topical alpha hydroxy acids.

Mustard Powder is powder made from the seeds of the mustard plant. Mustard baths have been used for centuries to stimulate sweat glands and increase circulation. This bath is perfect to ease sore muscles and your achy body.

N

Neat is a term used for applying essential oils undiluted to the skin, however essential oils should always be diluted before being applied to the skin.

Neem tincture is under-utilized in the Western culture. In India neem is very popular and commonly used as an antibacterial, antiviral, antifungal, antiseptic, anti-parasitic agent in toiletries, soap, toothpaste and skin/hair care products.

Neurotoxins are substances with an adverse effect on the nervous system.

O

Olfactory is relating to the sense of smell.

Organic Chemistry is the study of the properties of the compounds of carbon that are organic.

P

Pheromones are naturally occurring odorless substances the fertile body excretes externally, conveying an airborne signal that provides information to, and triggers responses from, the opposite sex of the same species.

Photosensitivity is the sensitivity to the sun.

Pituitary gland is about the size of a pea and is located at the base of the brain. It is sometimes called the "master" gland of the endocrine system, because it controls the functions of the other endocrine glands. The pituitary gland is attached to the by nerve fibers.

Polysorbate 20 is a non-ionic surfactant that is used to disperse and emulsify oils into water. It is indispensable oil-dispersant in body mists and spritzers. Polysorbate 20 is made from lauric acid (olive oil source) connected to a sugar (sorbitol) and this compound is then ethoxylated (grain based alcohol) to make it water dispersable. It is non-irritating. It is critical that an emulsifier used with essential is nonionic, because it does not disrupt the properties of the essential oils by creating ionic bonds which are formed when two or more atoms give up electrons. A nonionic bond does not borrow electrons which is preferable when using essential oils. Ionic bonds are stronger and do not separate in solution, but they do disrupt the properties of the essential oils. For this reason I recommend Polysorbate 20 over any other emusifier on the market.

As you know oil and water don't mix, but in cosmetic chemistry the solution to blending two immiscible (unblendable) liquids are emulsions. Oil simply can't form a strong bond with water on its own. Emulsifiers work by forming a sort of skin around small droplets of oil which allows the oil droplets to remain suspended in a solution of water in an oil-in-water (O/W) formula.

The opposite is true in a water-in-oil (W/O) solution. Emulsifiers have a large lipophilic end (attracted to oil) and a hydrophilic end (attracted to water). These lipophilic and hydrophilic ends create a game of tug-of-war between the oil and water which keeps the oil suspended in a water solution.

R

Ringworm is a skin infection due to a fungus.

S

Sebum is produced by the sebaceous glands in the skin. Sebum comes out of the glands in the skin and coats the hair follicles.

Shekels are any of several ancient units of weight, especially a Hebrew unit equal to about a half ounce.

Shelf Life is the length of time that food, drink, medicine, chemicals, essential oils and many other perishable items are given before they are considered unsuitable for sale, use, or consumption.

Sodium C14-16 Olefin Sulfonate (a Sodium Alpha-Olefin Sulfonate) is a mixture of long chain sulfonate salts prepared by the sulfonation of alpha olefins. The numbers (14-16) indicate the average lengths of the carbon chains of the alpha olefins. It is most commonly used in shampoos and bath and shower products. Sodium C14-16 Olefin Sulfonate helps clean the skin and hair by helping the water from your shower or bath to mix with the oil and dirt on your body and hair so they can be rinsed away.

The FDA reviewed the safety of Sodium C14-16 Olefin Sulfonate as indirect food additives, as components of adhesives, and as emulsifiers and/or surface-active agents. The safety of Sodium C14-16 Olefin Sulfonate has been assessed by the CIR Expert Panel and they concluded that it was safe as used in rinse-off products and safe up to 2% in leave-on products.

The CIR Expert Panel noted that Sodium Alpha-Olefin Sulfonates are poorly absorbed through normal skin but significantly absorbed through damaged skin. Short-term toxicity studies showed no consistent effects. High concentrations produced moderate to mild ocular irritation. At doses that were maternally toxic they found fetal abnormalities in animal studies. Genotoxicity, oral and dermal studies were negative.

Some studies found irritation and sensitization. This sensitization was attributed to low level gamma sultone residues. Because gamma sultones were sensitizers at very low levels, it was concluded that any product containing Sodium Alpha-Olefin Sulfonates should have very little gamma sultone residues. The gamma sultone levels should not exceed 10 ppm for saturated (alkane) sultones, 1 ppm for chlorosultones, and 0.1 ppm for unsaturated sultones. Sodium Alpha-Olefin Sulfonates are otherwise considered safe for use in rinse-off products. The use of Sodium Alpha-Olefin Sulfonates in leave-on products is limited to 2% in a formula.

According to the general provisions of the Cosmetics Directive of the European Union, Sodium C14-16 Olefin Sulfonate may be used in cosmetics and personal care products marketed in Europe.

Sodium Laureth Sulfate (SLES) is a very effective cleansing agent that belongs to the chemical class of alkyl ether sulfates. It is a salt of sulfated ethoxylated fatty alcohol and is the most commonly used of the alkyl ether sulfates that are used in cleansing products, including bubble baths, bath soaps and detergents and shampoos.

SLES exhibits emulsifying properties and imparts "softness" to the skin. As a cleansing agent the anionic surfactant SLES wets body surfaces, emulsifies or solubilize oils and suspends soil. It also contributes to the lathering properties and excellent viscosity response in cleansing products and bubble baths formulas. Sodium Laureth Sulfate exhibits a high degree of foaming. SLES was formulated to improved mildness over Sodium Lauryl Sulfate (SLS).

The safety of SLES was assessed in 1983 and re-reviewed in 2002 by the CIR Expert Panel and they concluded SLES is safe for use in cosmetics and personal care products in the present practices of use and concentration when formulated to be non-irritating. It can cause mild to moderate skin irritation in some people.

According to the general provisions of the Cosmetics Directive of the European Union, Sodium Laureth Sulfate may be used in cosmetics and personal care products that are marketed in Europe. SLES did not result in adverse effects in numerous safety studies including acute, sub-chronic and chronic oral exposure, reproductive and developmental toxicity, carcinogenic, photosensitization studies and SLES readily biodegrades.

Despite internet rumors SLES is not a carcinogenic substance. The World Health Organization, the International Agency for the Research of Cancer, US Environment Protection Agency and the European Union are all organizations that classify and register all substances that are known to be carcinogenic. None of these organizations have classified SLES as a carcinogen.

Sodium Lauryl Sulfoacetate: From a chemical standpoint, sodium lauryl sulfoacetate is a very unique surfactant. It demonstrates outstanding performance in cleansing, foaming, wetting, viscosity building, mildness and emulsification. It is an excellent surfactant for any water hardness and is biodegradable making it a versatile ingredient in cosmetic formulation. Sodium lauryl sulfoacetate was specifically developed to be mild to the skin. It is commonly the surfactant of choice for formulators developing products that are designed for those who have sensitivity to other soaps. The sodium lauryl sulfoacetate molecule is a valuable and unique molecule that has been in use for over 30 years in cosmetics.

Some common characteristics of sodium lauryl sulfoacetate are that it is relatively non-hygroscopic (it does not absorb or retain moisture from the air) and is resistant to hydrolysis (it does not react with water to produce other compounds) even at high temperatures. It is especially stable at the common cosmetic pH range of 5.5 to 7.8. Sodium lauryl sulfoacetate is biodegradable and has shown in laboratory studies to undergo both primary and ultimate biodegradation. This product has a good toxicological profile which makes it an ingredient of choice for dentifrice (toothpastes), shampoos, cleansing creams, sensitive skin soap bars and shower gels. To add to its track record, sodium lauryl sulfoacetate is registered in the United States, Japan, Canada, and Australia and is compliant with the EU regulations.

The safety and mildness of sodium lauryl sulfoacetate lies in the absence of a sulfate ion head, which is commonly found in many other surfactants. The sulfate ion, which originates in sulfuric acid, is replaced with the more stable sulfonated ester. This sulfate free surfactant is made with lauryl alcohol, derived from palm kernel oil, which is then condensed with a sulfonated form of acetic acid, or vinegar. It is this charged sulfonated acetate group which gives this molecule its mild surfactant properties.

Figure 1) Sodium lauryl sulfoacetate   Figure 2) Sodium lauryl sulfate

Note in figure 1 and 2 that the molecules posses an identical charge on their head and contain an equal number of carbon atoms attached to their functional group, making them very similar in physical appearance and overall function. The sodium lauryl sulfoacetate however, lacks the potentially harmful sulfate head attached to the carbon chain.

Solvent is a substance that dissolves another to form a solution.

Specific Gravity is the ratio of density of a substance compared to the density of fresh water at 4°C (39° F).

Stimulant is an substance that produces a temporary increase of the functional activity or efficiency of an organism or any of its parts.

Stimuli are events in the environment that influence behavior.

Surfactants are a vehicle used in cosmetic chemistry. They are important building blocks in personal care products. Surfactants allow cosmetics to slip across, onto or to clean the skin by breaking up and separating from the skin oils, fats, makeup, dirt, pollution and other debris.

There are four basic types of surfactants used in cosmetics.

- Anionic surfactants have a negative ionic charge. (Sodium Laureth Sulfate, Sodium Lauryl Sulfate, Stearic Acid,)
- Cationic surfactants have a postive ionic charge. (Cetearyl Alcohol, Stearalkonium Chloride)
- Amphoteric surfactants may have either a postive or negative ionic charge. Amphoeteric surfactants adapt to the pH of the water used in the formula. (Cocamidopropyl betaine, Sodium-Cocoamphoacetate)
- Nonionic surfactants has no charge. (Decyl Glucoside, Polysorbate)

Surfactants by definition lower the surface tension of the skin and/or of the water in a formula. Surfactants are both hydrophilic (water loving) and lipophilic (oil loving) which gives them the ability to reduce surface tension in a water and oil formula. Surfactants are commonly used in products that are designed to cleanse (shampoo, shower gel, face cleanser, hand soap), emulsify water and oil (lotion, creme), solubilize (polysorbate solubizing essential oil into a toner, body mist) or condition (hair conditioner).

Synergetic blend is when essential oils are blended and create a combination is more than the sum of its parts, which increases the potency without increasing the dosage.

T

Tartaric Acid is an organic alpha hydroxy acid found in many plants and known to the early Greeks and Romans as tartar, the acid potassium salt derived as a deposit from fermented grape juice.

Triethanolamine (TEA) is a clear, viscous liquid used to reduce the surface tension in emulsions. This allows the water-soluble and oil-soluble ingredients in a formula to blend better. It is a strong base, which makes it useful in adjusting the pH of a cosmetic formula. TEA is completely soluble in water and is rapidly biodegradable.

TEA neutralizes fatty acids and solubilizes oils and other ingredients that are not completely soluble in water. TEA combines the properties of both amines and alcohols and can undergo reactions common to both groups. As an amine, TEA reacts with acids because it is mildly alkaline, and forms soaps. When TEA acts as an alcohol it is hygroscopic and can cause the esterification of free fatty acids.

The FDA includes TEA on its list of indirect food additives, which means TEA may be used in adhesives in contact with food and to assist in the washing or peeling of fruits and vegetables. The safety of TEA has been assessed by the CIR Expert Panel and they concluded that TEA is safe for use in cosmetics and personal care products designed for discontinuous, brief use followed by thorough rinsing from the surface of the skin. In products intended for prolonged contact with the skin, the concentration of TEA should not exceed 5%.

Turbinado Sugar, also known as sugar in the raw, is natural cane turbinado sugar that is grown and cut in the tropics and less processed than refined sugar.

V

Viscous is substances having a thick, sticky consistency between solid and liquid; having a high viscosity.

Volatile: evaporating rapidly, readily vaporizable at a relatively low temperature.

W

Water activity is the amount of water that is available to microorganisms.

References

Every effort has been made to credit resources, however, 13 years of knowledge from reading books, industry magazines, websites, training material, material safety data sheets, certificate of analysis, industry sales material, personal communications and taking continuing education course has contributed to the writing of this book. If any unwitting omissions have occurred the author apologizes in advance.

Alliance of International Aromatherapists. Safety Statement, *http://www.alliance-aromatherapists.org/standardsofpractice.htm#standards*

Alliance of International Aromatherapists. Standards of Practice, *http://www.alliance-aromatherapists.org/standardsofpractice.htm#standards*

Alliance of International Aromatherapists. Code of Ethics, *http://www.alliance-aromatherapists.org/standardsofpractice.htm#code*

American Medical Association. Committee on Coetaneous Health. *http://www.ama-assn.org/*

Arranging Fine Perfume Compositions. Glen O. Brechbill, Fragrance Books Inc., New Jersey, USA, 2009

Australian Tea Tree Oil. ISO4730 and AS 2782-1997 Standards, *http://www.attia.org.au/standards.php*

Battaglia, Salvatore. The Complete Guide to Aromatherapy. 2nd Edition: The International Centre of Holistic Aromatherapy; 2003

Bike, Robert L. Biblical Aromatherapy: A comprehensive guide to buying, blending and using essential oils for healing with plants mentioned in the Bible. First Manuscript Printing: November, 1999. (Eugene, OR)

Buckle, Jane. Clinical Aromatherapy, Essential Oils in Practice. Churchill Livingstone, An Imprint of Elsevier Science; 2003.

Burfield, Tony. Cropwatch, Updated List of Threatened Aromatic Plants Used in Aroma and Cosmetic Industries, v 1.10, Jan. 2009. Tony Burfield for Cropwatch 2003-2009, *http://www.cropwatch.org/Threatened %20Aromatic %20Species %20v1.10.pdf*

California Department of Public Health. NDMA and Other Nitrosamines - Drinking Water Issues, *http://www.cdph.ca.gov/certlic/drinkingwater/Pages/NDMA.aspx*

City of Portland. Bureau of Emergency Communications, Administration SOP 00.20.050, Standard Operating Procedures, Fragrance Free Policy.

Collins, Jim. Good to Great, *Why Some Companies Make the Leap...and Others Don't.* Harper Business, 1st edition; 2001.

Cosmetic Ingredient Review. CIR Annual Report, CIR Compendium, CIR Ingredient Reports, *http://www.cir-safety.org/publications.shtml*

Cosmetic Ingredient Review. Quick Reference Table, Cosmetics Ingredient Reports through June 2010, *http://www.cir-safety.org/staff_files/PublicationsListDec2009.pdf*

Cosmetic Ingredient Review. Quick Reference Table, Cosmetics Ingredient Reports through June 2010, *http://www.cir-safety.org/staff_files/PublicationsListDec2009.pdf*

Cosmetics and Toiletries. Cosmetics Registration in California and the FDA's Electronic-only Drug Registration, David Steinberg, Vol.124, No.10/October 2009

Daily Mail. Tozer, James, Midwife struck off after her error led to pregnant patient drinking aromatherapy oils, August 7, 2009, *http://www.dailymail.co.uk/news/article-1205011/Midwife-struck-giving-pregnant-woman-cup-aromatherapy-oils-DRINK-headache-cure.html*

Davis, Patricia. Aromatherapy an A-Z. C.W. Daniel Company Limited, United Kingdom; 1988.

Fitzsimmons, Judith. Aromatherapy Answers. Author House: Bloomington, IN; 2005

Epsom Salt Council. About Epsom Salt, The Science of Epsom Salt, *http://www.epsomsaltcouncil.org/about/*

Essential U blog. various *http://www.essentialublog.com*

Essential Wholesale. MSDS and Certificate of Analysis Databases.

European Commission, Health and Consumers, Cosmetics-CosIng, *http://ec.europa.eu/consumers/cosmetics/cosing/*

European Commission, Health and Consumers, Cosmetics-CosIng, Annexes, *http://ec.europa.eu/consumers/cosmetics/cosing/index.cfm?fuseaction=ref_data.annexes_v2*

European Commission, Health and Consumers, Cosmetics-CosIng, Regulations and Directives, *http://ec.europa.eu/consumers/cosmetics/cosing/index.cfm?fuseaction=ref_data.regulations*

Facebook. Statistics, *http://www.facebook.com/press/info.php?statistics*

FDA, U.S. Food and Drug Administration. Cosmetics, *http://www.fda.gov/Cosmetics/default.htm*

FDA, U.S. Food and Drug Administration. Cosmetics Labeling and Label Claims, *http://www.fda.gov/Cosmetics/CosmeticLabelingLabelClaims/default.htm*

FDA, U.S. Food and Drug Administration. Federal Food, Drug, and Cosmetics Act (FDandC Act), *http://www.fda.gov/RegulatoryInformation/Legislation/FederalFoodDrugandCosmeticActFDCAct/default.htm*

FDA, U.S. Food and Drug Administration. Good Manufacturing Practice (GMP) Guildelines/Inspections Checklist, *http://www.fda.gov/Cosmetics/GuidanceComplianceRegulatoryInformation/GoodManufacturingPracticeGMPGuidelinesInspectionChecklist/default.htm*

FDA, U.S. Food and Drug Administration. Guidance, Compliance and Regulatory Information, *http://www.fda.gov/Cosmetics/GuidanceComplianceRegulatoryInformation/default.htm*

FDA, U.S. Food and Drug Administration. Is It a Cosmetic, a Drug, or Both? (Or Is It Soap?), *http://www.fda.gov/Cosmetics/GuidanceComplianceRegulatoryInformation/ucm074201.htm*

FDA, U.S. Food and Drug Administration. Product and Ingredient Safety, *http://www.fda.gov/Cosmetics/ProductandIngredientSafety/default.htm*

Flavors and Off-Flavors. Edit. G. Charalambous, Elsevier Sci. Publ. BV, Amsterdam, pp. 511-542 (1989).

Florida Department of Business and Professional Regulations, *http://www.myfloridalicense.com/dbpr/*

Fritz, Rene. Chief Executive Forum, Coaching, *http://www.ceforum.com/default.asp*

Gattefossé, Rene-Maurice. Gattefossé's Aromatherapy, The First Book on Aromatherapy, Tisserand, Robert, Editor. Random House UK, 2nd edition; 2004.

Grosjean, Nelly. Veterinary Aromatherapy. Edited and revised English-language edition; C.W. Daniel Company Limited, United Kingdom; 1994\

GroupM. GroupM Search, *http://groupmsearch.com/blog/*

Health Canada. List of Prohibited and Restricted Cosmetic Ingredients ("Hotlist"), *http://www.hc-sc.gc.ca/cps-spc/cosmet-person/indust/hot-list-critique/index-eng.php*

Health Canada. Cosmetics and Your Health, *http://www.hc-sc.gc.ca/hl-vs/iyh-vsv/prod/cosmet-eng.php*

Health Canada. Consumer Product Safety, *http://www.hc-sc.gc.ca/cps-spc/cosmet-person/indust/index-eng.php*

Health Canada. Cosmetics and Personal Care, For Consumers and For Industry and Professionals, *http://www.hc-sc.gc.ca/cps-spc/cosmet-person/index-eng.php*

Homan Christian Standard Bible. Homan Bible Publishers, Nashville, Tennessee, 1999

International Fragrance Association. Ingredients, *http://www.ifraorg.org/en-us/Ingredients_2*

International Organization for Standardization. *http://www.iso.org/iso/home.html*

Jager W, Buchbauer G, Jirovetz L, Fritzer M 1992 Percutaneous absorption of lavender oil from massage oil. Journal of Society of Cosmetic Chemists 43(1) (January-February): 49-54

Johnson, Donna Maria Coles, Essential U blog Interview

Lis-Balchin, Maria, BSc, PhD. Aromatherapy Science, A guide for healthcare professionals, Pharmaceutical Press, London; 2006

Merriam-Webster Online Dictionary, 2011 Merriam-Webster, Incorporated, *http://www.merriam-webster.com*

Lees, Mark PhD; Milady's Skin Care Reference Guide, Milady Publishing Company, New York; 1994

Malawian Air Fouling Legislations. Local Courts, Malawi Parliament, February 2011.

Millionaire Mom: *The Art of Raising a Business and a Family at the Same Time,* Joyce Bone, Morgan James Publishing, March 1, 2010

Mintel. Mintel Predicts Global Beauty Trends 2010 Press Release, *http://www.mintel.com/press-centre/press-releases/440/mintel-predicts-global-beauty-trends-for-2010*

National Association of Holistic Aromatherapy. Approved Schools and Educators, *http://www.naha.org/education.htm*

National Association of Holistic Aromatherapy. Code of Ethics, *http://www.naha.org/ethics.htm*

National Association of Holistic Aromatherapy. Consumers Cautions and Safety, *http://www.naha.org/consumer.htm*

National Association of Holistic Aromatherapy. Raindrop Therapy, *http://www.naha.org/safety.htm*

National Association of Holistic Aromatherapy. Scope of Practice, *http://www.naha.org/rdt_statement.htm*

National Association of Holistic Aromatherapy. Standards of Educaton/Training, *http://www.naha.org/standards.htm*

New International Version Bible. Zondervan, 2011 *http://www.thenivbible.com/*

NPCS Board of Consultants and Engineers. The Complete Technology Book on Flavours, Fragrances and Perfumes, NIIR Project Consultancy Services, 2007.

Official Journal of the European Union. Directive 2003/15/EC of the European Parliament and of the Council of 27 February 2003, amending Council Directive 76/768/ECC on the approximation of the laws of the Member States relating to cosmetic products, 11.3.2003, L 66/26 *http://eur-lex.europa.eu/LexUriServ/LexUriServ.do?uri=OJ:L:2003:066:0026:0035:en:PDF*

Online Sunshine. Official Internet Site of the Florida Legislature. The 2011 Florida Statutes, Regulation of Trade, Commerce, Investments, and Solicitations, Drug, Cosmetic, and Household Products, Chapter 499. *http://www.leg.state.fl.us/statutes/index.cfm?App_mode=Display_Statute&URL=0400-0499/0499/0499.html*

Pappas, Dr. Robert S., Chemistry of Essential Oils Continuing Education Course, Dr. Robert S. Pappas, The Atlantic Institute of Aromatherapy

Personal Care Products Council. Consumer Commitment Code, *http://www.ctfa.org/about-us/personal-care-products-council-consumer-commitment-code*

Price, Len and Price, Shirley. Aromatherapy For Health Professionals. Churchill Livingstone: London; 1999.

PubMed.gov. U.S. National library of Medicine, National Institute of Health, *http://www.ncbi.nlm.nih.gov/pubmed/*

Regulatory Toxicology and Pharmacology. Official Journal of the International Society for Regulatory Toxicology and Pharmacology, Elsevier Science, Gio B. Gori, DSc, MPH, ATS

Rodgers, Lisa. Personal Care, The Cosmetics Ingredient Review and Safe Cosmetics, August, 5, 2001, *http://personalcaretruth.com/2011/08/the-cosmetic-ingredient-review-and-safe-cosmetics/*

Rodgers, Lisa. Personal Care, Voluntary Cosmetic Registration Program (VCRP) and Safe Cosmetics, August 8, 2011, *http://personalcaretruth.com/2011/08/voluntary-cosmetic-registration-program-vcrp-and-safe-cosmetics/*

Rommelt H., Zuber A., Dirnagl K, Drexel H., 1974 Munchener medezine Wochenschrift 116:537 In: Price, Len and Price, Shirley. Aromatherapy For Health Professionals. Churchill Livingstone: London; 1999.

Rose, Jeanne. 375 Essential Oils and Hydrosols. Frog, Ltd: Berkeley, CA; 1999.

Schilcher H. 1985 Effects and side effects of essential oils In: Price, Len and Price, Shirley. Aromatherapy For Health Professionals. Churchill Livingstone: London; 1999.

Schnaubelt (Ph.D.), Kurt. Advanced Aromatherapy. Healing Arts Press: Cologne, Germany; 1998.

Schnaubelt (Ph.D.), Kurt. Medical Aromatherapy, Healing with Essential Oils. Frog, Ltd.; 1999.

Science Dictionary. Chemistry Terms and Definitions Listed Alphabetically, Science Dictionary - Scientific Definitions 2003-2006, *http://www.sciencedictionary.org/chemistry/*

Sellar, Wanda. The Directory of Essential Oils. C.W. Daniel Company Limited: United Kingdom; 1992.

Sense of Smell Institute. *http://www.senseofsmell.org/resources/index.php*

Sheppard-Hanger, Sylla. Principles of Perfumery Continuing Education Course, The Atlantic Institute of Aromatherapy

Sheppard-Hanger, Sylla. The Aromatherapy Practitioner Reference Manual. Atlantic Institute of Aromatherapy; Tampa, Florida; 2000.

Smell and Taste. *http://www.smellandtaste.org/*

Sundale Research. State of the Industry: Cosmetics and Toiletries in the U.S., March, 2011, 3rd Edition.

The Center for Drug Evaluation and Research (CDER). *http://www.fda.gov/Drugs/default.htm*

The International Organization for Standardization. *http://www.iso.org/iso/home.html*

The Daily Smell. Portland now first US city to voluntary ban fragrance, Genevive Bjorn, *http://dev.thedailysmell.com/2011/02/24/portland-becomes-the-first-fragrance-free-city-in-the-us/*

Tisserand, Maggie. Aromatherapy for Women. Healing Arts Press: Rochester, VA; 1985.

Tisserand, Robert. Aromatherapy: To heal and tend the body. Lotus Press: Wilmot, WI; 1988.

Tisserand, Robert. Essential Oils in Soap: Interview with Kevin Dunn, June 25, 2011 *http://roberttisserand.com/2011/06/essential-oils-in-soap-interview-with-kevin-dunn/*

Tisserand, Robert. Gattefossé's Burn, April 22, 2011, *http://roberttisserand.com/2011/04/gattefosses-burn/*

Tisserand, Robert. Is Clary Sage Estogenic? April 25, 2010, *http://roberttisserand.com/2010/04/is-clary-sage-oil-estrogenic/*
Twitter. Twitter blog, #numbers, http://blog.twitter.com/2011/03/numbers.html

Tisserand, Robert. Tea Tree and Lavender Not Linked To Gynecomastia, 2008, *http://roberttisserand.com/articles/TeaTreeAndLavenderNotLinkedToGynecomastia.pdf*

Valnet (MD), Jean. The Practice of Aromatherapy: A classic compendium of plant medicines and their healing properties. Healing Arts Press: Rochester, VA; 1980.

U.S. Consumer Product Safety Commission. Office of Compliance, Requirements under the Federal Hazardous Substances Act: Labeling and Banning Requirements for Chemical and Other Hazardous Substances, 15 U.S.C, 161 and 16 C.F.R. Part 1500, *http://www.cpsc.gov/BUSINFO/regsumfhsa.pdf*

U.S. Consumer Product Safety Commission. Office of Compliance, Requirements under the Poison Prevention Packaging Act, 16 C.F.R. 1700, *http://www.cpsc.gov/BUSINFO/regsumpppa.pdf*

Watt, Martin. Essential Oils in Aromatherapy, Martin Watt publisher, *http://www.aromamedical.com/ordering.html*

Watt, Martin. Plant Aromatics, A Data and Reference Manual on Essential Oils and Aromatic Extracts; Martin Watt publisher; 1994.

Wildwood, Chrissie. Encyclopedia of Aromatherapy. Healing Arts Press, Rochester, Vermont; 2000.

Williams, David G. The Chemistry of Essential Oils. Micelle Press; England; 1996, 1997.

Worwood, Susan. Essential Aromatherapy: A pocket guide to essential oils and aromatherapy. New World Library: Novato, CA; 1995.

Worwood, Valerie Ann. Aromatherapy for the Healthy Child. New World Library: Novato, CA; 2000.

Worwood, Valerie Ann. The Complete Book of Essential Oils and Aromatherapy. New World Library: Novato, CA; 1991.

Worwood, Valerie Ann. The Fragrant Mind: Aromatherapy for Personality, Mind, Mood, and Emotion. New World Library: Novato, CA; 1996.

Index

F

Family Blending 48
Fixative 46, 49-50, 206, 293
Flame Ionization Detector (FID) 151
Folded Essential Oils 46
Fragrance Oils 82, 88, 120, 124-135, 155, 292
Frankincense 20-21, 23, 44, 48, 50, 195, 199, 207, 212-215, 221, 226, 231, 257
Functional Groups 40, 43

G

Gas Chromatography 151
Geranium 41, 43, 48, 50, 76-77, 87-89, 153, 195, 202, 204, 215-217, 226, 233, 238, 243
Ginger 48, 50, 80, 153, 195, 216-219, 223, 251
Glycerin 79, 294
Glycolic 79, 289, 294-295
Goat Milk 78, 98
Grapefruit 42, 46, 48, 50, 70, 76-77, 88, 90, 119, 152, 156-157, 195, 199, 214, 220-222, 228, 251

H

Headspace 46, 197, 221, 229, 236
Hippocampus 35, 295
Hyaluronic Acid 75, 126, 295-296
Hydrosol 26, 45, 87, 140, 296, 265
Hypoallergenic 59, 62, 131, 296

I

Integumentary System 39

L

Lactose 104
Laurel Leaf 79, 88, 102, 195, 222-224

M

Lavender 26, 28-29, 32, 37-37, 41-43, 48, 50, 70, 75-77, 79-81, 87-89, 96, 101, 103, 105, 112, 115, 150-153, 155, 157, 160, 190, 195, 199, 202-204, 207, 214, 217, 219, 221, 223-227, 231, 233, 238, 240, 245, 251
Lemon 41-42, 45-46, 48, 50, 71, 76, 80, 90, 106, 119, 152-153, 156-157, 195-196, 199, 204, 214, 221, 227-229, 231, 247, 251, 298
Limbic System 35, 269, 289, 297
Lymphatic System 39, 88, 90, 221

M

Malic Acid 78, 297
Mass Spectrometry 151
Material Safety Data Sheets (MSDS) 129, 158-159
Middle Note 47-49
MSM 78, 98, 298
Multiple Fruit Blend Tincture 79, 298
Muscular System 38
Mustard Powder 88, 99, 308
Myrrh 20-23, 48, 51, 157, 195, 199, 207, 212, 214-215, 221, 229, 230-232

N

Neat 75, 82, 160, 298
Neem Tincture 37, 299
Neroli 48, 51, 76-77, 125, 150, 160, 195, 226, 232-234, 238
Nervous System 38, 196, 204, 208-209, 233, 237, 299

O

Oil, Avocado 54, 63, 72
Oil, Borage 55
Oil, Broccoli 55
Oil, Carrot 56